Prevalence and Risk Factors of Obesity and Hypertension

Prevalence and Risk Factors of Obesity and Hypertension

Guest Editors

Piotr Matłosz

Justyna Wyszyńska

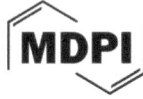

Basel • Beijing • Wuhan • Barcelona • Belgrade • Novi Sad • Cluj • Manchester

Guest Editors

Piotr Matłosz	Justyna Wyszyńska
Medical College of Rzeszów University	Medical College of Rzeszów University
Rzeszów	Rzeszów
Poland	Poland

Editorial Office
MDPI AG
Grosspeteranlage 5
4052 Basel, Switzerland

This is a reprint of the Special Issue, published open access by the journal *Journal of Clinical Medicine* (ISSN 2077-0383), freely accessible at: https://www.mdpi.com/journal/jcm/special_issues/prevalence_risk_obesity_hypertension.

For citation purposes, cite each article independently as indicated on the article page online and as indicated below:

Lastname, A.A.; Lastname, B.B. Article Title. *Journal Name* **Year**, *Volume Number*, Page Range.

ISBN 978-3-7258-2943-9 (Hbk)
ISBN 978-3-7258-2944-6 (PDF)
https://doi.org/10.3390/books978-3-7258-2944-6

© 2025 by the authors. Articles in this book are Open Access and distributed under the Creative Commons Attribution (CC BY) license. The book as a whole is distributed by MDPI under the terms and conditions of the Creative Commons Attribution-NonCommercial-NoDerivs (CC BY-NC-ND) license (https://creativecommons.org/licenses/by-nc-nd/4.0/).

Contents

Anna Bartosiewicz, Justyna Wyszyńska, Edyta Łuszczki, Anna Lewandowska, Małgorzata Zatorska-Zoła, Piotr Sulikowski and Piotr Matłosz
Impact of Consumption of Specific Food Groups on Metabolic and Cardiovascular Disorders among Nurses: Framingham's Multifactorial Predictive Model
Reprinted from: *J. Clin. Med.* **2024**, *13*, 5568, https://doi.org/10.3390/jcm13185568 1

Irena A. Dykiert, Krzysztof Kraik, Lidia Jurczenko, Paweł Gać, Rafał Poręba and Małgorzata Poręba
The Effect of Obesity on Repolarization and Other ECG Parameters
Reprinted from: *J. Clin. Med.* **2024**, *13*, 3587, https://doi.org/10.3390/jcm13123587 15

Muhammad Asif, Hafiz Ahmad Iqrash Qureshi, Saba Mazhar Seyal, Muhammad Aslam, Muhammad Tauseef Sultan, Maysaa Elmahi Abd Elwahab, et al.
Assessing Disparities about Overweight and Obesity in Pakistani Youth Using Local and International Standards for Body Mass Index
Reprinted from: *J. Clin. Med.* **2024**, *13*, 2944, https://doi.org/10.3390/jcm13102944 33

Eduardo Meaney, Enrique Pérez-Robles, Miguel Ortiz-Flores, Guillermo Perez-Ishiwara, Alejandra Meaney, Levy Munguía, et al.
Overweight, Obesity, and Age Are the Main Determinants of Cardiovascular Risk Aggregation in the Current Mexican Population: The FRIMEX III Study
Reprinted from: *J. Clin. Med.* **2024**, *13*, 2248, https://doi.org/10.3390/jcm13082248 42

Małgorzata Biernikiewicz, Małgorzata Sobieszczańska, Ewa Szuster, AnnaPawlikowska-Gorzelańczyk, Anna Janocha, Krystyna Rożek-Piechura, et al.
Erectile Dysfunction as an Obesity-Related Condition in Elderly Men with Coronary Artery Disease
Reprinted from: *J. Clin. Med.* **2024**, *13*, 2087, https://doi.org/10.3390/jcm13072087 56

Katarzyna Helon, Małgorzata Wisłowska, Krzysztof Kanecki, Paweł Goryński, Aneta Nitsch-Osuch and Krzysztof Bonek
Time Trend Analysis of Comorbidities in Ankylosing Spondylitis: A Population-Based Study from 53,142 Hospitalizations in Poland
Reprinted from: *J. Clin. Med.* **2024**, *13*, 602, https://doi.org/10.3390/jcm13020602 67

Blanca Estela Ríos-González, Ana Míriam Saldaña-Cruz, Sergio Gabriel Gallardo-Moya and Aniel Jessica Leticia Brambila-Tapia
Sex Differences in the Relationship between Personal, Psychological and Biochemical Factors with Blood Pressure in a Healthy Adult Mexican Population: A Cross-Sectional Study
Reprinted from: *J. Clin. Med.* **2024**, *13*, 378, https://doi.org/10.3390/jcm13020378 80

Irina Mihaela Abdulan, Veronica Feller, Andra Oancea, Alexandra Mașaleru, Anisia Iuliana Alexa, Robert Negru, et al.
Evolution of Cardiovascular Risk Factors in Post-COVID Patients
Reprinted from: *J. Clin. Med.* **2023**, *12*, 6538, https://doi.org/10.3390/jcm12206538 102

Maciej Kochman, Marta Brzuszek and Mirosław Jabłoński
Changes in Metabolic Health and Sedentary Behavior in Obese Children and Adolescents
Reprinted from: *J. Clin. Med.* **2023**, *12*, 5456, https://doi.org/10.3390/jcm12175456 114

Barbara Siewert, Agata Kozajda, Marta Jaskulak and Katarzyna Zorena
Examining the Link between Air Quality (PM, SO_2, NO_2, PAHs) and Childhood Obesity: A Systematic Review
Reprinted from: *J. Clin. Med.* **2024**, *13*, 5605, https://doi.org/10.3390/jcm13185605 . . . . **126**

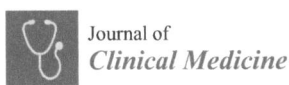

Article

Impact of Consumption of Specific Food Groups on Metabolic and Cardiovascular Disorders among Nurses: Framingham's Multifactorial Predictive Model

Anna Bartosiewicz [1,*], Justyna Wyszyńska [1], Edyta Łuszczki [1], Anna Lewandowska [2], Małgorzata Zatorska-Zoła [3], Piotr Sulikowski [4] and Piotr Matłosz [5]

1. Institute of Health Sciences, Medical College of Rzeszow University, 35-959 Rzeszow, Poland; jwyszynska@ur.edu.pl (J.W.); eluszczki@ur.edu.pl (E.Ł.)
2. Faculty of Healthcare, State Academy of Applied Sciences in Jaroslaw, 37-500 Jaroslaw, Poland; am.lewandowska@poczta.fm
3. Independent, Public Healthcare Complex, John Paul II Municipal Hospital, 35-241 Rzeszow, Poland; mzola1@poczta.onet.pl
4. Faculty of Computer Science and Information Technology, West Pomeranian University of Technology, 71-210 Szczecin, Poland; piotr.sulikowski@zut.edu.pl
5. Institute of Physical Culture Science, Medical College of Rzeszow University, 35-959 Rzeszow, Poland; pmatlosz@ur.edu.pl
* Correspondence: abartosiewicz@ur.edu.pl

Abstract: Objective: This study aimed to analyze the relationship between the consumption of selected food products and the risk of prevalence of selected metabolic and cardiovascular disorders among nurses. **Methodology:** This cross-sectional study was conducted among 405 nurses. To achieve the study objective, body composition analysis (Tanita MC-980), blood pressure measurement (Welch Allyn 4200B), anthropometric measurements, lipid profile, fasting blood glucose (CardioChek PA), and surveys regarding the consumption of specific food groups were conducted. **Results:** More than half of the respondents were overweight or/and obese, and almost 40% had elevated blood pressure levels. The results obtained from logistic regression models indicated that the consumption of specific food product groups may predispose to/increase the risk of hypertension, abdominal obesity, overweight, obesity, body fat accumulation, and the risk of cardiovascular events. **Conclusions:** These findings highlight the importance of targeted nutritional strategies to enhance the health and professional efficacy of nursing staff, paving the way for improved healthcare practices.

Keywords: dietary consumption; Framingham Risk Score; metabolic and cardiovascular disorders; nurses

1. Introduction

In recent years, with evolving trends in public health, there has been a growing interest in the impact of diet on various health indicators [1,2]. Numerous scientific studies have unequivocally shown that dietary habits significantly influence our health and well-being, and a proper diet plays a crucial role in preventing many chronic diseases and improving overall health status [2–4]. According to research by Willett and Stampfer et al., a well-balanced diet rich in diverse nutrients can substantially reduce the risk of developing conditions such as type 2 diabetes, cardiovascular diseases, certain types of cancer, and neurodegenerative diseases [5]. Regular consumption of vegetables, fruits, whole grains, low-fat proteins, and healthy fats is associated with lower cholesterol levels, better blood sugar regulation, and a reduced risk of many chronic diseases [6]. The Mediterranean and DASH diets, often cited as models of healthy eating, have been proven effective in enhancing cardiovascular health and longevity [7–11]. Previous studies have already emphasized that fruit and vegetable consumption may reduce the risk of coronary heart disease in part through the lowering of C-reactive protein (CRP) [12,13]. Esmaillzadeh et al. examined how fruit and vegetable consumption correlate with CRP levels and the occurrence of metabolic syndrome. Their research demonstrated that greater consumption of fruits and vegetables is linked to a reduced risk of metabolic syndrome, possibly due to decreased CRP levels. These results reinforce existing dietary guidelines that advocate for higher daily consumption of fruits and vegetables to prevent cardiovascular disease effectively [14].

The assessment of cardiovascular disease risk using the Framingham Risk Score is recognized as a crucial tool in cardiological prevention [15,16]. In studies conducted by Wilson et al., the use of this tool allowed for an effective prediction of cardiovascular events over the next ten years [15]. This study follows these findings, analyzing how the consumption of specific groups of products can impact the Framingham Risk Score and other key health indicators among nurses [16]. Nurses, as a professional group, represent a particularly interesting subject for study in this context, especially since numerous studies indicate that their health condition is worse compared to other professions [17,18]. Specific occupational demands and risks combined with irregular shift work significantly hinder proper and regular nutrition, thereby impacting the health of this professional group [19,20].

Given the critical role of nurses in society, there is an obligation for scientific entities to conduct research in this area to develop effective preventive and intervention strategies tailored to the specifics of nursing work [21]. It is particularly concerning that the life expectancy of Polish nurses is much shorter than that of the general population of Polish women [22].

Proper nutrition can help manage stress levels, improve concentration, and increase energy levels, which are essential for individuals working in such a demanding profession [23]. This study focusing on specific food groups provides valuable data on their impact on overall health and can contribute to a better understanding of the dietary needs of this professional group. The findings of such studies are expected to offer valuable insights for healthcare workers, dietitians, and policymakers, thereby contributing to enhanced work performance and overall well-being of nurses [23]. Furthermore, research indicates that health professionals who do not follow their own health advice are less likely to promote healthy lifestyle choices among their patients [24,25].

This study aimed to analyze the relationship between the consumption of selected food groups and the risk of prevalence of selected metabolic and cardiovascular disorders among nurses.

To the best of our knowledge, this study is one of the first to evaluate how the consumption of selected food products affects the prevalence of metabolic and cardiovascular disorders among such an important occupational group. This study fills a gap in existing research by utilizing advanced measurement techniques and statistical analysis.

2. Materials and Methods

2.1. Study Participants

This study was conducted in 2022 among 405 nurses working at a hospital in southeastern Poland, after obtaining the hospital director's consent to conduct measurements. All measurements (body mass analysis, anthropometric assessments, lipid profile, fasting blood glucose, and blood pressure checks) were performed in the morning. Participation in the study was voluntary and without charge. The recruitment criteria included professionally active nurses who had no symptoms of infection in the last two weeks, who were not aware of any health issues, and who were willing to participate in the project. The exclusion criteria included individuals with a pacemaker or other electronic implants (due to the possibility that the current used in the study could interfere with the operation of these devices), pregnancy (as bioimpedance testing is generally not recommended for pregnant women because the effects of electrical current on the fetus have not been fully investigated), and individuals with metal implants (since metal can affect electrical conductivity in the body and impact the quality of the results). The age of the subjects was not a criterion for participation in the measurements. Data from the measurements of 405 nurses underwent statistical analysis. All measurements were performed by qualified personnel, after a short rest and after signing the consent to participate in the study.

When analyzing the data, the following criteria and cut-offs were adopted:

Body mass index (BMI): <17—severely underweight; 17–18.49—underweight; 18.5–24.99—normal body weight; 25–29.99—overweight; 30–34.99—first-degree obesity; 35–39.99—second-degree obesity; >40—third-degree obesity [26].

Waist–hip ratio (WHR) was calculated by dividing the waist circumference by the hip circumference. A score of 0.83 or higher in women and 0.96 or higher in men was considered to indicate an android body type. In contrast, a coefficient of 0.83 or less in women and 0.96 or less in men indicated a gynoid body type [27].

Waist-to-height ratio (WHtR)

Men and women:

A value of <0.5 indicates an index within normal limits;

Values in the range of 0.5–0.6 indicate increased cardiometabolic risk;

Values ≥ 0.6 indicate significantly increased cardiometabolic risk [28].

Blood pressure: optimal SBP <120 mmHg and DBP <80 mmHg; normal blood pressure 120–129 mmHg (SBP) and/or 80–84 mmHg (DBP); normal high pressure 130–139 mmHg (SBP) and/or 85–89 mmHg (DBP); grade 1 hypertension 140–159 mmHg (SBP) and/or 90–99 mmHg (DBP); grade 2 hypertension 160–179 mmHg (SBP) and/or 100–109 mmHg (DBP); grade 3 hypertension ≥ 180 mmHg (SBP) and/or ≥ 110 mmHg (DBP); isolated systolic hypertension ≥ 140 (SBP) and <90 mmHg (DBP) [29,30].

Lipid profile

TC: 150–190 mg/dL;

LDL cholesterol: less than 115 mg/dL;

HDL cholesterol: men above 40 mg/dL, women over 48 mg/dL;

TRG: below 150 mg/dL [31].

Fasting glucose

Less than 70 mg/dL—hypoglycemia;

Values 70 to 99 mg/dL—normal glucose level;

Values 100 to 125 mg/dL—elevated glucose levels—pre-diabetes;

Values ≥ 126 mg/dL in at least two measurements—diabetes mellitus [32].

Body fat (BFP—assessed using bioelectrical impedance analysis)

Body fat within normal limits: men: 10–25% fat tissue, women: 20–35% fat tissue;

Increased body fat: men: above 25% fat tissue, women: above 35% fat tissue;

Excessive fatness: men: above 30% fat tissue, women: above 40% fat tissue [33,34].

2.2. Questionnaire

Questionnaires were distributed in paper format, accompanied by an envelope to ensure that participants could submit their responses securely and confidentially. The survey gathered sociodemographic information and explored various health-related behaviors and conditions. It included questions about the respondents' most commonly consumed food groups, salt consumption, participation in preventive health checks, weight management practices, smoking habits, work patterns, and self-rated health status.

2.3. Framingham Risk Score

The Framingham Risk Score (FRS) was utilized to assess cardiovascular risk among the study participants. This predictive model, derived from data collected in the Framingham Heart Study—a long-standing epidemiological study conducted in the United States—estimates the likelihood of experiencing a cardiovascular event within the next 10 years. The FRS calculation incorporates several established cardiovascular risk factors: age, gender, levels of HDL (high-density lipoprotein) and LDL (low-density lipoprotein) cholesterol, systolic blood pressure, smoking status, and diabetes status. Each factor contributes to a composite score that quantifies the overall cardiovascular risk for an individual [15,16].

The study methodology and the cut-off points used during the study have been published in detail in *BMC Public Health*, 2024 [35].

2.4. Statistical Analysis

The analysis was performed using the R program, version 4.2.1 [36]. The analysis of qualitative variables (i.e., not expressed in numbers) was performed by calculating the number and percentage of occurrences of each value. Single- and multifactor analyses were performed using logistic regression. The results are presented as values of odds ratio (OR) parameters with a 95% confidence interval. The variables for the multivariate analysis were selected based on their significance in the one-factor analyses.

The EPV (events per variable) index for the analysis was as follows: hypertension = 16.1; abdominal obesity according to WHR = 21.9; cardiometabolic risk according to WHtR = 14.8; overweight according to BMI = 13.75; obesity according to BMI = 10.8; increased amount of adipose tissue = 21.5; Framingham Risk Score = 10.6.

The quality of the multivariate models was assessed using the ROC (receiver operating characteristic) curves and the areas under the curve (AUCs). The analysis adopted a significance level of 0.05. Thus, all p-values below 0.05 were interpreted as significant associations.

3. Results

A total of 405 nurses took part in the measurements, with a significant majority being women (n = 380; 93.83%). The average age of the participants was about 48.5 years. Detailed characteristics of the study group are shown in Table 1.

Table 1. Characteristics of the study group [35].

Variable		Total (n = 405) n (%)
Sex *	Female	380 (93.8)
	Male	25 (6.1)
Age (years)	Average ± SD	48.4 (10.37)
	Median (quartiles)	51 (42–55)
Place of residence *	City	209 (51.6)
	Village	196 (48.4)
Type of work *	Staff management/administration	60 (14.8)
	Hospital ward	344 (85.1)
Work system *	One shift work	140 (34.5)
	Shift work and night duty	265 (65.4)
More than one job *	No	238 (58.7)
	Yes	167 (41.2)
Education *	Basic nursing education	131 (32.3)
	Bachelor	95 (23.4)
	Master's degree	179 (44.2)
Participation in preventive examinations other than obligatory *	No	293 (72.3)
	Yes	112 (27.6)
Cigarettes smoking *	No	305 (75.3)
	Yes	100 (24.6)
Adding sugar to coffee/tea *	No	175 (43.2)
	Yes	230 (56.7)

Table 1. Cont.

Variable		Total (n = 405) n (%)
Salting dishes *	I do not use salt at all	6 (1.4)
	Rarely or never add salt to food	71 (17.5)
	I taste the food and add salt as needed	234 (57.7)
	I add salt to my food without trying it first	94 (23.2)
Weight self-control *	Every day	16 (3.9)
	Once a week	69 (17.0)
	Twice a week	46 (11.3)
	Once a month	100 (24.6)
	Hardly ever	72 (17.7)
	I do not check my weight regularly	102 (25.1)
Self-assessment of the material situation *	Very good	30 (7.4)
	Good	208 (51.3)
	Average	158 (39.0)
	Bad	9 (22.2)
BMI * (kg/m^2)	Underweight	7 (1.7)
	Normal body mass	158 (39.0)
	Overweight	132 (32.6)
	Obesity	108 (26.7)
	Median (quartiles)	26.2 (23–30)
WHR *	Normal	208 (51.4)
	Abdominal obesity	197 (48.6)
	Median (quartiles)	0.83 (0.78–0.88)
WHtR *	Normal	178 (43.9)
	Increased cardiometabolic risk	164 (40.5)
	Significantly increased cardiometabolic risk	63 (15.6)
	Median (quartiles)	0.51 (0.46–0.57)
BP * (mmHg)	Normal	173 (42.7)
	Elevated	71 (17.5)
	Hypertension	161 (39.8)
	SBP Median (quartiles)	121.6 (110–132)
	DBP Median (quartiles)	75.6 (69–81)
BFP category * (%)	Normal	233 (57.5)
	Elevated	172 (42.5)
	Median (quartiles)	31.9 (26–36.8)
FG * (mg/dL)	Normal	276 (68.1)
	Elevated	123 (30.4)
	Abnormal glucose—suspicion of diabetes	6 (1.5)
	Median (quartiles)	97 (90–102)

Table 1. Cont.

Variable		Total (n = 405) n (%)
HDL * (mg/dL)	Decreased	94 (23.2)
	Normal	311 (76.8)
	Median (quartiles)	57 (49–66)
LDL * (mg/dL)	Elevated	207 (51.1)
	Normal	198 (48.9)
	Median (quartiles)	117 (88–144)

Data presented as follows: *—n (%); BMI—body mass index; WHR—waist–hip ratio; WHtR—waist-to-height ratio; BP—blood pressure; SBP—systolic blood pressure; DBP—diastolic blood pressure; BFP category—body fat percentage category; LDL—low-density lipoprotein cholesterol; HDL—high-density lipoprotein cholesterol; FG—fasting glucose.

The reported daily consumption rates for specific food product groups are as follows: white bread 56.3%, dark bread 25.4%, fish and seafood 1.7%, red meat and sausages 19.2%, sour milk products 27.9%, cheese 25.1%, cottage cheese 22.2%, fruits and vegetables 70.1%, sweets and salty snacks 27.4%, and fast food products 4.6%. Detailed frequencies for the consumption of selected food product groups are presented in Table 2.

Table 2. Consumption frequency of specific groups of products [35].

Group of Products	Frequency of Consumption				
	I Don't Eat n (%)	A Few Times a Month n (%)	2–4 Times a Week n (%)	Once a Week n (%)	Every Day n (%)
White bread	36 (8.8)	45 (11.1)	49 (12.1)	47 (11.6)	228 (56.3)
Wholemeal bread	66 (16.3)	69 (17.0)	88 (21.7)	79 (19.5)	103 (25.4)
Fishes and seafood	60 (14.8)	193 (47.6)	35 (8.6)	110 (27.1)	7 (1.7)
Red meat, ham, sausages	35 (8.6)	111 (27.4)	117 (28,8)	64 (15.8)	78 (19.2)
Sour milk products	44 (10.8)	50 (12.3)	119 (29.3)	79 (19.5)	113 (27.9)
Cheese	22 (5.4)	114 (28.1)	85 (20.9)	82 (20.2)	102 (25.1)
Cottage cheese	12 (2.9)	73 (18.0)	141 (34.8)	89 (21.9)	90 (22.2)
Vegetables/fruit	3 (0.7)	11 (2.7)	76 (18.7)	31 (7.6)	284 (70.1)
Sweets/salty snacks	13 (3.2)	65 (16.0)	132 (32.5)	84 (20.7)	111 (27.4)
Fast food products	168 (41.4)	159 (39.2)	28 (6.9)	31 (7.6)	19 (4.6)

The results obtained from logistic regression models indicated that the consumption of specific food product groups may predispose to/increase the risk of hypertension, abdominal obesity, overweight, obesity, body fat accumulation, and the risk of cardiovascular events. The adjusted regression models revealed that significant predictors for the prevalence of abdominal obesity according to WHR were male gender (OR = 0.317) and age (OR = 1.087), while for cardiometabolic risk according to WHtR, the predictors were male gender (OR = 5.082), age (OR = 1.099), sweetening coffee/tea (OR = 1.614), and consuming red meat and sausages 2–4 times a week (OR = 1.898). Significant predictors for the prevalence of overweight were age (OR = 1.066), consuming fish and seafood a few times a month (OR = 0.44), and consuming red meat and sausages 2–4 times a week (OR = 2.208), while for obesity, they were age (OR = 1.095) and sweetening coffee/tea (OR = 1.978). In the case of increased body fat accumulation and the risk of cardiovascular events, significant predictors were male gender (OR = 3.296; OR = 126.311) and age (OR = 1.093; OR = 1.751), (Table 3).

Table 3. Significant predictors of the odds of hypertension, abdominal obesity, cardiometabolic risk, overweight, obesity, increased body fat, and cardiovascular risk—univariate and multiple regression models.

Variable		Parameter **						
		Univariate Model				Multiple Model		
		OR	95% CI		p	OR	95% CI	p
Consumption of specific groups of products and the prevalence of hypertension								
Age	(ears)	1.068	1.043	1.093	<0.001 *	1.072	1.047	1.098	<0.001 *
Salting dishes	Rarely or never add salt to food	1	ref.			1	ref.	
	I taste the food and add salt as needed	0.58	0.344	0.98	0.042 *	0.528	0.299	0.93	0.027 *
	I add salt to my food without trying it first	1.091	0.597	1.995	0.776	1.089	0.553	2.141	0.806
Consumption of specific groups of products and the prevalence of abdominal obesity according to WHR								
Sex	Female	1	ref.			1	ref.	
	Male	0.312	0.122	0.8	0.015 *	0.317	0.116	0.864	0.025 *
Age	(years)	1.089	1.063	1.115	<0.001 *	1.087	1.061	1.115	<0.001 *
Consumption of specific groups of products and the prevalence of cardiometabolic risk according to WHtR								
Sex	Female	1	ref.			1	ref.	
	Male	2.619	1.023	6.702	0.045 *	5.082	1.583	16.319	0.006 *
Age	(years)	1.095	1.07	1.122	<0.001 *	1.099	1.071	1.127	<0.001 *
Adding sugar to coffee/tea	No	1	ref.			1	ref.	
	Yes	1.449	0.975	2.155	0.067	1.614	1.013	2.571	0.044 *
Red meat, ham, sausages	A few times a month or less	1	ref.			1	ref.	
	2–4 times a week	1.682	1.082	2.614	0.021 *	1.898	1.135	3.174	0.015 *
	Every day	1.646	0.942	2.875	0.08	1.556	0.823	2.944	0.174
Consumption of specific groups of products and the prevalence of overweight according to BMI								
Age	(years)	1.067	1.044	1.089	<0.001 *	1.066	1.042	1.091	<0.001 *
Fishes and seafood	I do not eat	1	ref.			1	ref.	
	A few times a month	0.442	0.238	0.822	0.01 *	0.44	0.219	0.882	0.021 *
	Once a week	0.824	0.432	1.572	0.557	0.597	0.284	1.255	0.174
Red meat, ham, sausages	A few times a month or less	1	ref.			1	ref.	
	2–4 times a week	2.184	1.394	3.423	0.001 *	2.208	1.347	3.618	0.002 *
	Every day	1.602	0.917	2.797	0.098	1.447	0.776	2.698	0.45
Consumption of specific groups of products and the prevalence of obesity according to BMI								
Age	(years)	1.091	1.06	1.124	<0.001 *	1.095	1.061	1.129	<0.001 *
Adding sugar to coffee/tea	No	1	ref.			1	ref.	
	Yes	2.082	1.303	3.326	0.002 *	1.978	1.19	3.289	0.009 *
Consumption of specific groups of products and the prevalence of increased body fat								
Sex	Female	1	ref.			1	ref.	
	Male	2.131	0.933	4.866	0.073	3.296	1.281	8.478	0.013 *
Age	(years)	1.088	1.061	1.115	<0.001 *	1.093	1.065	1.121	<0.001 *
Consumption of specific groups of products and the prevalence of and increased cardiovascular risk—Framingham Risk Score								
Sex	Female	1	ref.			1	ref.	
	Male	3.134	1.369	7.177	0.007 *	126.311	11.981	1331.671	<0.001 *
Age	(years)	1.623	1.455	1.811	<0.001 *	1.751	1.535	1.997	<0.001 *

* Statistically significant relationship ($p < 0.05$); p—single and multivariate linear regression; OR—odds ratio; CI—confidence interval; OR (95% CI)—odds ratio with a 95% confidence interval; ** adjusted to white bread, wholemeal bread, sour milk products, cheese, cottage cheese, vegetables/fruit, sweets/salty snacks, and fast food products.

Details of univariate and multivariate regression analyses are available in the Supplementary Materials Tables S1–S7.

Additionally, the quality and effectiveness of multifactorial models in predicting the impact of specific product groups on selected health indicators and the Framingham Risk Score were assessed in the study group of nurses. ROC curves and AUCs for models A–F showed good predictive accuracy for hypertension (AUC = 0.724, $p < 0.001$); abdominal obesity measured by WHR (AUC = 0.741, $p < 0.001$); cardiometabolic risk according to WHtR (AUC = 0.777, $p < 0.001$); overweight (AUC = 0.734, $p < 0.001$) and obesity (AUC = 0.756, $p < 0.001$) determined by BMI; and excessive body fat (AUC = 0.741, $p < 0.001$) (Figure 1).

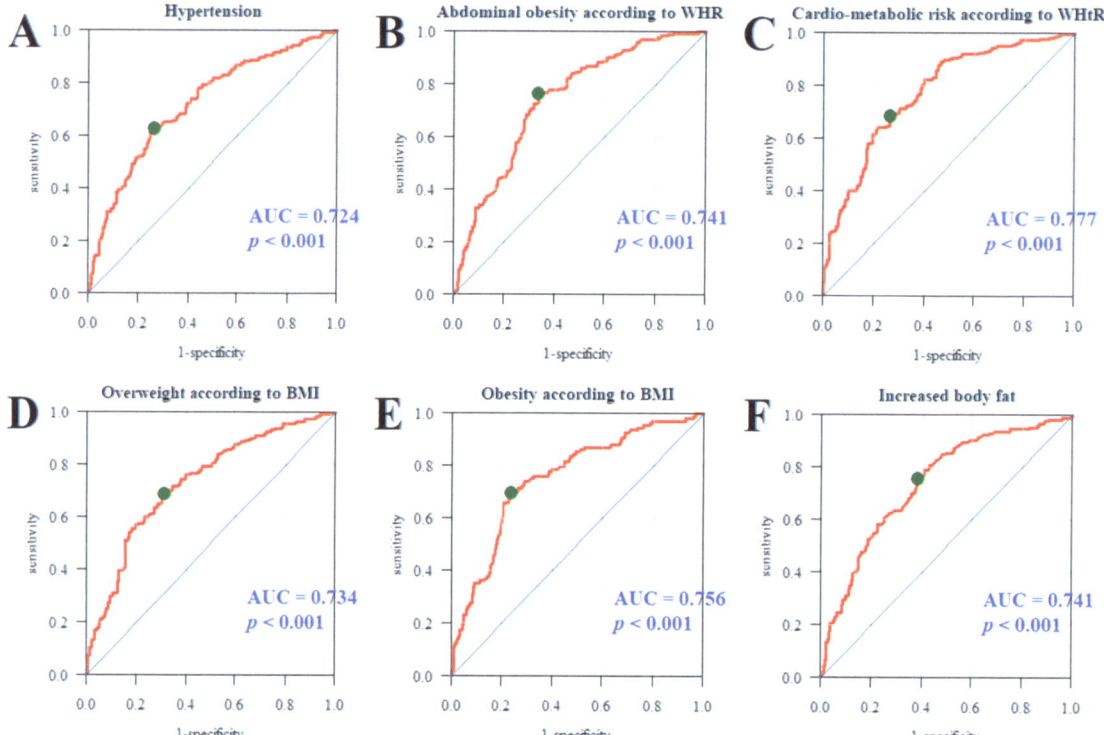

Figure 1. ROC curve and AUC value: hypertension (**A**), abdominal obesity according to WHR (**B**), cardiometabolic risk according to WHtR (**C**), overweight (**D**), obesity (**E**), and increased body fat (**F**). Line red—ROC curve for the analyzed model. Line blue—ROC curve for the random model (depicting a line with a 45-degree slope, indicating no predictive ability). Green dot—optimal cutpoint on the red curve, which is the point closest to the top-left corner of the plot, representing the best trade-off between sensitivity and specificity.

In the case of model G, which predicted the Framingham Risk Score, which estimates the likelihood of experiencing a cardiovascular event within the next 10 years, the AUC was 0.959, $p < 0.001$, indicating that the multifactorial model almost perfectly predicts cardiovascular risk (Figure 2).

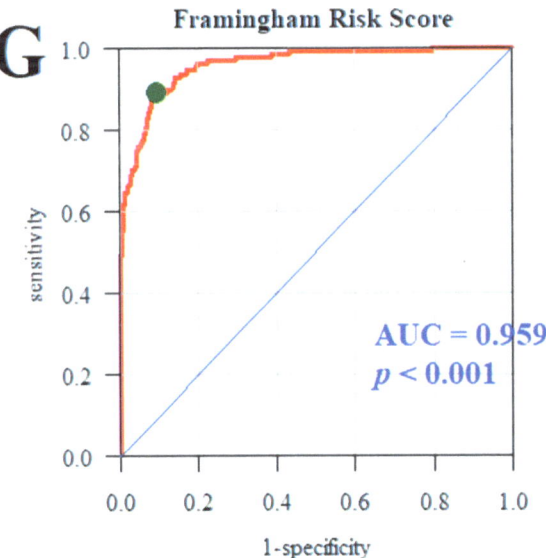

Figure 2. Likelihood of experiencing a cardiovascular event within the next 10 years according to Framingham Risk Score. Line red—ROC curve for the analyzed model. Line blue—ROC curve for the random model (depicting a line with a 45-degree slope, indicating no predictive ability). Green dot—optimal cutpoint on the red curve, which is the point closest to the top-left corner of the plot, representing the best trade-off between sensitivity and specificity.

This study demonstrated that the diet of nurses significantly impacts the risk of developing metabolic and cardiovascular disorders, with clear associations between specific food groups and health outcomes such as abdominal obesity, overweight, and cardiometabolic risk. Multifactorial modeling using the Framingham Risk Score effectively predicts cardiovascular risk (AUC = 0.959), confirming the potential of diet as a critical tool in health prevention among this professional group.

4. Discussion

This study demonstrates the influence of dietary patterns on metabolic and cardiovascular disorders among 405 predominantly female nurses, with a mean age of 48.5 years. Consumption data show a significant preference for fruits and vegetables (70.1%) and white bread (56.3%), consumed every day, while fish and seafood were the least consumed (1.7%). Logistic regression analyses highlighted significant predictors of health risks, such as hypertension, obesity, and cardiovascular events, to be notably male gender, increased age, and the consumption of red meat and sweetening coffee/tea. Importantly, the models exhibited strong predictive accuracy for cardiovascular risk, with an AUC of 0.959 for the Framingham Risk Score. These findings reinforce a significant link between dietary choices and health outcomes, emphasizing the need for targeted nutritional interventions to mitigate diet-related risks and promote overall health among nurses, who must be aware of the impact of their dietary habits impact of their health and well-being. The Global Burden of Disease study underscores the profound influence of diet on the incidence of major health conditions [37]. Despite guidance from health organizations like The European Society of Cardiology, adherence to dietary recommendations remains low, contributing to cardiovascular disease being a leading cause of death in Europe. This trend is exacerbated by inadequate nutritional knowledge and the influence of unhealthy dietary patterns increasingly adopted globally [38–40]. Nurses are pivotal in promoting healthy lifestyles and reducing cardiovascular risk [41]; however, their nutritional knowledge is often insufficient. A study involving 506 nurses revealed that only 58.4%, correctly understood nutrition related to obesity and cardiovascular disease [41,42]. Despite recognizing the benefits of certain nutrients, many lacked detailed knowledge about low-cholesterol diets and sources of water-soluble fiber, fatty acids, and specific cardioprotective foods [43].

Warber et al. observed a 66% accuracy rate in nutritional knowledge among nurse practitioners, underscoring the need to promote current, evidence-based nutrition education. This knowledge enhances their capacity to educate patients and integrate healthy practices into their own lives [44]. A study conducted by Kilar et al. found that 60% of nurses engaged in preventive examinations, and 70% prioritized family with health and work following closely. However, nurses with chronic conditions had lower health behavior levels than their healthy counterparts, highlighting the need for targeted health interventions within this group [45]. The findings of this study highlight the need for specific interventions to improve the health of nurses with chronic illnesses and to promote a more proactive approach to personal health management within the nursing profession. Research on the association between dietary patterns and the risk of metabolic syndrome or cardiovascular disease among nurses is limited and inconsistent. A study of 346 pre-registered UK nurses and midwives found a high prevalence of overweight or obese (33.8%) and poor dietary habits, with 67.6% not meeting the five-a-day fruit and vegetable guideline. Such participants were also less likely to view health professionals as role models, associating negative perceptions with health promotion [46]. Similarly, another study showed that over 50% of nurses did not meet recommended physical activity levels, and more than 75% did not consume adequate amounts of fruits and vegetables, with nearly 20% reporting current smoking habits [47]. Our study revealed a higher prevalence of smoking among nurses, with 24.6% reporting this habit. A significant majority of respondents (70.1%) indicated a daily consumption of fruits and vegetables; however, the survey did not assess whether they met the recommended intake of five servings per day. In contrast, studies in different regions like Australia and Brazil show varying adherence to dietary guidelines among nurses, indicating a complex relationship between professional health knowledge and personal health practices [48,49].

A nutritious diet is crucial for overall well-being and longevity; however, many nurses struggle to maintain healthy eating habits despite their role as advocates for health education. Research indicates a significant and growing trend of overweight and obesity among nurses, with a prevalence study in Scotland revealing that 69% of nurses were overweight or obese—rates notably higher than other healthcare professionals and those in non-health-related jobs [50,51]. In our study, the prevalence of excess weight based on BMI was nearly 60%, with 32.6% of participants classified as having obesity. Significant predictors for the prevalence of obesity included age (OR = 1.095) and the practice of sweetening coffee or tea (OR = 1.978). This trend may be linked to low physical activity and diets deficient in fruits and vegetables but high in sugar, exacerbated by shift work [52–54]. Although no single intervention has shown strong effectiveness against obesity, integrating tailored lifestyle interventions into nurses' routines is essential for addressing their unique challenges in maintaining a healthy lifestyle [55].

A study of 403 female nurses examined the links between dietary habits, alcohol use, and shift work on the risk of metabolic syndrome, finding a prevalence of 5.6%. The key risk factors included late-night calorie intake, carbonated drink consumption, family history of diabetes, and non-shift work [56]. Conversely, a cross-sectional study of 420 female Iranian nurses found a metabolic syndrome prevalence of 3.6%, with no significant correlations to waist circumference, blood pressure, triglycerides, HDL cholesterol, or fasting blood sugar, after controlling confounding factors [57]. A global systematic review and meta-analysis of 22 articles encompassing 117,922 nurses identified a sedentary lifestyle and lack of physical activity as the most prevalent cardiovascular disease risk factors, observed in 46.3% of participants. Additional risk factors included a family history of cardiovascular disease (41.9%), being overweight (33.3%), and alcohol consumption (24.6%). Among shift-working nurses, nearly all risk factors were more pronounced, suggesting worse conditions compared to their daytime counterparts [58]. These findings highlight the need for targeted interventions to mitigate cardiovascular disease risk among nurses, particularly those in shift work environments.

Future research should explore interventions aimed at improving dietary quality and increasing physical activity among nurses, assessing their long-term impact on health outcomes. Universities must prioritize health promotion initiatives, improving access to resources for nursing students and staff to foster a culture of well-being and resilience that enhances educational outcomes and patient care. The key initiatives could include promoting regular rest breaks, providing on-site fruits and vegetables, and incorporating brief exercise sessions into daily routines. Educational programs need to emphasize workplace well-being and self-care, addressing both personal and environmental factors affecting health-related decisions.

Strengths, Limitations, and Future Research

Based on our understanding, this study represents one of the earliest comprehensive efforts in Poland to explore how consumption of certain food groups affects the risk of prevalent metabolic and cardiovascular disorders within this professional group. It is important to acknowledge several potential limitations of this study that may affect the interpretation of its findings. The study's geographical reach was restricted and should be expanded to include more medical facilities across different regions. Given its cross-sectional design, it is inappropriate to infer causality or temporal relationships from the results. Additionally, some variables, such as alcohol consumption, physical activity, and menopausal and hormonal status, were not included in the selection criteria, although we acknowledge their potential impact on health. Further research involving a larger population that considers age-specific factors and other lifestyle variables is necessary.

5. Conclusions

This study reveals significant relationships between dietary habits and various health risks, particularly related to hypertension, obesity, and cardiovascular events. The key findings indicate that the consumption of certain food groups, particularly red meat and processed meats like sausages, 2 to 4 times per week is associated with an elevated prevalence of overweight and cardiometabolic risk. Factors such as male gender and age were significantly associated with abdominal obesity and cardiometabolic risk. Age was also a significant factor in the prevalence of overweight and obesity; moreover, sweetening coffee/tea was identified as a significant factor associated with obesity and cardiometabolic risk. These results underline the importance of dietary patterns in managing health outcomes among nurses.

Supplementary Materials: The following supporting information can be downloaded at: https://www.mdpi.com/article/10.3390/jcm13185568/s1, Table S1: Consumption of specific food groups and prevalence of hypertension. Univariate and multiple regression models. Table S2: Consumption of specific food groups and prevalence of abdominal obesity according to WHR. Univariate and multiple regression models. Table S3: Consumption of specific group of products and the prevalence of cardiometabolic risk according to WHtR. Univariate and multiple regression models. Table S4: Consumption of specific group of products and the prevalence of overweight according to BMI. Univariate and multiple regression models. Table S5: Consumption of specific group of products and the prevalence of obesity according to BMI. Univariate and multiple regression models. Table S6: Consumption of specific group of products and the prevalence of increased body fat. Univariate and multiple regression models. Table S7: Consumption of specific group of products and the prevalence of and increased cardiovascular risk-Framingham Risc Score. Univariate and multiple regression models.

Author Contributions: Conceptualization, A.B.; data curation, A.B., J.W., E.Ł. and P.M.; formal analysis, A.B.; funding acquisition, J.W.; investigation, A.B.; methodology, A.B.; software, A.B. and P.S.; writing—original draft preparation, A.B. and J.W.; writing—review and editing, A.B., J.W., A.L. and M.Z.-Z. All authors have read and agreed to the published version of the manuscript.

Funding: This research received no external funding.

Institutional Review Board Statement: This study was conducted according to the guidelines of the Declaration of Helsinki and approved by the University of Rzeszow Bioethics Commission (Resolution No. 2022/088, dated 5 October 2022). We confirm that written consent was obtained voluntarily from all respondents. No information allows the respondents to be identified.

Informed Consent Statement: Informed consent was obtained from all the subjects involved in the study.

Data Availability Statement: All the data generated or analyzed during this study are included in this published article.

Conflicts of Interest: The authors declare no conflicts of interest.

References

1. Yeung, S.S.; Kwan, M.; Woo, J. Healthy diet for healthy ageing. *Nutrients* **2021**, *13*, 4310. [CrossRef] [PubMed]
2. Lim, S. Eating a balanced diet: A healthy life through a balanced diet in the age of longevity. *J. Obes. Metab. Syndr.* **2018**, *27*, 39. [CrossRef] [PubMed]
3. Torquati, L.; Pavey, T.; Kolbe-Alexander, T.; Leveritt, M. Promoting diet and physical activity in nurses: A systematic review. *Am. J. Health Prom.* **2017**, *31*, 19–27. [CrossRef] [PubMed]
4. De Ridder, D.; Kroese, F.; Evers, C.; Adriaanse, M.; Gillebaart, M. Healthy diet: Health impact, prevalence, correlates, and interventions. *Psychol. Health* **2017**, *32*, 907–941. [CrossRef] [PubMed]
5. Willett, W.C.; Stampfer, M.J. *Rebuilding the Food Pyramid*; Scientific American: New York, NY, USA, 2003.
6. Hu, F.B. Plant-based foods and prevention of cardiovascular disease: An overview. *Am. J. Clin. Nutr.* **2003**, *78*, 544–551. [CrossRef]
7. Estruch, R.; Ros, E.; Salas-Salvadó, J.; Covas, M.I.; Corella, D.; Arós, F.; Gómez-Gracia, E.; Ruiz-Gutiérrez, V.; Fiol, M.; Lapetra, J.; et al. Primary prevention of cardiovascular disease with a Mediterranean diet. *N. Engl. J. Med.* **2013**, *368*, 1279–1290. [CrossRef]
8. Guasch-Ferré, M.; Willett, W.C. The Mediterranean diet and health: A comprehensive overview. *J. Int. Med.* **2021**, *290*, 549–566. [CrossRef]
9. Martinez-Lacoba, R.; Pardo-Garcia, I.; Amo-Saus, E.; Escribano-Sotos, F. Mediterranean diet and health outcomes: A systematic meta-review. *Eur. J. Public Health* **2018**, *28*, 955–961. [CrossRef]
10. Steinberg, D.; Bennett, G.G.; Svetkey, L. The DASH diet, 20 years later. *JAMA* **2017**, *317*, 1529–1530. [CrossRef]
11. Craddick, S.R.; Elmer, P.J.; Obarzanek, E.; Vollmer, W.M.; Svetkey, L.P.; Swain, M.C. The DASH diet and blood pressure. *Curr. Atherosc. Rep.* **2003**, *5*, 484–491. [CrossRef]
12. Watzl, B.; Kulling, S.E.; Möseneder, J.; Barth, S.W.; Bub, A. A 4-wk intervention with high intake of carotenoid-rich vegetables and fruit reduces plasma C-reactive protein in healthy, nonsmoking men. *Am. J. Clin. Nutr.* **2005**, *82*, 1052–1058. [CrossRef] [PubMed]
13. Gao, X.; Bermudez, O.I.; Tucker, K.L. Plasma C-reactive protein and homocysteine concentrations are related to frequent fruit and vegetable intake in Hispanic and non-Hispanic white elders. *J. Nutr.* **2004**, *134*, 913–918. [CrossRef] [PubMed]
14. Esmaillzadeh, A.; Kimiagar, M.; Mehrabi, Y.; Azadbakht, L.; Hu, F.B.; Willett, W.C. Fruit and vegetable intakes, C-reactive protein, and the metabolic syndrome. *Am. J. Clin. Nutr.* **2006**, *84*, 1489–1497. [CrossRef] [PubMed]
15. Wilson, P.W.; D'Agostino, R.B.; Levy, D.; Belanger, A.M.; Silbershatz, H.; Kannel, W.B. Prediction of coronary heart disease using risk factor categories. *Circulation* **1998**, *97*, 1837–1847. [CrossRef]
16. Mirashrafi, S.; Kafeshani, M.; Hassanzadeh, A.; Entezari, M.H. Cross-sectional Relationships Between Alternate Healthy Eating Index (AHEI) with General and Abdominal Obesity and Blood Pressure in Iranian Hospital Employees. *Endocr. Metab. Immune Disord.-Drug Targets* **2021**, *21*, 2281–2288. [CrossRef]
17. Domingues, J.G.; Silva, B.B.; Bierhals, I.O.; Barros, F.C. Noncommunicable diseases among nursing professionals at a charitable hospital in Southern Brazil. *Epidemiol. Serv. Saude* **2019**, *28*, e2018298.
18. Dutheil, F.; Baker, J.S.; Mermillod, M.; De Cesare, M.; Vidal, A.; Moustafa, F.; Pereira, B.; Navel, V. Shift work, and particularly permanent night shifts, promote dyslipidaemia: A systematic review and meta-analysis. *Atherosclerosis* **2020**, *313*, 156–169. [CrossRef]
19. Sooriyaarachchi, P.; Jayawardena, R.; Pavey, T.; King, N.A. Shift work and the risk for metabolic syndrome among healthcare workers: A systematic review and meta-analysis. *Obes. Rev.* **2022**, *23*, e13489. Available online: https://onlinelibrary.wiley.com/doi/full/10.1111/obr.13489 (accessed on 14 April 2024). [CrossRef]
20. World Health Organization (WHO). *State of World's Nursing 2020: Investing in Education, Jobs and Leadership*; WHO: Geneva, Switzerland, 2020. Available online: https://www.who.int/publications/i/item/9789240003279 (accessed on 20 May 2024).
21. Van der Heijden, B.; Brown Mahoney, C.; Xu, Y. Impact of job demands and resources on nurses' burnout and occupational turnover intention towards an age-moderated mediation model for the nursing profession. *Int. J. Environ. Res. Public Health* **2019**, *16*, 2011. [CrossRef]
22. Naczelna Izba Pielęgniarek i Położnych. *Raport Naczelnej Rady Pielęgniarek i Położnych: Pielęgniarka, Położna Zawody Deficytowe w Polskim Systemie Ochrony Zdrowia*; NIPiP: Warszawa, Poland, 2022. Available online: https://nipip.pl/wp-content/uploads/2022/06/2022_Raport-NIPiP-struktura-wiekowa-kadr.pdf (accessed on 14 April 2024).

23. Nedeltcheva, A.V.; Kilkus, J.M.; Imperial, J.; Schoeller, D.A.; Penev, P.D. Insufficient sleep undermines dietary efforts to reduce adiposity. *Ann. Intern. Med.* **2010**, *153*, 435–441. [CrossRef]
24. Blake, H.; Patterson, J. Paediatric nurses' attitudes towards the promotion of healthy eating. *Br. J. Nurs.* **2015**, *24*, 108–112. [CrossRef] [PubMed]
25. Esposito, E.M.; Fitzpatrick, J.J. Registered nurses' beliefs of the benefits of exercise, their exercise behaviour and their patient teaching regarding exercise. *Int. J. Nurs. Pract.* **2011**, *17*, 351–356. [CrossRef] [PubMed]
26. Silveira, E.A.; Pagotto, V.; Barbosa, L.S.; Oliveira, C.D.; Pena, G.D.; Velasquez-Melendez, G. Accuracy of BMI and waist circumference cut-off points to predict obesity in older adults. *Cienc. Saude Coletiva* **2020**, *25*, 1073–1082. [CrossRef]
27. Nishida, C.; Ko, G.; Kumanyika, S. Body fat distribution and noncommunicable diseases in populations: Overview of the 2008 WHO Expert Consultation on Waist Circumference and Waist–Hip Ratio. *Eur. J. Clin. Nutr.* **2010**, *64*, 2–5. [CrossRef] [PubMed]
28. Gibson, S.; Ashwell, M. A simple cut-off for waist-to-height ratio (0·5) can act as an indicator for cardiometabolic risk: Recent data from adults in the Health Survey for England. *Br. J. Nutr.* **2020**, *123*, 681–690. [CrossRef] [PubMed]
29. Williams, B.R.; Mancia, G.; Spiering, W.; Rosei, E.A.; Azizi, M.; Burnier, M.; Clement, D.L.; Coca, A.; de Simone, G.; Dominiczak, A.; et al. Guidelines for the management of arterial hypertension. *Kardiol. Pol. (Pol. Heart J.)* **2019**, *77*, 71–159. [CrossRef]
30. Pęksa, J. Prawidłowe wykonywanie pomiarów ciśnienia tętniczego w gabinecie lekarskim. *Lek. POZ* **2022**, *8*, 130–136.
31. Banach, M.; Burchardt, P.; Chlebus, K.; Dobrowolski, P.; Dudek, D.; Dyrbuś, K.; Gąsior, M.; Jankowski, P.; Jóźwiak, J.; Kłosiewicz-Latoszek, L.; et al. Wytyczne PTL/ KLRWP/PTK diagnostyki i leczenia zaburzeń lipidowych w Polsce 2021. *Nadciśnienie Tętnicze W Prakt.* **2021**, *7*, 113–122.
32. American Diabetes Association. Classification and diagnosis of diabetes: Standards of medical care in diabetes—2021. *Diabetes Care* **2021**, *44*, 15–33. [CrossRef]
33. Imboden, M.T.; Welch, W.A.; Swartz, A.M.; Montoye, A.H.; Finch, H.W.; Harber, M.P.; Kaminsky, L.A. Reference standards for body fat measures using GE dual energy x-ray absorptiometry in Caucasian adults. *PLoS ONE* **2017**, *12*, e0175110. [CrossRef]
34. Tanita. Professional Product. Guide. Available online: https://tanita.es/media/pdf/documents/professional/EN%20-%20Medical%20Product%20Guide%20DIGITAL.pdf (accessed on 22 April 2024).
35. Bartosiewicz, A.; Wyszyńska, J.; Matłosz, P.; Łuszczki, E.; Oleksy, Ł.; Stolarczyk, A. Prevalence of dyslipidaemia within Polish nurses. Cross-sectional study-single and multiple linear regression models and ROC analysis. *BMC Public Health* **2024**, *24*, 1002.
36. R Core Team. *R: A Language and Environment for Statistical Computing*; R Foundation for Statistical Computing: Vienna, Italy, 2018. Available online: https://www.R-project.org (accessed on 3 February 2024).
37. Anand, S.S.; Hawkes, C.; De Souza, R.J.; Mente, A.; Dehghan, M.; Nugent, R.; Zulyniak, M.A.; Weis, T.; Bernstein, A.M.; Krauss, R.M.; et al. Food Consumption and its Impact on Cardiovascular Disease: Importance of Solutions Focused on the Globalized Food System: A Report From the Workshop Convened by the World Heart Federation. *J. Am. Coll. Cardiol.* **2015**, *66*, 1590–1614. [CrossRef]
38. Visseren, F.L.; Mach, F.; Smulders, Y.M.; Carballo, D.; Koskinas, K.C.; Bäck, M.; Benetos, A.; Biffi, A.; Boavida, J.M.; Capodanno, D.; et al. 2021 ESC Guidelines on cardiovascular disease prevention in clinical practice. *Eur. Heart J.* **2022**, *43*, 4468. [CrossRef] [PubMed]
39. European Society of Cardiology, Fact Sheets for Press. Available online: https://www.escardio.org/The-ESC/Press-Office/Fact-sheets (accessed on 14 August 2024).
40. Waśkiewicz, A.; Piotrowski, W.; Sygnowska, E.; Broda, G.; Drygas, W.; Zdrojewski, T.; Kozakiewicz, K.; Tykarski, A.; Biela, U. Quality of nutrition and health knowledge in subjects with diagnosed cardio-vascular diseases in the Polish population-National Multicentre Health Survey (WOBASZ). *Kardiol. Pol.* **2008**, *66*, 507–513.
41. Zheng, X.; Yu, H.; Qiu, X.; Chair, S.Y.; Wong, E.M.; Wang, Q. The effects of a nurse-led lifestyle intervention program on cardiovascular risk, self-efficacy and health promoting behaviours among patients with metabolic syndrome: Randomized controlled trial. *Int. J. Nurs. Stud.* **2020**, *109*, 103638. [CrossRef]
42. Zhu, B.; Haruyama, Y.; Muto, T.; Yamasaki, A.; Tarumi, F. Evaluation of a community intervention program in Japan using Framingham risk score and estimated 10-year coronary heart disease risk as outcome variables: A non-randomized controlled trial. *BMC Public Health* **2013**, *13*, 219. [CrossRef]
43. Park, K.A.; Cho, W.I.; Song, K.J.; Lee, Y.S.; Sung, I.S.; Choi-Kwon, S.M. Assessment of nurses' nutritional knowledge regarding therapeutic diet regimens. *Nurse Educ. Today* **2011**, *31*, 192–197. [CrossRef] [PubMed]
44. Warber, J.I.; Warber, J.P.; Simone, K.A. Assessment of general nutrition knowledge of nurse practitioners in New England. *J. Am. Diet. Assoc.* **2000**, *100*, 368–370. [CrossRef] [PubMed]
45. Kilar, R.; Harpula, K.; Nagórska, M. Health behaviors in professionally active nurses–preliminary research. *Eur. J. Clin. Exp. Med.* **2019**, *17*, 214–220. [CrossRef]
46. Blake, H.; Watkins, K.; Middleton, M.; Stanulewicz, N. Obesity and Diet Predict Attitudes towards Health Promotion in Pre-Registered Nurses and Midwives. *Int. J. Environ. Res. Public Health* **2021**, *18*, 13419. [CrossRef]
47. Blake, H.; Malik, S.; Mo, P.K.; Pisano, C. 'Do as say, but not as I do': Are next generation nurses role models for health? *Perspect. Public Health* **2011**, *131*, 231–239. [CrossRef] [PubMed]
48. Perry, L.; Xu, X.; Gallagher, R.; Nicholls, R.; Sibbritt, D.; Duffield, C. Lifestyle Health Behaviors of Nurses and Midwives: The 'Fit for the Future' Study. *Int. J. Environ. Res. Public Health* **2018**, *15*, 945. [CrossRef] [PubMed]

49. Hidalgo, K.D.; Mielke, G.I.; Parra, D.C.; Lobelo, F.; Simões, E.J.; Gomes, G.O.; Florindo, A.A.; Bracco, M.; Moura, L.; Brownson, R.C.; et al. Health promoting practices and personal lifestyle behaviors of Brazilian health professionals. *BMC Public Health* **2016**, *16*, 1114. [CrossRef] [PubMed]
50. Davies, R. Promoting and supporting healthy eating among nurses. *Nurs. Stand.* **2020**, *35*, 45–50. [CrossRef] [PubMed]
51. Kyle, R.G.; Neall, R.A.; Atherton, I.M. Prevalence of overweight and obesity among nurses in Scotland: A cross-sectional study using the Scottish Health Survey. *Int. J. Nurs. Stud.* **2016**, *53*, 126–133. [CrossRef]
52. Blake, H.; Harrison, C. Health behaviours and attitudes towards being role models. *Br. J. Nurs.* **2013**, *22*, 86–94. [CrossRef]
53. Happell, B.; Gaskin, C.J.; Reid-Searl, K.; Dwyer, T. Physical and psychosocial wellbeing of nurses in a regional Queensland hospital. *Collegian* **2014**, *21*, 71–78. [CrossRef]
54. Liu, Q.; Shi, J.; Duan, P.; Liu, B.; Li, T.; Wang, C.; Li, H.; Yang, T.; Gan, Y.; Wang, X.; et al. Is shift work associated with a higher risk of overweight or obesity? A systematic review of observational studies with meta-analysis. *Int. J. Epidemiol.* **2018**, *47*, 1956–1971. [CrossRef]
55. Kelly, M.; Wills, J. Systematic review: What works to address obesity in nurses? *Occup. Med.* **2018**, *68*, 228–238. [CrossRef]
56. Jung, H.; Dan, H.; Pang, Y.; Kim, B.; Jeong, H.; Lee, J.E.; Kim, O. Association between Dietary Habits, Shift Work, and the Metabolic Syndrome: The Korea Nurses' Health Study. *Int. J. Environ. Res. Public Health* **2020**, *17*, 7697. [CrossRef]
57. Ghosn, B.; Falahi, E.; Keshteli, A.H.; Yazdannik, A.R.; Azadbakht, L.; Esmaillzadeh, A. Lack of association between nuts and legumes consumption and metabolic syndrome in young Iranian nurses. *Clin. Nutr. ESPEN* **2021**, *46*, 173–178. [CrossRef] [PubMed]
58. Khani, S.; Rafiei, S.; Ghashghaee, A.; Masoumi, M.; Rezaee, S.; Kheradkhah, G.; Abdollahi, B. Cardiovascular risk factors among nurses: A global systematic review and meta-analysis. *PLoS ONE* **2024**, *19*, e0286245. [CrossRef] [PubMed]

Disclaimer/Publisher's Note: The statements, opinions and data contained in all publications are solely those of the individual author(s) and contributor(s) and not of MDPI and/or the editor(s). MDPI and/or the editor(s) disclaim responsibility for any injury to people or property resulting from any ideas, methods, instructions or products referred to in the content.

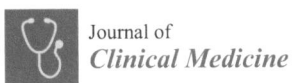

Article

The Effect of Obesity on Repolarization and Other ECG Parameters

Irena A. Dykiert [1], Krzysztof Kraik [2], Lidia Jurczenko [2], Paweł Gać [3,*], Rafał Poręba [4] and Małgorzata Poręba [5]

[1] Department of Physiology and Pathophysiology, Division of Pathophysiology, Wroclaw Medical University, 50-368 Wrocław, Poland
[2] Students' Scientific Association of Cardiovascular Diseases Prevention, Wroclaw Medical University, 50-368 Wrocław, Poland
[3] Department of Population Health, Division of Environmental Health and Occupational Medicine, Wroclaw Medical University, 50-372 Wrocław, Poland
[4] Department of Internal Medicine, Occupational Diseases, Hypertension and Clinical Oncology, Wroclaw Medical University, 50-556 Wrocław, Poland
[5] Department of Paralympic Sport, Wroclaw University of Health and Sport Sciences, 51-617 Wrocław, Poland
* Correspondence: pawel.gac@umw.edu.pl or pawelgac@interia.pl

Abstract: Background: Overweight and obesity are important risk factors in the development of cardiovascular diseases. New repolarization markers, such as the Tpeak-Tend interval and JTpeak intervals, have not yet been profoundly studied in obese patients. The study aims to analyze whether, in patients with obesity and overweight, repolarization markers, including the Tpeak-Tend interval, are prolonged and simultaneously check the frequency of other ECG pathologies in a 12-lead ECG in this group of patients. **Methods**: A study group consisted of 181 adults (90 females and 91 males) with overweight and first-class obesity. The participants completed a questionnaire, and the ECG was performed and analyzed. **Results**: When analyzing the classic markers, only QT dispersion was significantly higher in obese people. The Tpeak-Tend parameter (97.08 ms ± 23.38 vs. 89.74 ms ± 12.88, respectively), its dispersion, and JTpeak-JTend parameters were statistically significantly longer in the obese group than in the controls. There were also substantial differences in P-wave, QRS duration, and P-wave dispersion, which were the highest in obese people. Tpeak-Tend was positively correlated with body mass and waist circumference, while JTpeak was with BMI, hip circumference, and WHR. Tpeak/JT was positively correlated with WHR and BMI. In backward stepwise multiple regression analysis for JTpeak-WHR, type 2 diabetes and smoking had the highest statistical significance. **Conclusions**: Only selected repolarization markers are significantly prolonged in patients with class 1 obesity and, additionally, in this group, we identified more pathologies of P wave as well as prolonged QRS duration,

Keywords: electrocardiography; repolarization markers; obesity; overweight

1. Introduction

Overweight and obesity are characterized by abnormal and excessive adipose tissue deposition in the body [1]. These states are important risk factors in the development of several diseases, including cardiovascular diseases, diabetes, and neoplastic diseases, which are leading causes of death worldwide [2]. They may also increase the risk of death by exacerbating symptoms of respiratory disorders [3] and infectious diseases, including COVID-19 [4,5]. Moreover, overweight and obesity often lead to lowering the quality of life as risk factors for diabetes mellitus, respiratory disorders, and musculoskeletal disease development. In connection with these risks, the governments of numerous countries allocate considerable resources to prevent and treat obesity; for example, the USA's healthcare system spends about USD 173 billion annually for that purpose only [6].

Nowadays, obesity is considered a separate disease entity, and its prevalence is common; sometimes, the term "a pandemic of obesity" is used [7]. In 2016, globally, about

13% of all adults were classified as obese, and 39% were classified as overweight [1]. The epidemiological situation regarding these states looks very pessimistic. The number of obese people has almost tripled in the last 50 years [7]. In Poland, there is also a continuing trend of increasing incidence of obesity. In 1975, the prevalence of obesity in Polish adults was estimated to be 10.6%, which grew by about 0.3% per year until 2006. After 2006, this trend accelerated to about 0.5% per year. In 2016, the prevalence of obesity in Poland was estimated to be 25.6%. The prevalence of obesity in Polish children and adolescents also become higher over the years, and in 2016, it was estimated to be 9.1%. Similarly, the prevalence of overweight and obesity among children and adolescents increased globally—in 1975, 4.3% were classified as overweight and 0.8% as obese, while in 2016, 18.4% were classified as overweight and 6.8% as obese [8].

A standard 12-lead ECG has numerous clinical applications, including screening for cardiac abnormalities in asymptomatic individuals, diagnosing and monitoring cardiac conditions, assessing response to treatment, guiding medical decisions, and evaluating perioperative risk in surgical patients. In the context of obesity, this condition may be associated with various ECG abnormalities [9–11]. ECG findings can provide valuable information for risk stratification, identifying potential complications, and guiding management strategies in obese individuals at risk for cardiovascular disease.

The evidence of the relationship between obesity and ECG findings is inconsistent across studies, showing conflicting results [12–15]. Until now, most commonly reported ECG findings in obese patients include increased heart rate, prolonged QT interval, increased QRS duration and R wave amplitude, and altered T wave morphology [9–11].

In recent years, new repolarization markers have been proposed. The new repolarization markers can be divided into early and late repolarization indices. Early repolarization indices include the JTpeak interval, while late repolarization indices include the Tpeak-Tend interval (Tp-e) and, additionally, the JTpeak/JT, Tp-e/Jtpeak, and Tpeak/JT ratios have been introduced as playing a role in the potential use in patients after myocardial infarction [16]. There are still not many studies establishing the role and clinical significance of the novel repolarization parameters regarding a group of people with obesity and overweight. The Tpeak to Tend interval is one of the most promising novel ventricular repolarization parameters. Tp-e is potentially helpful as a predictor of mortality in patients with heart failure [17,18], as a predictor of cardiac events in long QT syndrome [19–21], and its prolongation may be used as a risk factor of ventricular arrhythmia in STEMI patients after percutaneous coronary interventions [22,23]. Current studies are inconsistent regarding whether Tp-e is HR (heart rate)-dependent [24,25]. For this reason, the Tp-e/QT ratio was proposed as an indicator independent of HR.

This study aims to analyze whether, in patients with obesity and overweight, the classic repolarization markers, as well as the novel ones, including the Tpeak-Tend interval, are prolonged. Additionally, we have attempted to determine if other ECG pathologies are present in this group of patients.

2. Materials and Methods

2.1. Study Population and Trial Design

The study was conducted at the Department of Pathophysiology of Wroclaw Medical University in 2020–2023. The Wroclaw Medical University Ethics Committee approved the study, which was conducted following Good Clinical Practice and the Declaration of Helsinki. The population of the examined patients included adult residents of Wroclaw and its vicinity. We created the initial study group of 303 people out of the adult volunteers who agreed to participate in the study and gave their written consent.

The inclusion criteria for the study group were age over 18 and BMI above 25. Adult patients with a BMI below or equal to 25 were recruited to the control group. We excluded seven patients due to the following causes: one was underage at the moment of recruitment, one person was an athlete, which could affect the ECG results, and for similar reasons, four patients with implantable devices and one person with a history of anorexia in the questionnaire. After collecting the data, we excluded 46 patients due to incomplete information in the questionnaire or the lack of ECG. Figure 1 presents the process of selection of participants, and the characteristics of the comorbidities are presented in Tables 1 and 2.

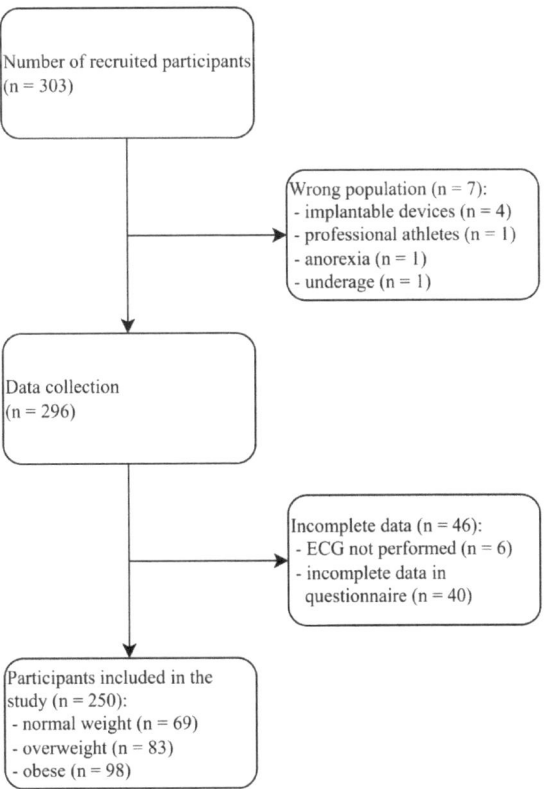

Figure 1. Flowchart presenting the selection of participants.

Table 1. Clinical characteristics of the entire study group.

Parameter	%/n or Mean ± SD
age (years)	59.94 ± 13.22
sex (%/n)	
Male	41.6/104
Female	58.4/146
height (cm)	167.37 ± 9.76
weight (kg)	80.42 ± 17.50
BMI (kg/m^2)	28.64 ± 4.99
waist circumference (cm)	95.99 ± 14.26
hip circumference (cm)	106.60 ± 12.16
WHR	0.95 ± 0.74
hypertension (%/n)	52.8/132
myocardial infarction (%/n)	6.4/16
stroke (%/n)	2.8/7
atrial fibrillation (%/n)	8.8/22
deep vein thrombosis (%/n)	3.6/9
type 2 diabetes (%/n)	13.2/33
thyroid disease (%/n)	16.4/41
smoking (%/n)	13.2/33

BMI—body mass index, WHR—waist-hip ratio.

Table 2. Clinical characteristics of the studied subgroups.

Parameter	Obesity (A, n = 98)	Overweight (B, n = 83)	Control Group (C, n = 69)	$p < 0.05$
age (years)	61.18 ± 11.07	53.40 ± 13.70	58.83 ± 15.33	ns
sex (%/n)				
Male	50.0/49	50.6/42	18.8/13	A, B vs. C
Female	50.0/49	49.4/41	81.2/56	A, B vs. C
height (cm)	168.14 ± 9.65	168.64 ± 10.36	164.76 ± 8.78	ns
weight (kg)	95.09 ± 13.24	78.39 ± 11.10	62.02 ± 7.99	A vs. B, C; B vs. C
BMI (kg/m^2)	33.62 ± 3.26	27.56 ± 1.34	22.86 ± 1.71	A vs. B, C; B vs. C
waist circumference (cm)	107.29 ± 10.16	95.29 ± 8.55	79.72 ± 7.55	A vs. B, C; B vs. C
hip circumference (cm)	115.23 ± 7.32	104.26 ± 5.23	93.83 ± 14.14	A vs. B, C; B vs. C
WHR	0.93 ± 0.08	0.91 ± 0.09	1.05 ± 1.56	ns
hypertension (%/n)	64.3/63	50.6/42	39.1/27	A, B vs. C
myocardial infarction (%/n)	7.1/7	7.2/6	4.3/3	ns
stroke (%/n)	2.0/2	3.6/3	2.9/2	ns
atrial fibrillation (%/n)	8.2/8	12.0/10	5.8/4	ns
deep vein thrombosis (%/n)	7.1/7	1.2/1	1.4/1	ns
type 2 diabetes (%/n)	21.4/21	10.8/9	4.3/3	A vs. C
thyroid disease (%/n)	16.3/16	13.2/11	20.3/14	ns
smoking (%/n)	9.2/9	15.8/13	15.9/11	ns

BMI—body mass index, WHR—waist-hip ratio, ns—not significant.

A research group of 181 adults (female/male 90/91) whose BMI exceeds 25 qualified for the study. Among this group, 83 participants were classified as overweight (BMI in the range of 25.0–29.9 kg/m^2; female/male 41/42), and 98 were classified as obese (BMI equal or higher than 30 kg/m^2; female/male 49/49). The control group consisted of 69 volunteers (females/males 56/13) with a normal BMI. The mean BMI of the obese patients was 33.6 kg/m^2, and all participants belonged to the class 1 obesity category; the mean in the group with overweight was 27.5 kg/m^2, and in the controls, 22.8 kg/m^2.

The first stage of the research was to fill out a proprietary questionnaire, including questions about physical activity, the use of stimulants, eating habits, comorbidities, and family and psychological history. In the next step, the basic anthropometric measurements were carried out: weight, height, heart rate, and blood pressure. Then, the appropriate calculations were made (including BMI and WHR). Then, a 12-lead ECG was performed. The analysis of electrocardiogram recordings included standard ECG measurements and the novel electrocardiographic markers currently used in literature.

2.2. Electrocardiographic Analysis

The standard electrocardiographic parameters such as heart rate, P-wave width, P dispersion, PQ interval, QRS complex width, QT interval, QTc interval, and QT dispersion were measured. Novel repolarization parameters measured were: Tpeak-Tend, (Tpeak-Tend) disp, (Tpeak-Tend)/QT, (Tpeak-Tend)/QTc, JTpeak, JT interval, JTpeak/JT, (Tpeak-Tend)/JTpeak, Tpeak, Tpeak/JT, JTpeak-Jtend, and (JTpeak-JTend) dispersion. The Tpeak-Tend was measured using the tangent method based on Rosenthal's method [26], as shown in Figure 2. All measured parameters are presented in Table 3.

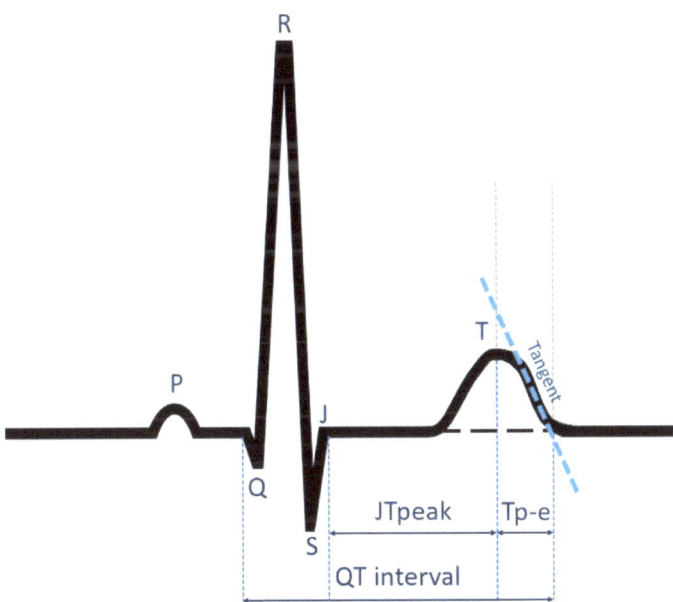

Figure 2. ECG repolarization intervals—QT, JTpeak, Tp-e.

Table 3. 12-lead ECG parameters in the entire study group.

Parameter	Mean	Confidence Interval −95.000%	Confidence Interval +95.000%	SD	Coefficients of Variability
HR (bpm)	66.73	66.25	68.21	11.87	17.79
P-wave width (ms)	109.63	107.18	112.08	19.65	17.92
P disp (ms)	34.45	31.91	36.99	20.38	59.16
PQ interval (ms)	168.19	164.37	172.01	30.68	18.24
QRS complex width (ms)	103.70	101.17	106.23	20.34	19.62
QT interval (ms)	389.79	385.72	393.86	32.69	8.39
QTc interval (ms)	408.54	405.37	411.71	25.46	6.23
QTd (ms)	35.02	31.97	38.06	24.45	69.82
QRS axis (°)	26.24	21.09	31.38	41.31	157.46
Sokolow–Lyon index LV (mm)	18.40	17.67	19.13	5.87	31.93
Sokolow–Lyon index RV (mm)	3.63	3.27	3.99	2.26	62.20
Tpeak-Tend (ms)	94.66	92.01	97.31	21.28	22.48
(Tpeak-Tend) disp (ms)	39.17	36.76	41.59	19.38	49.46
(Tpeak-Tend)/QT	0.24	0.23	0.24	0.05	23.28
(Tpeak-Tend)/QTc	0.22	0.22	0.23	0.04	19.35
JTpeak (ms)	199.89	195.92	203.85	31.83	15.92
JT interval (ms)	293.54	289.39	297.70	33.34	11.36
JTpeak/JT	0.69	0.68	0.69	0.07	10.03
(Tpeak-Tend)/JTpeak	0.42	0.40	0.44	0.17	40.93
Tpeak (mV)	0.40	0.37	0.43	0.24	61.05
Tpeak/JT (mV/ms)	0.00	0.00	0.00	0.00	62.92
JTpeak-JTend (ms)	95.93	92.37	99.49	28.57	29.79
(JTpeak-JTend) disp (ms)	44.90	41.23	48.56	29.34	65.36

HR—heart rate, P disp—P wave dispersion, QTc interval—corrected QT interval, QTd—QTd interval dispersion, Sokolow–Lyon index LV—Sokolow–Lyon criteria for left ventricular hypertrophy, Sokolow–Lyon index RV—Sokolow–Lyon criteria for right ventricular hypertrophy, (Tpeak-Tend) disp—Tpeak-Tend dispersion, (JTpeak-JTend) disp—Jtpeak-JTend dispersion.

The electrocardiography was performed using the CardioExpress SL 12 (Spacelabs Health Care Ltd., Hertford, UK) employing the Sentinel cardiology information management system (Spacelabs Health Care 2017 (Sentinel v10.5.0.8939). The 12-lead ECG was performed with a standard chart speed of 25 mm/s and a 10 mm/mV voltage. The acquisition mode of the ECG was 10 s of 12-lead simultaneous recording. The calibration signal input was 1 mV ± 2%, and the sample frequency—1000 Hz. The filters used included an enabled network filter, 0.15 Hz isoline filter, 25 Hz muscle filter, and 100 Hz low-pass filter.

The ECG recordings included between 7 and 21 full ECG cycles, depending on the patient's heart rate. Two independent researchers, medical students and a physician blinded to the clinical status, performed the ECG measurements. Two qualified cardiologists were in the group of researchers; in any case of problematic ECG recording, the cardiologist finally accepted the results.

2.3. Statistical Analysis

The statistical package "Dell Statistica 13.1" (Dell Inc., Round Rock, TX, USA) was used for statistical analysis. The arithmetic means and standard deviations of the estimated parameters were calculated for the quantitative variables. For the 12-lead ECG parameters in the whole study group, the values of the −95.000% confidence interval, +95.000% confidence interval, and coefficients of variability were also calculated. The distribution of variables was examined using the Lilliefors test and the W-Shapiro–Wilk test. The results for qualitative (nominal) variables were expressed as percentages. In comparative analyses, three subgroups of patients were compared: obese, overweight, and normal body mass. Therefore, multiple comparison was used. ANOVA was used for further statistical analysis in the case of quantitative independent variables with a normal distribution. The homogeneity of variances was checked using Levene and Brown–Forsyth tests. In the absence of homogeneity of variances, the Kruskal–Wallis ANOVA test was used to compare the significance of mean differences in 3 subgroups. In the case of variables with a distribution other than normal, the Kruskal–Wallis ANOVA test, a non-parametric equivalent of the analysis of variance, was used for quantitative independent variables. Statistically significant differences between individual arithmetic means were then determined with the Newman–Keuls post hoc test. For independent qualitative variables, multi-way tables and the maximum likelihood chi-square test were used for further statistical analysis. Correlation and regression analyses were performed to determine the relationship between the analyzed variables. In the case of quantitative variables with a normal distribution, Pearson's r correlation coefficients were determined, and in the case of quantitative variables with a non-normal distribution, Spearman's r coefficients were determined. The parameters of the models obtained in the backward stepwise multivariable regression analysis were estimated using the least squares method. The results were statistically significant at $p < 0.05$.

3. Results
3.1. Baseline Characteristic

The mean age in the entire study group was 59.94 ± 13.22, with a BMI of 28.64 ± 4.99. In the study group, 104 patients (41.6%) were men, and 146 were female (58.4%). The mean BMI was 28.64 ± 4.99. The comorbidities in the study group are shown in Table 1. When divided into subgroups, obesity A vs. overweight B and control group C, the mean BMI for the subgroups were 33.62, 27.56, and 22.86, respectively. There were no statistically significant differences in WHR. However, significant differences were noted in waist values: 107.29, 95.29, and 79.72, respectively, and in hip circumference: 115.23, 104.26, and 93.83, respectively. In the subgroups with obesity and overweight, hypertension was significantly more commonly present even in 64.3% of patients with obesity as well as type 2 diabetes, and the highest incidence was in patients with obesity, ranging to 21.4%.

Tables 1 and 2 summarize the study group and subgroups' baseline characteristics. On analyzing the regular medication use in the whole study group, it was found that 16.4% (41 persons) of participants were on thyroid hormones, 27% (68 persons) were on beta-blockers, 14.5 (36 persons) were on dihydropyridine calcium channel blockers, and 36.4% (91 persons) declared the use of other drugs. Among them, there were patients after stroke and myocardial infarction who declared acetylsalicylic acid, patients with paroxysmal atrial fibrillation 8% (22 patients) were on NOAC treatment, 13.2% (33 patients) were on oral medication for diabetes treatment, mainly biguanides; few patients declared other drugs such ACE inhibitors and proton-pump inhibitors.

3.2. Analysis of 12-Lead ECG Parameters in Studied Subgroups

Statistically significant differences were found in subsequent subgroups in P-wave width, with the highest values for obesity and overweight groups (A 113.12 ± 19.98 ms, B 111.66 ± 17.92 ms) as well as in the case of P-wave dispersion, which was the highest for obese people (A 40.08 ± 19.39 ms, B 31.01 ± 21.58 ms, 30.59 ± 18.66 ms). There were also differences in the PQ interval, which was the longest for the obese people but still within the norm (A 177.45 ± 29.74 ms, B 167.73 ± 28.92 ms, C 155.58 ± 29.86 ms). QRS complex width was the highest for obese people and statistically longer than in controls (A 107.24 ± 21.34 ms, B 102.47 ± 23.26 ms, C 100.14 ± 13.42 ms, p A vs. C).

When analyzing the classic depolarization and repolarization markers, slight differences in QT and QTc intervals were observed. However, they were not significant, and only QT dispersion was significantly higher in obese people when compared to patients with overweight and normal body mass (A 39.63 ± 23.14 ms, 32.02 ± 27.95 ms, C 32.06 ± 20.77 ms). All data are presented in Table 4.

Table 4. Parameters of the 12-lead ECG recording in the studied subgroups.

Parameter	Obesity (A, n = 98)	Overweight (B, n = 83)	Control Group (C, n = 69)	$p < 0.05$
HR (bpm)	66.50 ± 11.45	66.04 ± 12.10	67.90 ± 12.26	ns
P-wave width (ms)	113.12 ± 19.98	111.66 ± 17.92	102.22 ± 19.45	A, B vs. C
P disp (ms)	40.08 ± 19.39	31.01 ± 21.58	30.59 ± 18.66	A vs. B, C
PQ interval (ms)	177.45 ± 29.74	167.73 ± 28.92	155.58 ± 29.86	A vs. B, C; B vs. C
QRS complex width (ms)	107.24 ± 21.34	102.47 ± 23.26	100.14 ± 13.42	A vs. C
QT interval (ms)	392.66 ± 25.77	390.19 ± 40.85	385.23 ± 30.32	ns
QTc interval (ms)	411.50 ± 23.43	406.95 ± 30.23	406.25 ± 21.61	ns
QTd (ms)	39.63 ± 23.14	32.02 ± 27.95	32.06 ± 20.77	A vs. B, C
QRS axis (°)	17.32 ± 38.36	27.05 ± 41.37	37.93 ± 42.80	ns
Sokolow-index LV (mm)	17.11 ± 5.15	19.77 ± 6.16	18.58 ± 6.15	ns
Sokolow-index RV (mm)	3.73 ± 2.23	3.32 ± 2.40	3.71 ± 2.22	ns
Tpeak-Tend (ms)	97.08 ± 23.38	95.88 ± 23.71	89.74 ± 12.88	A vs. C
(Tpeak-Tend) disp (ms)	43.29 ± 24.14	37.34 ± 17.75	35.52 ± 11.03	A vs. B, C
(Tpeak-Tend)/QT	0.23 ± 0.05	0.25 ± 0.07	0.23 ± 0.03	ns
(Tpeak-Tend)/QTc	0.22 ± 0.04	0.23 ± 0.05	0.22 ± 0.03	ns
JTpeak (ms)	205.92 ± 28.04	198.77 ± 32.39	192.67 ± 34.88	A vs. C
JT interval (ms)	292.82 ± 28.67	295.52 ± 36.14	292.20 ± 36.25	ns
JTpeak/JT	0.69 ± 0.07	0.67 ± 0.07	0.69 ± 0.05	ns
(Tpeak-Tend)/JTpeak	0.46 ± 0.16	0.35 ± 0.21	0.45 ± 0.11	ns
Tpeak (mV)	0.39 ± 0.26	0.40 ± 0.25	0.41 ± 0.21	ns
Tpeak/JT (mV/ms)	0.00 ± 0.00	0.00 ± 0.00	0.00 ± 0.00	ns
JTpeak-JTend (ms)	99.55 ± 34.53	95.98 ± 29.64	90.72 ± 13.54	A vs. C
(JTpeak-JTend) disp (ms)	48.22 ± 37.60	44.04 ± 26.32	41.19 ± 16.33	ns

HR—heart rate, P disp—P wave dispersion, QTc interval—corrected QT interval, QTd—QTd interval dispersion, Sokolow–Lyon index LV—Sokolow–Lyon criteria for left ventricular hypertrophy, Sokolow–Lyon index RV—Sokolow–Lyon criteria for right ventricular hypertrophy, (Tpeak-Tend) disp—Tpeak-Tend dispersion, (JTpeak-JTend) disp—Jtpeak-JTend dispersion; ns—not significant.

Taking into account the novel electrocardiographic parameters, we found that in the whole study group, the mean Tpeak to Tend interval was 94.66 ± 21.28 ms, (Tpeak-Tend) dispersion was 39.17 ± 19.38 ms, (Tpeak-Tend)/QT was 0.24 ± 0.05 ms and (Tpeak-Tend)/QTc was 0.22 ± 0.04 ms. All the novel parameters of repolarization are presented in Table 3, together with classical parameters. Confidence intervals and coefficients of variability of ECG parameters in the entire study group were also presented in Table 3. Tpeak-Tend and its dispersion were statistically significantly longer in the obese group than in the control group. Additionally, the JTpeak-JTend parameter was significantly longer in obese patients than in people with normal body mass.

The differences in repolarization markers are shown in Table 4.

3.3. Linear Relationship between Body Mass Parameters and 12-Lead ECG Parameters in the Entire Study Group

There were positive linear correlations between both atrial parameters, P-wave and PQ interval, and some body mass parameters, that is, body mass, BMI, waist and hip circumference, and between P dispersion and BMI, waist and hip circumferences. Moreover, a relationship existed between QRS complex width and body weight, BMI, and waist circumference.

Amongst novel electrocardiographic parameters, Tpeak-Tend was positively correlated with body mass and waist circumference, while JTpeak was associated with BMI, hip circumference, and WHR. Additionally, Tpeak was correlated with WHR. Also, Tpeak/JT was positively correlated with WHR and BMI. The correlations are summarized in Table 5.

Table 5. Linear relationships between body weight parameters and 12-lead ECG parameters in the entire study group.

Parameter	Body Weight (kg)	BMI (kg/m^2)	Waist Circumference (cm)	Hip Circumference (cm)	WHR
HR (bpm)	ns	ns	ns	ns	ns
P-wave width (ms)	0.31	0.25	0.30	0.20	ns
P disp (ms)	ns	0.15	0.16	0.17	ns
PQ interval (ms)	0.38	0.33	0.40	0.32	ns
QRS complex width (ms)	0.16	0.16	0.14	ns	ns
QT interval (ms)	ns	ns	ns	ns	ns
QTTc interval (ms)	ns	ns	ns	ns	ns
QTd (ms)	ns	ns	ns	ns	ns
QRS axis (°)	ns	ns	ns	ns	ns
Sokolow-index LV (mm)	ns	ns	ns	ns	ns
Sokolow-index RV (mm)	ns	ns	ns	ns	ns
Tpeak-Tend (ms)	0.16	ns	0.16	ns	ns
(Tpeak-Tend) disp (ms)	ns	ns	ns	ns	ns
(Tpeak-Tend)/QT	ns	ns	ns	ns	ns
(Tpeak-Tend)/QTc	ns	ns	ns	ns	ns
JTpeak (ms)	ns	0.15	ns	0.19	0.18
JT interval (ms)	ns	ns	ns	ns	ns
JTpeak/JT	ns	ns	ns	ns	ns
(Tpeak-Tend)/JTpeak	ns	ns	ns	ns	ns
Tpeak (mV)	ns	ns	ns	ns	0.16
Tpeak/JT (mV/ms)	ns	0.15	ns	ns	0.16
JTpeak-JTend (ms)	ns	ns	ns	ns	ns
(JTpeak-JTend) disp (ms)	ns	ns	ns	ns	ns

HR—heart rate, P disp—P wave dispersion, QTc interval—corrected QT interval, QTd—QTd interval dispersion, Sokolow–Lyon index LV—Sokolow–Lyon criteria for left ventricular hypertrophy, Sokolow–Lyon index RV—Sokolow–Lyon criteria for right ventricular hypertrophy, (Tpeak-Tend) disp—Tpeak-Tend dispersion, (JTpeak-JTend) disp—Jtpeak-JTend dispersion, ns—not significant.

3.4. Backward Stepwise Multiple Regression Model

After implementing a backward stepwise multivariable regression model for JTpeak and Tpeak/JT as dependent variables, we assessed the specific models presented in Tables 6 and 7.

Table 6. Backward stepwise multivariable regression model in the entire study group for JTpeak (ms) as the dependent variable.

	Age	WHR	Type 2 Diabetes	Smoking
Regression coefficient (RC)	0.439	17.563	13.064	6.259
SEM of Rc	0.163	3.032	6.081	2.803
p	<0.01	<0.001	<0.05	<0.05
p for the model			$p < 0.001$	

Table 7. Backward stepwise multivariable regression model in the entire study group for Tpeak/JT (mV/ms) as the dependent variable.

	Male	BMI (kg/m^2)	β-Blockers
Regression coefficient (RC)	0.001	0.001	−0.001
SEM of Rc	0.000	0.000	0.000
p	<0.001	<0.001	<0.05
p for the model		$p < 0.001$	

For the 12-lead ECG JTpeak, age, WHR, type 2 diabetes, and smoking had the highest statistical significance (p for the model $p < 0.001$), as for the Tpeak/JT as the dependent variable, male sex and BMI had a positive effect on the model. B-blockers had a negative impact on the model (p for the model $p < 0.001$).

The backward stepwise multivariable regression model is summarized in Tables 6 and 7.

The summary of the results of our research and the effects of obesity and overweight on repolarization and other ECG parameters are presented in Figure 3.

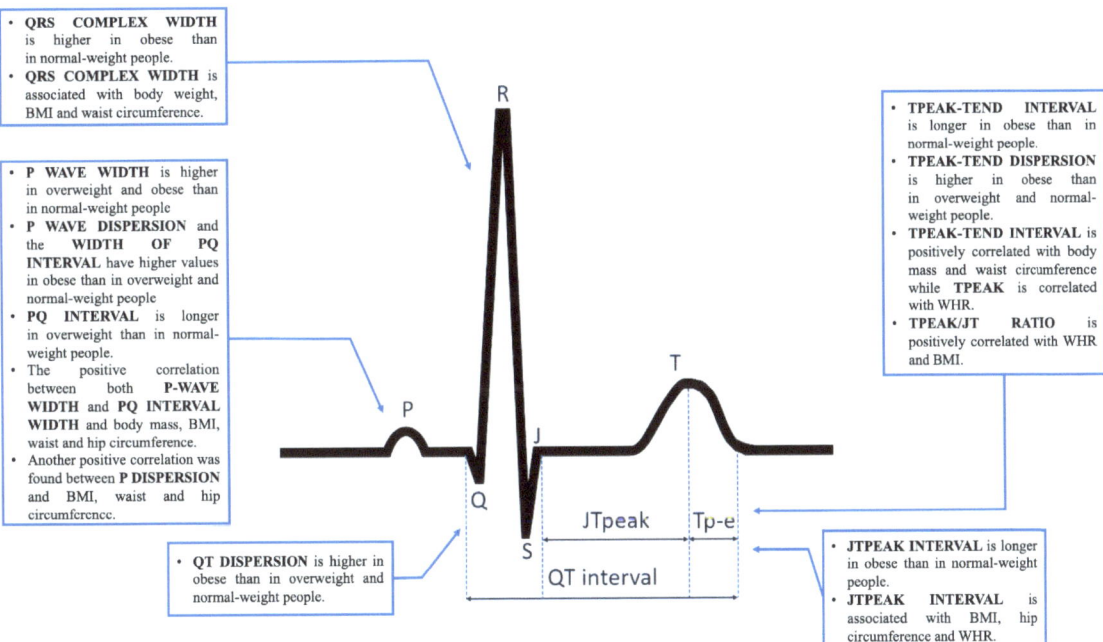

Figure 3. Effects of obesity and overweight on repolarization and other ECG parameters in our study.

4. Discussion

The current study investigated the alterations of ECG parameters in people with overweight and obesity, especially the ones concerning repolarization parameters. We found an increase in P-wave dispersion and QRS complex width in obese individuals and an increase in P-wave width and PQ interval in both overweight and obese individuals. Moreover, taking into consideration classic repolarization parameters, we found that obese individuals have significantly higher values of QT dispersion, and analyzing novel repolarization parameters, we found that Tp-e interval, Tp-e dispersion, and JTpeak-JTend have substantially higher values in obese individuals. Our study found that alterations in repolarization parameters in obese individuals are marked mostly in novel rather than classic repolarization parameters. This may indicate the potential clinical use of parameters such as Tp-e interval, Tp-e dispersion, and JTpeak-JTend after standardizing the normal values of these parameters. We also found positive linear correlations between ECG parameters (P-wave width, PQ interval, QRS complex width, Tp-e interval, JTpeak, Tpeak amplitude) and body mass parameters (body mass, BMI, waist circumference, hip circumference, WHR), which may be related to electrophysiological changes present in obese people secondary to remodeling of the myocardium in both atria and ventricles.

Other studies investigating ECG changes in obese people also reported an increased prevalence of left ventricular hypertrophy, left atrial enlargement, and left axis deviation in obese patients, which may indicate structural changes in the heart [9,10]. These findings suggest potential alterations in cardiac electrophysiology, myocardial function, and ventricular repolarization in obese individuals. We did not observe the criteria for left ventricular hypertrophy, which is more common in obese people, even though hypertension was the most common in this group. However, the study group should be highlighted as being comprised mainly of class 1 obesity patients. The most significant electrocardiographic changes could be expected in patients from classes 2 and 3, where chamber overload and enlargements are higher, more comorbidities are identified, and cardiovascular risk is higher.

Regarding classic repolarization parameters, Omran et al.'s meta analysis found that obesity or overweight is related to an increase in the length of QT and QTc intervals and QTc dispersion. Moreover, weight loss was able to revert these alterations [11]. Seyfeli et al. also associated increased QTc dispersion with obesity in women [27]. In Kumar et al.'s study, obese adults aged 18–40 had significantly higher width of QT intervals than adults without obesity. Moreover, Kumar et al. associated prolongation of QT interval with a higher risk of left ventricular hypertrophy and ventricular fibrillation [10].

Furthermore, Waheed et al. found that obese people have wider QTc interval than normal-weight people and associated this prolongation with increased cardiovascular and all-cause mortality [28]. Our study showed slight differences in QT and QTc intervals between BMI groups. However, the trend of these changes was consistent with the conclusions of the previously mentioned studies. On the contrary, Braschi et al. found no significant differences in classical repolarization parameters between normal-weight people and people with uncomplicated overweight or obesity. Moreover, they found a trend in QT dispersion that increased with BMI without reaching the significance condition [14]. Our study also found this trend, and it was statistically significant. Furthermore, Guo et al. associated the prolongation of QTc with metabolic syndrome, which often co-exists with obesity [29]. Analyzing the abovementioned studies to estimate the potential risk, we should consider the class of obesity and co-existing comorbidities, which increase with the increase in body mass.

There are still not many research studies investigating the changes in novel repolarization parameters in overweight and obese individuals. The results of previous studies on these parameters are not consistent. Inanir et al.'s study found that the novel repolarization parameters Tp-e interval, Tp-e/QT, Tp-e/QTc, Tp-e/JT, and Tp-e/JTc are significantly higher in individuals with BMI $\geq$ 40 than in individuals with normal body weight [12]. Moreover, Bağcı et al. found that the alterations concerning the Tp-e interval and Tp-e/QT and Tp-e/QTc ratios progress gradually with the growth of BMI [13]. Our study partly supports these results regarding Tp-e interval width. However, we found no significant differences between BMI groups regarding Tp-e/QT, Tp-e/QTc, and Tp-e/JT ratios. Contrary to these studies and ours, a study conducted by Al-Mosawi et al. found that Tp-e interval width decreased with the growth of BMI, although this change did not reach significance [15]. Al-Mosawi et al.'s study is the only study we have found with this negative relationship between Tp-e width and BMI. Furthermore, Braschi et al.'s study found no significant changes in Tp-e interval, Tp-e dispersion, and Tp-e/QT ratio between groups of normal-weight people, people with uncomplicated overweight, and people with uncomplicated obesity [14].

Kosar et al. found that P-wave dispersion was increased in obese individuals and that P-wave dispersion was correlated positively with BMI. They also found that obese people had higher values of maximal P-wave duration than normal-weight people. They hypothesized that obesity might be a factor leading to the development of atrial fibrillation [30]. Moreover, Cosgun et al.'s study associated obesity with no other comorbidities to the increase in maximal values of P-wave width and the prolongation of P-wave dispersion [31]. Bocchi et al.'s study also associated BMI and abdominal obesity with an increase in P-wave dispersion [32], and Seyfeli et al.'s study associated obesity with an increase in P-wave dispersion [27]. Our research also found that P-wave duration and dispersion have higher values in overweight and obese people. Therefore, our study supports previously mentioned studies.

Furthermore, Russo et al. found that P-wave dispersion can be significantly reduced by bariatric surgery in morbidly obese patients without comorbidities [33]. Similarly, weight loss due to diet and medical therapy or diet only resulted in decreased P-wave duration and dispersion [34,35]. Prolonging P-wave width or dispersion is associated with a higher risk of developing supraventricular arrhythmias, including atrial fibrillation [36–44].

Another alteration reported in obese people's ECG is a prolongation of QRS complex in comparison to normal-weight people [45,46]. Furthermore, a recent study by Sobhani et al. also found that higher BMI was associated with prolonged QRS complex [47]. Our study supports these findings. We also observed that obese people have a statistically significant increase in QRS complex duration compared with people with normal weight.

Additionally, children and adolescents with abdominal obesity were revealed to have longer PQ intervals, wider QRS complex, and leftward shifts in frontal P-wave, QRS, and T-wave axes in comparison to normal-weight children adolescents. In this group, a positive correlation between PQ interval and QRS duration and BMI, waist circumference, and WHR was also found [48]. We found similar changes in the adult population: an increase in PQ interval and QRS complex width in obese and similar positive correlations between ECG and body weight parameters.

Apart from the ECG parameters examined in this study, there are others that are potentially useful in practice, which we did not take under study. Among them is a microvolt T-wave alternans, potentially useful for patients with coronary artery disease [49]. However, this method has several limitations. Applying this method requires special equipment and the proper heart rate.

There are multiple theories explaining the changes in ECG repolarization parameters due to obesity. Firstly, the changes in P-wave and T-wave morphology may be associated with myocardial fibrosis of ventricles or within the atria [50]. Secondly, obesity may affect ion channels, which may change the potential of myocytes [51]. Obesity may influence I_{Na}, $I_{Ca,L}$, and I_{to} ion channels, increasing the risk of long QT syndrome and atrial fibrillation in obese patients. According to Aromolaran et al., the candidates for modulation by obesity are cardiac, such as the abovementioned ion channels and Ca handling proteins. However, the underlying mechanisms of such interactions remain incompletely understood [51]. In research studies on the relationships between obesity and atrial fibrillation in mice, it has been found that the process was partly mediated by a combined effect of sodium, potassium, and calcium channel remodeling and atrial fibrosis [52].

Moreover, mitochondrial antioxidant therapy reduced atrial fibrillation burden, restoring I_{Na}, $I_{Ca,L}$, and I_{Kur}, resulting in shorter action potential duration and reversed atrial fibrosis. Obesity may be connected with fibrosis and the increased secretion of pro-inflammatory cytokines, hyperglycemia, and insulin resistance, leading to electrical remodeling and thus predisposing to arrhythmias [51]. Additionally, the adipose tissue is associated with subcutaneous and visceral fat accumulation, causing distinct signaling mechanisms. Eventually, some differences may be present in the regional distribution of fat deposits, affecting ion channel/Ca handling protein expression. Other authors found that cardiomyocytes of obese and diabetic patients have increased lipid accumulation, which contributes to the pathophysiology of heart failure and arrhythmia [53,54]. It is known that diabetes quite commonly co-exists with obesity; even in our study subgroup with class 1 obesity, it was identified in 21% of patients. Morrow et al. demonstrated on transgenic models that cardiac lipid overload causes spontaneous arrhythmias, and Purohit et al. revealed that oxidative stress may partly mediate the arrhythmogenic effect [55,56]. Furthermore, in other studies, authors have found that cardiomyocyte lipid overload may increase oxidative stress by activating the protein NOX2, causing mitochondrial dysfunction and abnormalities of internal calcium handling, promoting arrhythmia [57]. More experimental studies in this area are needed.

Obesity may affect survival, and it has been proven in numerous studies that it is associated with the increased risk of several diseases and death, particularly from cardiovascular diseases and cancer; however, only grade 2 and 3 obesity was associated with significantly higher all-cause mortality [58–60]. Interestingly, in a comprehensive meta-analysis, it was shown that patients with low weight and overweight had a higher mortality risk during acute coronary syndrome than normal-weight patients [61]. The results showed the U-shaped nonlinear association detected between body mass index and mortality risk with higher mortality risk for BMI < 21.5 kg/m^2 and >40 kg/m^2. In contrast, the lowest mortality risk was detected at approximately 30 kg/m^2, called the "obesity paradox" effect. Additionally, it has been clearly shown that the most severe clinical complications and increase in risk are dedicated to class 3 obesity, which is also called high-risk obesity. In such patients, we may expect the most frequent remodeling of the heart muscle and, secondarily, ECG changes and arrhythmias. From this point of view, class 1 obesity and overweight are theoretically connected with not-severe initial stages changes within the cardiovascular system and heart muscle, resulting in less frequent and minor ECG pathologies.

The association between obesity and cardiovascular diseases has been widely studied. However, this issue is still not fully understood and is complex. Discussing briefly several methods determining cardiovascular risk in obese people, several data present the risk of obese patients in the context of coronary artery disease. Even metabolically healthy obese subjects have a higher incidence of subclinical coronary artery atherosclerosis when compared to normal-weight individuals, which was diagnosed by the calcium scores in cardiac computer tomography (CCT). Furthermore, every 1 kg/m^2 increase in BMI led to a 5–7% increase in the incidence of CAD across all BMI categories [62,63]. CCT has relatively good sensitivity and specificity; however, even using modern and up-to-date equipment could not always guarantee high image quality for overweight or obese patients [64]. Echocardiography also needs a good visualization, which may be impaired in this group of patients. In uncomplicated obesity cases, the enlarged left ventricular mass in echocardiography might often be an early adaptation of cardiac function, compensating for the greater hemodynamic and metabolic demand. It should be underlined that increased body mass leads to increased metabolic requirements, which may be a step towards the development of CAD [65]. Single-photon emission CT (SPECT) is used in lower-weight patients and avoided in patients whose BMI is more than 35 kg/m^2 [66]. However, in some studies in which obese people were participating, it was found that, although the obese had a higher risk profile than their non-obese counterparts, obesity was not an independent predictor of abnormal MPS (myocardial perfusion SPECT), raising the possibility that other risk factors associated with obesity (e.g., diabetes) have a much higher impact on the occurrence of coronary artery disease than obesity per se [67]. Nevertheless, there are some limitations of this technique in the obese. Electrocardiography is extensively available and cheap, so it is the first-line test. The common ECG changes in obese people have been commented on within this article, mainly including the increased heart rate, which has not been proven in our study, as we only noted insignificant differences. Other typical pathologies include increased QRS and QT interval. In light of CAD, there are no specific parameters in obese people that could be proposed as specific prognostic markers, especially for obese people. It is noteworthy that the baseline ECG may be influenced by obesity, especially in more advanced obesity stages. ST-T changes are found due to ventricular hypertrophy and overload, which may perplex the diagnostic process [68]. For this reason, non-invasive testing for CAD often has a suboptimal performance.

It is also worth mentioning that being overweight or obese is not the only factor that impacts changes in repolarization parameters. Other factors include the effects of the autonomic nervous system, hormonal metabolism, especially steroid hormones and sex hormones, hyper- and hypokalemia, other electrolyte disorders, using medications, medical procedures performed, and metabolic diseases [69,70]. Moreover, the influence of genetic factors is also possible, e.g., by modifying the operation of ion channels, as in congenital long QT syndrome (LQTS). There are also reports of the potential impact of hyperventilation on disturbances in ventricular repolarization [71]. The influence of air pollution, especially $PM_{2.5}$, cytokines, stress and emotions, and the menstrual cycle's influence on ventricular repolarization cannot be definitively denied [69,72–74].

A growing number of drugs are influencing ventricular repolarization and prolonging the QT interval, potentially also new electrocardiographic repolarization markers. In this group, there are numerous medications, including noncardiac ones. In our study group, patients did not declare any anti-arrhythmic drugs having a significant impact on repolarization; however, some minor relations could have happened, which may have been a confounding factor to some extent. As presented in Table 2, 64%, 50%, and 39% of patients had hypertension, consecutively in obesity, overweight, and normal-weight subgroups. However, only a few participants were treated with ACE inhibitors, which may have a beneficial and protective effect on repolarization and affect the results. Sixty-eight patients (27.2%) were treated with beta-blockers, which also have beneficial activity.

Moreover, we found a negative relation in regression analysis between beta-blockers and one of the repolarization markers (Tpeak/JT) [75,76]. It may explain slight differences in some repolarization parameters between the studied subgroups. It is also possible that some other agents used by patients could affect the repolarization. The majority of agents may have a potential influence on repolarization; one example may be varenicline, approved to help in smoking cessation, which led to prolongation of ventricular repolarization parameters QTc, Tp-e, and Tp-e/QTc ratio [77]. However, in our study group, no one declared the use of this drug. Additionally, 16% of our study group also proclaimed the use of thyroid hormones and 14% of calcium channel blockers, mainly nifedipine and lercanidipine, which may have some effect. More and more evidence is gathered on the relationship between various medications and repolarization markers; however, when patients use various drugs and agents in real-life clinical conditions, the ultimate effect may be complex and unpredictable.

The significance of our study assumes that it may increase our knowledge of pathophysiological changes in the cardiovascular system, especially within the heart and its electrical system function in people with obesity and overweight, as there are still some controversies. Mainly, we have found more pathologies connected to repolarization in patients with class 2 obesity, and probably further studies should employ more patients with class 3 obesity, in whom we expect more cardiovascular and non-cardiovascular complications. The study may contribute to improving the understanding of the role of repolarization indices with the increase in body weight even in the setting of the usual physician's practice, as the analysis of the electrocardiogram is frequently rather superficial. Numerous studies, including this one, are focused on the detailed ECG examination. It is possible that in the future, Tp-e and its derivates will also be included in computed electrocardiogram analysis, and all the markers, including the classic and the novel ones, will be presented in the report.

4.1. Limitations

Our study also has some limitations. We analyzed the 12-lead ECG only once for every participant. Therefore, we could not observe changes in ECG in the long term. Furthermore, the Polish population is mostly ethnically monogenic and does not include minorities. Therefore, we cannot guarantee that the results of our study are universal for all populations. The other limitation mentioned in the last paragraph of the Discussion addresses the medications used by some of the study participants, mainly antihypertensive ones. Potentially, it may constitute a confounding factor.

4.2. Future Perspectives

Despite emerging trends and relationships, current research still has many inconsistencies regarding novel repolarization parameters. There is a need for studies with large-scale research and control groups. Thanks to large-scale studies, it would be possible to distinguish subgroups based on age and smaller ranges of BMI (e.g., distinction of alterations in every obesity class). Especially within the study group, there should be more patients with class 2 and 3 obesity in the future perspective.

Furthermore, examining these relationships in more homogenous subgroups, such as diabetes mellitus and hypertension, would also allow for a better understanding of studied ECG alterations. Eventually, ECG, as a simple and easily feasible, as well as widely available, technique, may serve as a first-line tool to estimate the initial pathologies and indicate the increasing cardiovascular risk in obese patients. Paying attention to even minor changes could help to select patients at higher risk.

5. Conclusions

We can hypothesize that considering all the limitations and confounding factors, the results we have analyzed may be addressed to class 1 obesity and overweight people.

In patients with class 1 obesity, only QT dispersion was significantly higher in obese people when compared to patients with overweight and normal body mass, and QTc was only insignificantly higher.

The novel repolarization indices, Tpeak-Tend, and its dispersion were statistically significantly longer in the obese group than in the control group, and the JTpeak-JTend parameter was considerably longer in obese patients. Additionally, Tpeak-Tend was positively correlated with body mass and waist circumference.

We revealed significant differences in P-wave and QRS duration and P-wave dispersion in obese people with class 1 obesity, with positive correlations between these parameters and anthropometric parameters such as BMI and waist and hip circumferences.

This study is the introduction for further research on novel electrocardiographic parameters in the future, that is, the Tpeak-Tend and its derivates, and especially interesting would be employing more patients with class 3 obesity, where the number of cardiovascular and non-cardiovascular complications increases.

Author Contributions: Conceptualization, I.A.D. and M.P.; methodology, I.A.D. and M.P.; software, P.G. and R.P.; validation, M.P. and P.G.; formal analysis, M.P.; investigation, I.A.D., K.K., L.J. and M.P.; resources, I.A.D., K.K. and L.J.; data curation, M.P. and R.P.; writing—original draft preparation, K.K. and L.J.; writing—review and editing, I.A.D. and M.P.; visualization, I.A.D. and M.P.; supervision, M.P.; project administration, M.P. and P.G.; funding acquisition, P.G. All authors have read and agreed to the published version of the manuscript.

Funding: This research received no external funding. APC was funded by Wroclaw Medical University (SUBZ.E264.24.033).

Institutional Review Board Statement: The study was conducted in accordance with the Declaration of Helsinki and approved by the Ethics Committee of Wroclaw Medical University (protocol code 710/2020 and date of approval 10 November 2020).

Informed Consent Statement: Informed consent was obtained from all subjects involved in the study.

Data Availability Statement: The data are not publicly available due to patients' privacy.

Conflicts of Interest: The authors declare no conflicts of interest.

References

1. World Health Organization. Obesity and Overweight. Available online: https://www.who.int/news-room/fact-sheets/detail/obesity-and-overweight (accessed on 12 August 2023).
2. Global Health Estimates: Leading Causes of Death. Available online: https://www.who.int/data/gho/data/themes/mortality-and-global-health-estimates/ghe-leading-causes-of-death (accessed on 12 August 2023).
3. Dixon, A.E.; Peters, U. The effect of obesity on lung function. *Expert. Rev. Respir. Med.* **2018**, *12*, 755–767. [CrossRef]
4. Yu, W.; Rohli, K.E.; Yang, S.; Jia, P. Impact of obesity on COVID-19 patients. *J. Diabetes Complicat.* **2021**, *35*, 107817. [CrossRef]
5. Williamson, E.J.; Walker, A.J.; Bhaskaran, K.; Bacon, S.; Bates, C.; Morton, C.E.; Curtis, H.J.; Mehrkar, A.; Evans, D.; Inglesby, P.; et al. Factors associated with COVID-19-related death using OpenSAFELY. *Nature* **2020**, *584*, 430–436. [CrossRef]
6. Centers for Disease Control and Prevention. Obesity is Common, Serious, and Costly. Available online: https://www.cdc.gov/obesity/php/about/index.html (accessed on 12 August 2023).
7. The Lancet Gastroenterology Hepatology. Obesity: Another ongoing pandemic. *Lancet Gastroenterol. Hepatol.* **2021**, *6*, 411. [CrossRef]
8. Global Health Observatory Data Repository. Overweight/Obesity. Available online: https://apps.who.int/gho/data/node.main.A896?lang=en (accessed on 15 August 2023).
9. Binu, A.J.; Srinath, S.C.; Cherian, K.E.; Jacob, J.R.; Paul, T.V.; Kapoor, N. A Pilot Study of Electrocardiographic Features in Patients with Obesity from a Tertiary Care Centre in Southern India (Electron). *Med. Sci.* **2022**, *10*, 56. [CrossRef]
10. Kumar, T.; Jha, K.; Sharan, A.; Sakshi, P.; Kumar, S.; Kumari, A. Study of the effect of obesity on QT-interval among adults. *J. Family Med. Prim. Care.* **2019**, *8*, 1626–1629.
11. Omran, J.; Firwana, B.; Koerber, S.; Bostick, B.; Alpert, M.A. Effect of obesity and weight loss on ventricular repolarization: A systematic review and meta-analysis. *Obes. Rev.* **2016**, *17*, 520–530. [CrossRef]
12. Inanir, M.; Sincer, I.; Erdal, E.; Gunes, Y.; Cosgun, M.; Mansiroglu, A.K. Evaluation of electrocardiographic ventricular repolarization parameters in extreme obesity. *J. Electrocardiol.* **2019**, *53*, 36–39. [CrossRef]
13. Bağcı, A.; Aksoy, F.; Baş, H.A.; Işık, İ.B.; Orhan, H. The effect of Systolic and diastolic blood pressure on Tp-e interval in patients divided according to World Health Organization classification for body mass index. *Clin. Exp. Hypertens.* **2021**, *43*, 642–646. [CrossRef]
14. Braschi, A.; Abrignani, M.G.; Francavilla, V.C.; Francavilla, G. Novel electrocardiographic parameters of altered repolarization in uncomplicated overweight and obesity. *Obesity* **2011**, *19*, 875–881. [CrossRef]
15. Al-Mosawi, A.A.; Nafakhi, H.; Hassan, M.B.; Alareedh, M.; Al-Nafakh, H.A. ECG markers of arrhythmogenic risk relationships with pericardial fat volume and BMI in patients with coronary atherosclerosis. *J. Electrocardiol.* **2018**, *51*, 569–572. [CrossRef]
16. Tse, G.; Yan, B.P. Traditional and novel electrocardiographic conduction and repolarization markers of sudden cardiac death. *Europace* **2017**, *19*, 712–721. [CrossRef]
17. Piccirillo, G.; Moscucci, F.; Corrao, A.; Carnovale, M.; Di Diego, I.; Lospinuso, I.; Caltabiano, C.; Mezzadri, M.; Rossi, P.; Magrì, D. Noninvasive Hemodynamic Monitoring in Advanced Heart Failure Patients: New Approach for Target Treatments. *Biomedicines* **2022**, *10*, 2407. [CrossRef]
18. Piccirillo, G.; Moscucci, F.; Carnovale, M.; Corrao, A.; Di Diego, I.; Lospinuso, I.; Caltabiano, C.; Mezzadri, M.; Rossi, P.; Magrì, D. Short-Period Temporal Dispersion Repolarization Markers in Elderly Patients with Decompensated Heart Failure. *Clin. Ter.* **2022**, *173*, 356–361.
19. Tse, G.; Gong, M.; Meng, L.; Wong, C.W.; Georgopoulos, S.; Bazoukis, G.; Wong, M.C.; Letsas, K.P.; Vassiliou, V.S.; Xia, Y.; et al. Meta-analysis of Tpeak-Tend and Tpeak Tend/QT ratio for risk stratification in congenital long QT syndrome. *J. Electrocardiol.* **2018**, *51*, 396–401. [CrossRef]
20. Tse, G.; Gong, M.; Meng, L.; Wong, C.W.; Bazoukis, G.; Chan, M.T.; Wong, M.C.; Letsas, K.P.; Baranchuk, A.; Yan, G.X.; et al. Predictive Value of T peak—T end Indices for Adverse Outcomes in Acquired QT Prolongation: A Meta-Analysis. *Front. Physiol.* **2018**, *9*, 1226. [CrossRef]
21. Markiewicz-Łoskot, G.; Moric-Janiszewska, E.; Mazurek, B.; Łoskot, M.; Bartusek, M.; Skierska, A.; Szydłowski, L. Electrocardiographic T-wave parameters in families with long QT syndrome. *Adv. Clin. Exp. Med.* **2018**, *27*, 501–507. [CrossRef]
22. Wang, X.; Zhang, L.; Gao, C.; Zhu, J.; Yang, X. Tpeak-Tend/QT interval predicts ST-segment resolution and major adverse cardiac events in acute ST-segment elevation myocardial infarction patients undergoing percutaneous coronary intervention. *Medicine* **2018**, *97*, e12943. [CrossRef]

23. Yu, Z.; Chen, Z.; Wu, Y.; Chen, R.; Li, M.; Chen, X.; Qin, S.; Liang, Y.; Su, Y.; Ge, J. Electrocardiographic parameters effectively predict ventricular tachycardia/fibrillation in acute phase and abnormal cardiac function in chronic phase of ST-segment elevation myocardial infarction. *J. Cardiovasc. Electrophysiol.* **2018**, *29*, 756–766. [CrossRef]
24. Andršová, I.; Hnatkova, K.; Šišáková, M.; Toman, O.; Smetana, P.; Huster, K.M.; Barthel, P.; Novotný, T.; Schmidt, G.; Malik, M. Heart Rate Dependency and Inter-Lead Variability of the T Peak—T End Intervals. *Front. Physiol.* **2020**, *11*, 595815. [CrossRef]
25. Gupta, P.; Patel, C.; Patel, H.; Narayanaswamy, S.; Malhotra, B.; Green, J.T.; Yan, G.X. T(p-e)/QT ratio as an index of arrhythmogenesis. *J. Electrocardiol.* **2008**, *41*, 567–574. [CrossRef]
26. Rosenthal, T.M.; Masvidal, D.; Abi Samra, F.M.; Bernard, M.L.; Khatib, S.; Polin, G.M.; Rogers, P.A.; Xue, J.Q.; Morin, D.P. Optimal method of measuring the T-peak to T-end interval for risk stratification in primary prevention. *Europace* **2018**, *20*, 698–705. [CrossRef]
27. Seyfeli, E.; Duru, M.; Kuvandik, G.; Kaya, H.; Yalcin, F. Effect of obesity on P-wave dispersion and QT dispersion in women. *Int. J. Obes.* **2006**, *30*, 957–961. [CrossRef]
28. Waheed, S.; Dawn, B.; Gupta, K. Association of corrected QT interval with body mass index, and the impact of this association on mortality: Results from the Third National Health and Nutrition Examination Survey. *Obes. Res. Clin. Pract.* **2017**, *11*, 426–434. [CrossRef]
29. Guo, X.; Li, Z.; Guo, L.; Yu, S.; Yang, H.; Zheng, L.; Pan, G.; Zhang, Y.; Sun, Y.; Pletcher, M.J. Effects of Metabolically Healthy and Unhealthy Obesity on Prolongation of Corrected QT Interval. *Am. J. Cardiol.* **2017**, *119*, 1199–1204. [CrossRef]
30. Kosar, F.; Aksoy, Y.; Ari, F.; Keskin, L.; Sahin, I. P-wave duration and dispersion in obese subjects. *Ann. Noninvasive Electrocardiol.* **2008**, *13*, 3–7. [CrossRef]
31. Cosgun, M.; Sincer, I.; Inanir, M.; Erdal, E.; Mansiroglu, A.K.; Gunes, Y. P-wave Duration and Dispersion in Lone Obesity. *J. Coll. Physicians Surg. Pak.* **2021**, *30*, 567–570.
32. Bocchi, F.; Marques-Vidal, P.; Pruvot, E.; Waeber, G.; Vollenweider, P.; Gachoud, D. Clinical and biological determinants of P-wave duration: Cross-sectional data from the population-based CoLaus|PsyCoLaus study. *BMJ Open.* **2020**, *10*, e038828. [CrossRef]
33. Russo, V.; Ammendola, E.; De Crescenzo, I.; Docimo, L.; Santangelo, L.; Calabrò, R. Severe obesity and P-wave dispersion: The effect of surgically induced weight loss. *Obes. Surg.* **2008**, *18*, 90–96. [CrossRef]
34. Duru, M.; Seyfeli, E.; Kuvandik, G.; Kaya, H.; Yalcin, F. Effect of weight loss on P wave dispersion in obese subjects. *Obesity* **2006**, *14*, 1378–1382. [CrossRef]
35. Falchi, A.G.; Grecchi, I.; Muggia, C.; Tinelli, C. Weight loss and P wave dispersion: A preliminary study. *Obes. Res. Clin. Pract.* **2014**, *8*, e614–e617. [CrossRef]
36. Chousou, P.A.; Chattopadhyay, R.; Tsampasian, V.; Vassiliou, V.S.; Pugh, P.J. Electrocardiographic Predictors of Atrial Fibrillation. *Med. Sci.* **2023**, *11*, 30. [CrossRef]
37. Wang, Y.S.; Chen, G.Y.; Li, X.H.; Zhou, X.; Li, Y.G. Prolonged P-wave duration is associated with atrial fibrillation recurrence after radiofrequency catheter ablation: A systematic review and meta-analysis. *Int. J. Cardiol.* **2017**, *227*, 355–359. [CrossRef]
38. Kawczynski, M.J.; Van De Walle, S.; Maesen, B.; Isaacs, A.; Zeemering, S.; Hermans, B.; Vernooy, K.; Maessen, J.G.; Schotten, U.; Bidar, E. Preoperative P-wave parameters and risk of atrial fibrillation after cardiac surgery: A meta-analysis of 20,201 patients. *Interact. Cardiovasc. Thorac. Surg.* **2022**, *35*, ivac220. [CrossRef]
39. Pranata, R.; Yonas, E.; Vania, R. Prolonged P-wave duration in sinus rhythm pre-ablation is associated with atrial fibrillation recurrence after pulmonary vein isolation-A systematic review and meta-analysis. *Ann. Noninvasive Electrocardiol.* **2019**, *24*, e12653. [CrossRef]
40. Nielsen, J.B.; Kühl, J.T.; Pietersen, A.; Graff, C.; Lind, B.; Struijk, J.J.; Olesen, M.S.; Sinner, M.F.; Bachmann, T.N.; Haunsø, S.; et al. P-wave duration and the risk of atrial fibrillation: Results from the Copenhagen ECG Study. *Heart Rhythm.* **2015**, *12*, 1887–1895. [CrossRef]
41. Pérez-Riera, A.R.; de Abreu, L.C.; Barbosa-Barros, R.; Grindler, J.; Fernandes-Cardoso, A.; Baranchuk, A. P-wave dispersion: An update. *Indian. Pacing Electrophysiol. J.* **2016**, *16*, 126–133. [CrossRef]
42. Intzes, S.; Zagoridis, K.; Symeonidou, M.; Spanoudakis, E.; Arya, A.; Dinov, B.; Dagres, N.; Hindricks, G.; Bollmann, A.; Kanoupakis, E.; et al. P-wave duration and atrial fibrillation recurrence after catheter ablation: A systematic review and meta-analysis. *Europace* **2023**, *25*, 450–459. [CrossRef]
43. Weng, L.C.; Hall, A.W.; Choi, S.H.; Jurgens, S.J.; Haessler, J.; Bihlmeyer, N.A.; Grarup, N.; Lin, H.; Teumer, A.; Li-Gao, R.; et al. Genetic Determinants of Electrocardiographic P-Wave Duration and Relation to Atrial Fibrillation. *Circ. Genom. Precis. Med.* **2020**, *13*, 387–395. [CrossRef]
44. Hari, K.J.; Nguyen, T.P.; Soliman, E.Z. Relationship between P-wave duration and the risk of atrial fibrillation. *Expert. Rev. Cardiovasc. Ther.* **2018**, *16*, 837–843. [CrossRef]
45. Dzikowicz, D.J.; Carey, M.G. Obesity and hypertension contribute to prolong QRS complex duration among middle-aged adults. *Ann. Noninvasive Electrocardiol.* **2019**, *24*, e12665. [CrossRef]
46. Rao, A.C.; Ng, A.C.; Sy, R.W.; Chia, K.K.; Hansen, P.S.; Chiha, J.; Kilian, J.; Kanagaratnam, L.B. Electrocardiographic QRS duration is influenced by body mass index and sex. *Int. J. Cardiol. Heart Vasc.* **2021**, *37*, 100884. [CrossRef]
47. Sobhani, S.; Sara, R.; Aghaee, A.; Pirzadeh, P.; Miandehi, E.E.; Shafiei, S.; Akbari, M.; Eslami, S. Body mass index, lipid profile, and hypertension contribute to prolonged QRS complex. *Clin. Nutr. ESPEN.* **2022**, *50*, 231–237. [CrossRef]

48. Sun, G.Z.; Li, Y.; Zhou, X.H.; Guo, X.F.; Zhang, X.G.; Zheng, L.Q.; Li, Y.; Jiao, Y.D.; Sun, Y.X. Association between obesity and ECG variables in children and adolescents: A cross-sectional study. *Exp. Ther. Med.* **2013**, *6*, 1455–1462. [CrossRef]
49. Figliozzi, S.; Stazi, A.; Pinnacchio, G.; Laurito, M.; Parrinello, R.; Villano, A.; Russo, G.; Milo, M.; Mollo, R.; Lanza, G.A.; et al. Use of T-wave alternans in identifying patients with coronary artery disease. *J. Cardiovasc Med.* **2016**, *17*, 20–25. [CrossRef]
50. Hekkanen, J.J.; Kenttä, T.V.; Holmström, L.; Tulppo, M.P.; Ukkola, O.H.; Pakanen, L.; Junttila, M.J.; Huikuri, H.V.; Perkiömäki, J.S. Association of electrocardiographic spatial heterogeneity of repolarization and spatial heterogeneity of atrial depolarization with left ventricular fibrosis. *Europace* **2023**, *25*, 820–827. [CrossRef]
51. Aromolaran, A.S.; Boutjdir, M. Cardiac Ion Channel Regulation in Obesity and the Metabolic Syndrome: Relevance to Long QT Syndrome and Atrial Fibrillation. *Front. Physiol.* **2017**, *8*, 431. [CrossRef]
52. McCauley, M.D.; Hong, L.; Sridhar, A.; Menon, A.; Perike, S.; Zhang, M.; da Silva, I.B.; Yan, J.; Bonini, M.G.; Ai, X.; et al. Ion Channel and Structural Remodeling in Obesity-Mediated Atrial Fibrillation. *Circ. Arrhythm. Electrophysiol.* **2020**, *13*, e008296. [CrossRef]
53. Sharma, S.; Adrogue, J.V.; Golfman, L.; Uray, I.; Lemm, J.; Youker, K.; Noon, G.P.; Frazier, O.H.; Taegtmeyer, H. Intramyocardial lipid accumulation in the failing human heart resembles the lipotoxic rat heart. *FASEB J.* **2004**, *18*, 1692–1700. [CrossRef]
54. Lopaschuk, G.D.; Ussher, J.R.; Folmes, C.D.; Jaswal, J.S.; Stanley, W.C. Myocardial fatty acid metabolism in health and disease. *Physiol. Rev.* **2010**, *90*, 207–258. [CrossRef]
55. Morrow, J.P.; Katchman, A.; Son, N.H.; Trent, C.M.; Khan, R.; Shiomi, T.; Huang, H.; Amin, V.; Lader, J.M.; Vasquez, C.; et al. Mice with cardiac overexpression of peroxi-some proliferator-activated receptor γ have impaired repolarization and spontaneous fatal ventricular ar-rhythmias. *Circulation* **2011**, *124*, 2812–2821. [CrossRef]
56. Purohit, A.; Rokita, A.G.; Guan, X.; Chen, B.; Koval, O.M.; Voigt, N.; Neef, S.; Sowa, T.; Gao, Z.; Luczak, E.D.; et al. Oxidized Ca(2+)/calmodulin-dependent protein kinase II triggers atrial fibrillation. *Circulation* **2013**, *128*, 1748–1757. [CrossRef]
57. Joseph, L.C.; Barca, E.; Subramanyam, P.; Komrowski, M.; Pajvani, U.; Colecraft, H.M.; Hirano, M.; Morrow, J.P. Inhibition of NAPDH Oxidase 2 (NOX2) Prevents Oxidative Stress and Mitochondrial Abnormalities Caused by Saturated Fat in Cardiomyocytes. *PLoS ONE* **2016**, *11*, e0145750. [CrossRef]
58. Abdelaal, M.; le Roux, C.W.; Docherty, N.G. Morbidity and mortality associated with obesity. *Ann. Transl. Med.* **2017**, *5*, 161. [CrossRef]
59. Prospective Studies Collaboration; Whitlock, G.; Lewington, S.; Sherliker, P.; Clarke, R.; Emberson, J.; Halsey, J.; Qizilbash, N.; Collins, R.; Peto, R. Body-mass index and cause-specific mortality in 900,000 adults: Collabo-rative analyses of 57 prospective studies. *Lancet* **2009**, *373*, 1083–1096.
60. Flegal, K.M.; Kit, B.K.; Orpana, H.; Graubard, B.I. Association of all-cause mortality with overweight and obesity using standard body mass index categories: A systematic review and meta-analysis. *JAMA* **2013**, *309*, 71–82. [CrossRef]
61. Şaylık, F.; Çınar, T.; Hayıroğlu, M.İ. Effect of the Obesity Paradox on Mortality in Patients with Acute Coronary Syndrome: A Comprehensive Meta-analysis of the Literature. *Balkan Med. J.* **2023**, *40*, 93–103. [CrossRef]
62. Chang, Y.; Kim, B.K.; Yun, K.E.; Cho, J.; Zhang, Y.; Rampal, S.; Zhao, D.; Jung, H.S.; Choi, Y.; Ahn, J.; et al. Metabolically-healthy obesity and coronary artery calcification. *J. Am. Coll. Cardiol.* **2014**, *63*, 2679–2686. [CrossRef]
63. Zhang, X.; Lv, W.Q.; Qiu, B.; Zhang, L.J.; Qin, J.; Tang, F.J.; Wang, H.T.; Li, H.J.; Hao, Y.R. Assessing causal estimates of the association of obesity-related traits with coronary artery disease using a Mendelian randomization approach. *Sci. Rep.* **2018**, *8*, 7146. [CrossRef]
64. Law, W.Y.; Huang, G.L.; Yang, C.C. Effect of Body Mass Index in Coronary CT Angiography Performed on a 256-Slice Multi-Detector CT Scanner. *Diagnostics* **2022**, *12*, 319. [CrossRef]
65. Bagi, Z.; Broskova, Z.; Feher, A. Obesity and coronary microvascular disease—Implications for adipose tissue-mediated remote inflammatory response. *Curr. Vasc. Pharmacol.* **2014**, *12*, 453–461. [CrossRef]
66. Powell-Wiley, T.M.; Poirier, P.; Burke, L.E.; Després, J.P.; Gordon-Larsen, P.; Lavie, C.J.; Lear, S.A.; Ndumele, C.E.; Neeland, I.J.; Sanders, P.; et al. Obesity and Cardiovascular Disease: A Scientific Statement From the American Heart Association. *Circulation* **2021**, *143*, e984–e1010. [CrossRef]
67. Zellweger, M.J.; Burger, P.C.; Mueller-Brand, J.; Pfisterer, M.E. Is obesity per se as weighty as other risk factors of coronary artery disease? *J. Nucl. Cardiol.* **2004**, *11*, S16. [CrossRef]
68. Poirier, P.; Giles, T.D.; Bray, G.A.; Hong, Y.; Stern, J.S.; Pi-Sunyer, F.X.; Eckel, R.H. Obesity and cardiovascular disease: Pathophysiology, evaluation, and effect of weight loss: An update of the 1997 American Heart Association scientific statement on obesity and heart disease from the Obesity Committee of the Council on Nutrition, Physical Activity, and Metabolism. *Circulation* **2006**, *113*, 898–918.
69. Salem, J.E.; Alexandre, J.; Bachelot, A.; Funck-Brentano, C. Influence of steroid hormones on ventricular repolarization. *Pharmacol. Ther.* **2016**, *167*, 38–47. [CrossRef]
70. Zukowski, M.; Biernawska, J.; Kotfis, K.; Kaczmarczyk, M.; Bohatyrewicz, R.; Blaszczyk, W.; Zegan-Baranska, M.; Ostrowski, M.; Brykczynski, M.; Ciechanowicz, A. Factors influencing QTc interval prolongation during kidney transplantation. *Ann. Transplant.* **2011**, *16*, 43–49. [CrossRef]
71. Alexopoulos, D.; Christodoulou, J.; Toulgaridis, T.; Sitafidis, G.; Manias, O.; Hahalis, G.; Vagenakis, A.G. Repolarization abnormalities with prolonged hyperventilation in apparently healthy subjects: Incidence, mechanisms and affecting factors. *Eur. Heart J.* **1996**, *17*, 1432–1437. [CrossRef]

72. Mirowsky, J.E.; Carraway, M.S.; Dhingra, R.; Tong, H.; Neas, L.; Diaz-Sanchez, D.; Cascio, W.E.; Case, M.; Crooks, J.L.; Hauser, E.R.; et al. Exposures to low-levels of fine particulate matter are associated with acute changes in heart rate variability, cardiac repolarization, and circulating blood lipids in coronary artery disease patients. *Environ. Res.* **2022**, *214 Pt 1*, 113768. [CrossRef]
73. Kazanski, V.; Mitrokhin, V.M.; Mladenov, M.I.; Kamkin, A.G. Cytokine Effects on Mechano-Induced Electrical Activity in Atrial Myocardium. *Immunol. Invest.* **2017**, *46*, 22–37. [CrossRef]
74. Piccirillo, G.; Magrì, D.; Matera, S.; Marigliano, V. Emotions that afflict the heart: Influence of the autonomic nervous system on temporal dispersion of myocardial repolarization. *J. Cardiovasc. Electrophysiol.* **2008**, *19*, 185–187. [CrossRef]
75. Wang, L. ACE inhibitors suppress ischemia-induced arrhythmias by reducing the spatial dispersion of ven-tricular repolarization. *Cardiology* **1999**, *92*, 106–109. [CrossRef]
76. Viitasalo, M.; Oikarinen, L.; Swan, H.; Väänänen, H.; Järvenpää, J.; Hietanen, H.; Karjalainen, J.; Toivonen, L. Effects of beta-blocker therapy on ventricular repolarization documented by 24-h electrocardiography in patients with type 1 long-QT syndrome. *J. Am. Coll. Cardiol.* **2006**, *48*, 747–753. [CrossRef]
77. Yıldırım, D.İ.; Hayıroğlu, M.İ.; Ünal, N.; Eryılmaz, M.A. Evaluation of varenicline usage on ventricular repolar-ization after smoking cessation. *Ann. Noninvasive Electrocardiol.* **2019**, *24*, e12609. [CrossRef]

Disclaimer/Publisher's Note: The statements, opinions and data contained in all publications are solely those of the individual author(s) and contributor(s) and not of MDPI and/or the editor(s). MDPI and/or the editor(s) disclaim responsibility for any injury to people or property resulting from any ideas, methods, instructions or products referred to in the content.

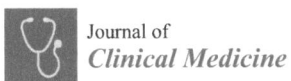

Article

Assessing Disparities about Overweight and Obesity in Pakistani Youth Using Local and International Standards for Body Mass Index

Muhammad Asif [1], Hafiz Ahmad Iqrash Qureshi [2], Saba Mazhar Seyal [3], Muhammad Aslam [4], Muhammad Tauseef Sultan [5], Maysaa Elmahi Abd Elwahab [6], Piotr Matłosz [7] and Justyna Wyszyńska [8,*]

1. Department of Statistics, Govt. Graduate College Qadir Pur Raan, Multan 60000, Pakistan; asifmalik722@gmail.com
2. The Children Hospital and Institute of Child Health, Multan 60000, Pakistan; iqrash1010@gmail.com
3. South City Hospital, District Headquarter (DHQ) Sadar, Multan 60000, Pakistan; usman-s86@yahoo.com
4. Department of Statistics, Bahauddin Zakariya University, Multan 60800, Pakistan; aslamasadi@bzu.edu.pk
5. Department of Human Nutrition, Bahauddin Zakariya University, Multan 60800, Pakistan; tauseefsultan@bzu.edu.pk
6. Department of Mathematical Sciences, College of Science, Princess Nourah bint Abdulrahman University, Riyadh 11671, Saudi Arabia; meabdelwahab@pnu.edu.sa
7. Institute of Physical Culture Sciences, Medical College of Rzeszow University, 35-959 Rzeszów, Poland; pmatlosz@ur.edu.pl
8. Institute of Health Sciences, Medical College of Rzeszow University, 35-959 Rzeszów, Poland
* Correspondence: justyna.wyszynska@onet.pl

Abstract: Background/Objectives: Obesity is currently considered a public health problem in both developed and developing countries. Gender- and age-specific body mass index (BMI) growth standards or references are particularly effective in monitoring the global obesity pandemic. This study aimed to report disparities in age-, gender- and ethnic-specific statistical estimates of overweight and obesity for 2–18 years aged Pakistani children and adolescents using the World Health Organization (WHO), the Center for Disease Control (CDC) 2000 references, the International Obesity Task Force (IOTF) and Pakistani references for BMI. **Methods**: The study used secondary data of 10,668 pediatric population, aged 2–18 years. Demographic information like age (years), gender, city and anthropometric examinations, i.e., height (cm) and weight (kg) were used in this study. The recommended age- and gender-specific BMI cut-offs of the WHO, CDC 2000 and the IOTF references were used to classify the children sampled as overweight and obese. For the Pakistani reference, overweight and obesity were defined as BMI-for-age ≥ 85th percentile and BMI-for-age ≥ 95th percentile, respectively. Cohen's κ statistic was used to assess the agreement between the international references and local study population references in the classification of overweight/obesity. **Results**: The statistical estimates (%) of the participants for overweight and obesity varied according to the reference used: WHO (7.4% and 2.2%), CDC (4.9% and 2.1%), IOTF (5.2% and 2.0%) and Pakistan (8.8% and 6.0%), respectively; suggesting higher levels of overweight and obesity prevalence when local study references are used. The Kappa statistic shows a moderate to excellent agreement (κ ≥ 0.6) among three international references when classifying child overweight and obesity and poor agreement between local references and the WHO (0.45, 0.52), CDC (0.25, 0.50) and IOTF references (0.16, 0.31), for overweight and obesity, respectively. **Conclusions**: The results of the study showed a visible difference in the estimates of excess body weight after applying the WHO, CDC, IOTF and local BMI references to the study population. Based on the disparity results and poor agreement between international references and the local study reference, this study recommends using local BMI references in identifying children with overweight and obesity.

Keywords: body mass index; CDC; IOTF; WHO; references; overweight; obesity

Citation: Asif, M.; Qureshi, H.A.I.; Seyal, S.M.; Aslam, M.; Sultan, M.T.; Elwahab, M.E.A.; Matłosz, P.; Wyszyńska, J. Assessing Disparities about Overweight and Obesity in Pakistani Youth Using Local and International Standards for Body Mass Index. *J. Clin. Med.* **2024**, *13*, 2944. https://doi.org/10.3390/jcm13102944

Academic Editors: Bernward Lauer and Attila Nemes

Received: 18 April 2024
Revised: 10 May 2024
Accepted: 14 May 2024
Published: 16 May 2024

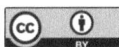

Copyright: © 2024 by the authors. Licensee MDPI, Basel, Switzerland. This article is an open access article distributed under the terms and conditions of the Creative Commons Attribution (CC BY) license (https://creativecommons.org/licenses/by/4.0/).

1. Introduction

Obesity has become a widespread public health concern globally, affecting both developed and developing nations. Studies have shown that excessive consumption of high-calorie foods, a lack of physical activity, and a sedentary lifestyle are prevalent among school-aged children, and these factors are the primary drivers of obesity [1,2]. The alarming increase in childhood obesity has been a major concern in recent years. According to worldwide data estimates, the prevalence of obesity in boys increased from 0.9% (0.5–13%) in 1975 to 7.8% (6.7–9.1%) in 2016, and in girls from 0.7% (0.4–1.2%) in 1975 to 5.6% (4.8–6.5%) in 2016 [3]. This public health issue has also been expended in developing countries including Pakistan. Data from several pieces of research in diverse contexts revealed that the prevalence of excess weight among Pakistani children has risen considerably, ranging between 5% and 20%, with rates higher in boys than in girls [4–6].

Epidemiological researchers regularly used the body mass index (BMI) as an internationally applicable indicator for assessing children's growth and addressing the overweight and obesity problems. A child's BMI is strongly linked to their body fat levels and future health risks, with a significant impact on long-term health outcomes during adolescence. Gender- and age-specific BMI growth standards or growth references are particularly effective for monitoring the global obesity pandemic. In 2000, the International Obesity Task Force (IOTF) used the data of children from six countries (n = 192,727): Brazil, Hong Kong, Singapore, Netherlands, Great Britain and the United States to establish a universally recognized definition for childhood overweight and obesity [7]. The World Health Organization (WHO) established a set of global growth standards for children from birth to five years old in 2006, using data from healthy pediatric populations from around the world [8]. The WHO introduced growth references for school-aged children and adolescents in 2007 [9], whereas the US Center for Disease Control (CDC) had already published its growth references in 2000 [10]. All three international obesity classification criteria are deemed valid, and one of them is usually employed in research or endorsed in local clinical practice guidelines. However, they raise the question of the comparability between them when applied to the same individual, and if they differ, which one is more precise. The selection of a reference is paramount, as it can have a significant impact on the accuracy of classification, and the use of an incorrect reference may lead to flawed conclusions and biased results.

Few studies [11–14] from developed countries have investigated the comparability of the WHO, IOTF and CDC references in evaluating the overweight and obesity status of children's population. But, in developing countries, efforts to explore the comparability of each of these three references to the other in categorizing overweight and obesity are scarce. A contentious issue in the categorization of overweight and obesity in developing countries is whether international references are applicable, given that children in these regions tend to have lower BMI distributions and mature later than the reference population. This concern is evident, particularly in South Asian developing countries, including Pakistan, where growth characteristics in the pediatric population are different due to genetic and environmental variations from the populations used to develop international references [15–18]. A multi-ethnic anthropometric survey (MEAS) study formulated BMI-for-age growth references specifically for Pakistani children and adolescents aged 2–18 years [18], providing a tailored BMI-for-age reference for the Pakistani population. Therefore, the aim of this study is to report the age- and gender-specific statistical estimates of overweight and obesity for the 2 to 18-year-old pediatric population in Pakistan using three international references and the Pakistani reference for BMI. This study also compares the agreement between the WHO, CDC 2000, IOTF and the Pakistani references in the categorization of overweight/obesity.

2. Materials and Methods

We analyzed a dataset of 10,668 children aged 2–18 years collected by the MEAS survey, which has been thoroughly documented in a separate study [19–21]. The study, conducted through the MEAS survey, focused on a group of children from four major cities including four major cities, i.e., Multan (located in the south of Punjab), Lahore (located in central Punjab), Rawalpindi (located in North Punjab) and Islamabad (the capital city of Pakistan) [18]. Data from children aged 5 to 18 were gathered from various public and private schools (n = 68 schools) across the respective cities. The selection of children from each class was carried out through simple random sampling. For subjects under five years old, data were collected from various public locations, such as parks, shopping malls, and markets, using non-probability convenience sampling methods.

For this study, the demographic variables related to information like age (years), gender (boys/girls), residential city (Multan/Lahore/Rawalpindi/Islamabad) and anthropometric examinations, i.e., height (cm) and weight (kg) were used. Body weight and height (using a portable stadiometer SECA: SCA 217) were performed with the subject standing upright, following standard protocols. The complete procedure was discussed in detail elsewhere [19–21]. BMI was calculated using the formula: BMI = weight (in kilograms) divided by height (in meters) squared. The researchers ensured that the entire study adhered to the highest ethical standards.

Statistical Analysis

The software "Statistical Package for Social Sciences (SPSS)" version 21.0 was used for data entry and performing all statistical analyses. Here is the revised text with corrected grammar: The normality of BMI data was assessed using the Kolmogorov–Smirnov test. Since the test revealed non-normality in the data, descriptive statistics were reported as the median and interquartile range (IQR). For comparisons between two groups, the Mann–Whitney U test was employed, while the Kruskal–Wallis test was utilized for comparisons involving more than two groups. Statistical estimates of overweight and obesity, categorized by age, gender, and residential city, were presented in frequency (n) along with corresponding percentages (%). For measuring overweight and obesity in children and adolescents, WHO growth standards for less than five years of age [8] and growth references for 5–19 years of age [9], CDC 2000 reference [10], IOTF growth references [7] and local BMI-for-age growth references developed by Asif et al. [18] were utilized. According to WHO growth standards or references, a subject having a BMI-for-age >1SD above the mean and >2SD above the mean was considered overweight and obese, respectively [8,9]. The USCDC 2000 growth reference system explained that a subject having BMI-for-age ≥ 85th percentile and BMI-for-age ≥ 95th percentile was considered to be overweight and obese, respectively [10]. The IOTF references provided percentile cut-offs corresponding to a BMI of 25.0 and 30.0 kg/m^2 at 18 years of age for overweight and obesity, respectively. According to this criterion, a boy having BMI-for-age ≥90.5th percentile and ≥98.9th percentile was considered overweight and obese. While, the cut-offs for detecting overweight and obesity in girls were; ≥89.3th percentile and ≥98.6th percentile, respectively [7]. The Pakistani references were employed to classify overweight and obesity, with definitions set as BMI-for-age ≥ 85th percentile and BMI-for-age ≥ 95th percentile, respectively. While these percentile cut-offs mirror those outlined by the USCDC, they yield different threshold values for the local population. For instance, in the case of a 10-year-old boy, the 85th percentile results in a BMI cut-off value of 19.32, according to the USCDC, whereas it is 17.97, as reported in Asif et al. [18].

Cohen's κ statistic was used to assess the agreement between the international references and our study population references in the classification of overweight and obesity. The values of κ < 0.6 and κ ≥ 0.90 were considered poor and excellent agreement, respectively [22]. A p-value < 0.05 was considered statistically significant. The study was approved by the Departmental Ethics Committee of Bahauddin Zakariya University, Multan, Pakistan (IRB# SOC/D/2715/19).

3. Results

The present study recruited 10,668 participants in the age range from 2 to 18 years {boys = 5539 (51.9%) and girls = 5129 (48.1%)}. Among those, the majority (26.61%) of the subjects were from Lahore city, followed by Rawalpindi or Islamabad city (16.53%) and Multan city (8.77%). The median BMI of the total subjects was 16.0 (14.40–18.29) kg/m². Boys had significantly higher BMI values than those of girls ($p < 0.001$). The average BMI value of both boys and girls belonging to different ethnicities was also significantly different ($p < 0.001$) (Table 1).

Table 1. Median (interquartile range (IQR)) body mass index and frequency (%) of overweight and obesity in boys by age and residential city area.

Age (Years)	n	Median (IQR)	Overweight n (%) [a]	n (%) [b]	n (%) [c]	n (%) [d]	Obesity n (%) [a]	n (%) [b]	n (%) [c]	n (%) [d]
2	19	12.49 (11.45–13.72)	2 (10.5)	1 (5.3)	1 (5.3)	1 (5.3)	1 (5.3)	--	--	--
3	100	14.34 (13.13–15.62)	15 (15.0)	3 (3.0)	3 (3.0)	4 (4.0)	8 (8.0)	6 (6.0)	6 (6.0)	4 (4.0)
4	208	14.42 (13.35–15.62)	18 (8.7)	11 (5.3)	6 (2.9)	5 (2.4)	5 (2.4)	5 (2.4)	6 (2.9)	3 (1.4)
5	240	14.61 (13.61–15.72)	16 (6.7)	18 (7.5)	14 (5.8)	8 (3.3)	19 (7.9)	19 (7.9)	21 (8.8)	17 (7.1)
6	292	14.61 (13.79–15.53)	14 (4.8)	14 (4.8)	14 (4.8)	15 (5.1)	16 (5.5)	16 (5.5)	16 (5.5)	11 (3.8)
7	279	14.62 (13.64–15.72)	20 (7.2)	23 (8.2)	18 (6.5)	23 (8.2)	21 (7.5)	21 (7.5)	20 (7.2)	7 (2.5)
8	273	14.81 (13.68–16.09)	12 (4.4)	14 (5.1)	9 (3.3)	13 (4.8)	18 (6.6)	17 (6.2)	16 (5.9)	8 (2.9)
9	247	15.14 (13.86–16.39)	17 (6.9)	20 (8.1)	17 (6.9)	19 (7.7)	16 (6.5)	11 (4.5)	8 (3.2)	3 (1.2)
10	420	15.38 (14.20–17.03)	47 (11.2)	34 (8.1)	25 (6.0)	25 (6.0)	19 (4.5)	12 (2.9)	8 (1.9)	--
11	439	15.68 (14.57–17.30)	40 (9.1)	40 (9.1)	27 (6.2)	25 (5.7)	27 (6.2)	10 (2.3)	6 (1.4)	--
12	675	16.02 (14.61–17.75)	54 (8.0)	64 (9.5)	43 (6.4)	35 (5.2)	45 (6.7)	6 (0.9)	2 (0.3)	--
13	593	16.42 (15.11–18.43)	49 (8.3)	58 (9.8)	28 (4.7)	27 (4.6)	42 (7.1)	--	--	--
14	563	17.33 (15.82–19.14)	60 (10.7)	37 (6.6)	25 (4.4)	26 (4.6)	30 (5.3)	--	--	--
15	546	17.85 (16.53–19.82)	52 (9.5)	32 (5.9)	18 (3.3)	19 (3.5)	35 (6.4)	--	--	--
16	381	18.59 (17.06–20.57)	40 (10.5)	13 (3.4)	2 (0.5)	5 (1.3)	22 (5.8)	--	--	--
17	169	19.38 (17.98–21.45)	31 (18.3)	--	--	--	7 (4.1)	--	--	--
18	95	19.57 (17.75–21.15)	13 (13.7)	--	--	--	4 (4.2)	--	--	--
Age-groups (years)										
2–10	2078	14.80 (13.66–16.07)	161 (7.7)	138 (6.6)	107 (5.1)	113 (5.4)	123 (5.9)	107 (5.1)	101 (4.9)	53 (2.6)
11–18	3461	17.12 (15.45–19.23)	339 (9.8)	244 (7.0)	143 (4.1)	137 (4.0)	212 (6.1)	16 (0.5)	8 (0.2)	--
02–18	5539	16.12 (14.58–18.26)	500 (9.0)	382 (6.9)	250 (4.5)	250 (4.5)	335 (6.0)	123 (2.2)	109 (2.0)	53 (1.0)
Residential city										
Lahore	2839	18.22 (14.57–18.36)	269 (9.5)	210 (7.4)	144 (5.1)	139 (4.9)	186 (6.6)	77 (2.7)	67 (2.4)	36 (1.3)
R. Pindi/Isl	1764	15.98 (14.48–18.03)	133 (7.5)	92 (5.2)	54 (3.1)	61 (3.5)	83 (4.7)	21 (1.2)	18 (1.0)	6 (0.3)
Multan	936	16.23 (14.79–18.30)	98 (10.5)	80 (8.5)	52 (5.6)	50 (5.3)	66 (7.1)	25 (2.7)	24 (2.6)	11 (1.2)

[a]: Overweight and obesity prevalence using local study reference; [b]: Overweight and obesity prevalence using WHO reference; [c]: Overweight and obesity prevalence using USCDC reference; [d]: Overweight and obesity prevalence using IOTF reference; SD: Standard deviation; R. Pindi: Rawalpindi; Isl: Islamabad.

Statistical estimates of overweight and obesity were substantially different across ages when three international and local references were applied. The results exhibited that 8.8% of the overall subjects (boys = 9.0% and girls = 8.5%) were overweight, and 6.0% (boys = 6.0% and girls = 5.9%) were obese by using the local study reference. By using the WHO, CDC and IOTF cut-offs, the overweight prevalence was 7.4% (boys = 6.9% and girls = 7.9%), 4.9% (boys = 4.5% and girls = 5.2%) and 5.2% (boys = 4.5% and girls = 5.8%), respectively and obesity was 2.2% (boys = 2.2% and girls = 2.2%), 2.1% (boys = 2.0% and girls = 2.3%) and 1.2% (boys = 1.0% and girls = 1.4%), respectively. We categorized our study population into two sub-age groups (2–10 years and 11–18 years) and three ethnicities (Lahore, Rawalpindi/Islamabad and Multan). Estimates of overweight and obesity prevalence based on local references were also higher among sub-age groups and ethnicities compared to the three international BMI cut-offs (Tables 1 and 2).

Table 2. Median (interquartile range (IQR)) body mass index and frequency (%) of overweight and obesity in girls by age and residential city area.

Age (Years)	n	Median (IQR)	Overweight n (%) [a]	Overweight n (%) [b]	Overweight n (%) [c]	Overweight n (%) [d]	Obesity n (%) [a]	Obesity n (%) [b]	Obesity n (%) [c]	Obesity n (%) [d]
2	43	13.00 (11.81–14.71)	3 (7.0)	2 (4.7)	--	--	1 (2.3)	1 (2.3)	1 (2.3)	1 (2.3)
3	170	14.33 (13.01–15.51)	10 (5.9)	5 (2.9)	3 (1.8)	4 (2.4)	10 (5.9)	8 (4.7)	8 (4.7)	6 (3.5)
4	313	14.57 (13.22–15.71)	31 (9.9)	17 (5.4)	13 (4.2)	12 (3.8)	20 (6.4)	14 (4.5)	18 (5.8)	13 (4.2)
5	381	14.42 (13.25–15.42)	23 (6.0)	26 (6.8)	21 (5.5)	20 (5.2)	29 (7.6)	19 (5.0)	25 (6.6)	17 (4.5)
6	405	14.35 (13.43–15.43)	25 (6.2)	28 (6.9)	23 (5.7)	23 (5.7)	12 (3.0)	9 (2.2)	11 (2.7)	8 (2.0)
7	381	14.72 (13.66–15.86)	27 (7.1)	31 (8.1)	25 (6.6)	29 (7.6)	19 (5.0)	15 (3.9)	15 (3.9)	9 (2.4)
8	376	14.88 (14.00–16.47)	31 (8.2)	41 (10.9)	31 (8.2)	36 (9.6)	25 (6.6)	18 (4.8)	15 (4.0)	10 (2.7)
9	336	15.33 (13.90–17.00)	36 (10.7)	41 (12.2)	28 (8.3)	34 (10.1)	18 (5.4)	11 (3.3)	11 (3.3)	5 (1.5)
10	459	15.83 (14.31–17.56)	44 (9.6)	45 (9.8)	23 (5.0)	28 (6.1)	17 (3.7)	9 (2.0)	8 (1.7)	4 (0.9)
11	325	16.56 (15.04–18.37)	21 (6.5)	32 (9.8)	28 (8.6)	35 (10.8)	30 (9.2)	11 (3.4)	7 (2.2)	--
12	436	16.89 (15.35–18.93)	42 (9.6)	53 (12.2)	32 (7.3)	35 (8.0)	31 (7.1)	--	--	--
13	460	17.58 (15.82–19.55)	51 (11.1)	44 (9.6)	24 (5.2)	24 (15.2)	26 (5.7)	--	--	--
14	341	18.26 (16.65–19.98)	--	--	--	--	--	--	--	--
15	257	18.67 (17.09–20.72)	--	--	--	--	--	--	--	--
16	191	18.92 (17.16–20.40)	--	--	--	--	--	--	--	--
17	129	18.97 (17.33–20.75)	--	--	--	--	--	--	--	--
18	126	19.26 (17.65–21.37)	--	--	--	--	--	--	--	--
Age-groups (years)										
2–10	2864	14.79 (13.65–16.15)	230 (8.0)	236 (8.2)	167 (5.8)	186 (6.5)	151 (5.3)	104 (3.6)	112 (3.9)	73 (2.5)
11–18	2265	17.86 (16.02–19.88)	208 (9.2)	167 (7.4)	102 (4.5)	114 (5.0)	153 (6.8)	11 (0.5)	7 (0.3)	--
02–18	5129	15.87 (14.27–18.31)	438 (8.5)	403 (7.9)	269 (5.2)	300 (5.8)	304 (5.9)	115 (2.2)	119 (2.3)	73 (1.4)
Residential city										
Lahore	2091	16.42 (14.47–18.75)	203 (9.7)	159 (7.6)	105 (5.0)	116 (5.5)	127 (6.1)	51 (2.4)	54 (2.6)	35 (1.7)
R. Pindi/Isl	1926	15.39 (14.05–17.57)	126 (6.5)	119 (6.2)	80 (4.2)	86 (4.5)	82 (4.3)	26 (1.3)	26 (1.3)	16 (0.8)
Multan	1112	16.11 (14.51–18.31)	109 (9.8)	125 (11.2)	84 (7.6)	98 (8.8)	95 (8.5)	38 (3.4)	39 (3.5)	22 (2.0)

[a]: Overweight and obesity prevalence using local study reference; [b]: Overweight and obesity prevalence using WHO reference; [c]: Overweight and obesity prevalence using USCDC reference; [d]: Overweight and obesity prevalence using IOTF reference; SD: Standard deviation; R. Pindi: Rawalpindi; Isl: Islamabad.

Cohen's kappa statistic findings for total participants revealed a poor agreement between local references and the WHO, CDC and IOTF references, i.e., κ = 0.45, 0.25, 0.16, respectively, for overweight and κ = 0.52, 0.50, 0.31, respectively, for obesity (Table 3).

Table 3. Agreement between international references in classifying overweight and obesity in a sample of Pakistani children.

Variable	Kappa Co-Efficient					
	Overweight			Obesity		
	IOTF	CDC	Pakistani Reference	IOTF	CDC	Pakistani Reference
Overall (n = 10,668)						
WHO	0.634	0.741	0.450	0.687	0.912	0.527
IOTF		0.808	0.160		0.707	0.316
CDC			0.258			0.503
Boys (n = 5539)						
WHO	0.595	0.722	0.775	0.597	0.912	0.522
IOTF		0.744	0.058		0.650	0.261
CDC			0.186			0.461
Girls (n = 5129)						
WHO	0.715	0.759	0.530	0.773	0.913	0.534
IOTF		0.864	0.266		0.756	0.373
CDC			0.336			0.548

IOTF: International Obesity Task Force, CDC: Centers for Disease Control and Prevention, WHO: World Health Organization.

4. Discussion

International references play a crucial role in facilitating comparisons between studies and countries, as well as in monitoring global trends of overweight and obesity. However, there is insufficient conclusive evidence to affirm their validity in developing countries [23]. It is widely observed that populations in developing countries often exhibit lower BMI reference values [15,18] compared to those outlined by the WHO, CDC, and other references from developed nations. This deviation may lead to overestimations in the prevalence of overweight and obesity if local references are not utilized. This observation was further supported by a recent study conducted in Pakistan by Qaisar and Karim [24], which revealed a significantly higher overall prevalence of overweight and obesity among girls when using local references compared to those from the WHO, CDC, and IOTF.

This study examines the prevalence of overweight and obesity among children and adolescents in Pakistan aged 2–18, providing gender- and ethnic-specific statistics. It also emphasizes the need to consider the suitability of global references for measuring overweight and obesity in Pakistani youth and their alignment with local cut-off points.

The MEAS data of 10,668 children and adolescents 2–18 years of age indicated that the estimates of overnutrition were found to be higher by the WHO references compared to the CDC and IOTF references (7.4% vs. 4.9% and 5.2% for overweight and 2.2% vs. 2.1% and 1.2% for obesity, respectively). The same trend was also observed among both boys (6.9% vs. 4.5% and 4.5% for overweight and 2.2% vs. 2.0% and 1.0% for obesity, respectively) and girls (7.9% vs. 5.2% and 5.8% for overweight and 2.2% vs. 2.3% and 1.4% for obesity, respectively). These findings were consistent with the earlier studies with the Algerian [25], Malaysian [26] and Saudi [27] child samples. A study in Lahore, Pakistan, found that 1860 schoolchildren had a higher prevalence of overweight and obesity when measured against the WHO reference compared to the IOTF and CDC references [28].

By using the local reference, the rates of overweight (8.8%) and obesity (6.0%) were higher compared to the aforementioned three different BMI classifications (i.e., WHO 2007, USCDC, and IOTF references). These results also support the previous study trend [24], showing that overweight and obesity rates among 8–16-year-old girls were higher when using local references compared to the results obtained by the three international references. The disparities in rates are largely attributed to variations in the criteria used to define and measure the threshold. The disparity in results may also be attributed to various related factors, including differences in the reference populations, such as the date of data collection, country of origin, study design, and genetic or environmental factors. The local study references were based on the cross-sectional data collected in 2016, while the IOTF references were constructed by using the dataset collected in six countries, mostly during the 1980s. In order to establish CDC references, two different datasets were collected in 1963–1965 and in 1976–1980 from the US children's settings. The development of WHO growth references for school-aged children and adolescents was also based on pooling three data sets collected from the Health and Nutrition Examination Survey (HANES) Cycle I and Cycle II and Cycle III from the Health Examination Survey (HES). The inconsistency in statistical data on overweight and obesity highlights the need to consider whether universal international standards are suitable for all populations, as they may not accurately reflect the specific characteristics of certain groups.

In Pakistan, numerous published studies [4–6,29–31] were undertaken at a regional level, encompassing various age groups in which the criteria of WHO or CDC reference was used to deliver the estimates of overweight and obesity in children. Results in different settings indicated that the estimates for overweight vary between 8% to 19% and for obesity between 5% to 8%. The most recent cross-sectional study by Tanveer et al. [32] conducted in seven districts of central Punjab province with 3551 school children aged 9 to 17 years showed that 5.8% of the children were overweight and 5.4% were obese. Our study findings were also akin to the earlier study results.

Overall and across genders, the three international references showed a moderate agreement ($0.6 \leq \kappa < 0.8$) among themselves when categorizing children as overweight. The agreement was moderate to excellent ($\kappa \geq 0.8$) when examining child obesity, particularly between the WHO and CDC references. These results were also consistent with the Algerian and Malaysian study results [25,26] revealing that the agreement was excellent between the WHO and CDC for examining childhood obesity. In contrast, a comparison between three international references and the population's own BMI reference showed a poor agreement (i.e., $\kappa < 0.6$), which is also parallel to earlier research results [24].

The study reveals that the choice of BMI reference can significantly impact estimates of overweight and obesity, ultimately affecting the strategies used by healthcare resources to address these issues and pediatricians' decisions to provide clinical advice and management. It is not reasonable to rely solely on a single reference standard for all populations. Instead, we propose that each country develop its own local anthropometric reference based on its unique population data. These references must be thoroughly validated to ensure their accuracy in predicting and addressing potential health risks early on.

The treatment of various obesity-related diseases like cardio-metabolic and certain types of cancers is much more expensive, and timely assessment of abnormal weight status assists in reducing the economic burden. These statistical estimates of overweight and obesity will be helpful for pediatricians to combat abnormal weight status in childhood.

These can inform the development of targeted health policies to mitigate the negative consequences of being overweight and obese in the long term. Although we analyzed large and multi-ethnic sample data for representing statistical estimates of overweight and obesity, this study still has some limitations. Given the limitations of the MEAS dataset, which is comprised of a predominantly urban and affluent population, future research should strive to include diverse cohorts with varying ages and socio-economic backgrounds to broaden the generalizability of our findings. Moreover, a sedentary lifestyle and dietary intake behavior also have great influences on the BMI of children [1,2]. Therefore, comparative studies should also plan to include these significant factors. Despite the study's limitations, we anticipate that our findings will contribute to the advancement of public health knowledge.

5. Conclusions

We observed a notable disparity in the estimates of overweight and obesity among Pakistani children and adolescents aged 2 to 18 when applying BMI references from the World Health Organization, Centers for Disease Control and Prevention, International Obesity Task Force, and local sources. The disparities uncovered and the limited agreement between international references and the local study reference suggest that this study advocates for the use of local BMI references to identify children with overweight and obesity. Population-specific BMI references undergo thorough validation to accurately assess health risks in the early stages, thereby aiding in the formulation of effective health policies to mitigate the long-term adverse effects of overweight and obesity.

Author Contributions: Data curation, M.A. (Muhammad Asif) and M.A. (Muhammad Aslam); Formal analysis, M.A. (Muhammad Asif) and M.A. (Muhammad Aslam); Methodology, J.W.; Resources, S.M.S., M.T.S. and J.W.; Software, M.A. (Muhammad Asif); Validation, P.M.; Visualization, H.A.I.Q.; Writing–original draft, M.A. (Muhammad Asif); Writing–review & editing, M.A. (Muhammad Asif), H.A.I.Q., S.M.S., M.T.S., M.E.A.E., P.M. and J.W. All authors have read and agreed to the published version of the manuscript.

Funding: This research did not receive any grant from funding agencies in the public, commercial or non-profit sectors.

Institutional Review Board Statement: The study was conducted in accordance with the Declaration of Helsinki and approved by the Departmental Ethics Committee of Bahauddin Zakariya University, Multan, Pakistan (IRB# SOC/D/2715/19).

Informed Consent Statement: Informed consent was obtained from all subjects involved in the study.

Data Availability Statement: https://data.mendeley.com/datasets/sxgymx5xjm/1 (accessed on 13 May 2024).

Conflicts of Interest: The authors declare no conflicts of interest.

References

1. Li, Y.; Zhai, F.; Yang, X.; Schouten, E.G.; Hu, X.; He, Y.; Luan, D.; Ma, G. Determinants of childhood overweight and obesity in China. *Br. J. Nutr.* **2007**, *97*, 210–215. [CrossRef] [PubMed]
2. Mushtaq, M.U.; Gull, S.; Mushtaq, K.; Shahid, U.; Shad, M.A.; Akram, J. Dietary behaviors, physical activity and sedentary lifestyle associated with overweight and obesity, and their socio-demographic correlates, among Pakistani primary school children. *Int. J. Behav. Nutr. Phys. Act.* **2011**, *8*, 130. [CrossRef] [PubMed]
3. Abarca-Gómez, L.; Abdeen, Z.A.; Hamid, Z.A.; Abu-Rmeileh, N.M.; Acosta-Cazares, B.; Acuin, C.; Adams, R.J.; Aekplakorn, W.; Afsana, K.; Aguilar-Salinas, C.A.; et al. Worldwide trends in body-mass index, underweight, overweight, and obesity from 1975 to 2016: A pooled analysis of 2416 population-based measurement studies in 128·9 million children, adolescents, and adults. *Lancet* **2017**, *390*, 2627–2642. [CrossRef] [PubMed]
4. Aziz, S.; Noorulain, W.; Zaidi, U.-R.; Hossain, K.; Siddiqui, I.A. Prevalence of overweight and obesity among children and adolescents of affluent schools in Karachi. *J. Pak. Med. Assoc.* **2009**, *59*, 35–38. [PubMed]
5. Mushtaq, M.U.; Gull, S.; Abdullah, H.M.; Shahid, U.; Shad, M.A.; Akram, J. Waist circumference, waist-hip ratio and waist-height ratio percentiles and central obesity among Pakistani children aged five to twelve years. *BMC Pediatr.* **2011**, *11*, 105. [CrossRef] [PubMed]
6. Ahmed, J.; Laghari, A.; Naseer, M.; Mehraj, V. Prevalence of and factors associated with obesity among Pakistani schoolchildren: A school-based, cross-sectional study. *East. Mediterr. Health J.* **2013**, *19*, 242–247. [CrossRef] [PubMed]
7. Cole, T.J. Establishing a standard definition for child overweight and obesity worldwide: International survey. *BMJ* **2000**, *320*, 1240. [CrossRef] [PubMed]
8. WHO Multicentre Growth Reference Study Group. WHO Child Growth Standards: Length/Height-for-Age, Weight-for-Age, Weight-for-Length, Weight-for-Height and Body Mass Index-for-age: Methods and Development. Available online: https://www.who.int/toolkits/child-growth-standards/standards/body-mass-index-for-age-bmi-for-age (accessed on 13 May 2024).
9. de Onis, M.; Onyango, A.W.; Borghi, E.; Siyam, A.; Nishida, C.; Siekmann, J. Development of a WHO growth reference for school-aged children and adolescents. *Bull. World Health Organ.* **2007**, *85*, 660–667. [CrossRef] [PubMed]
10. Kuczmarski, R.J.; Ogden, C.L.; Guo, S.S.; Grummer-Strawn, L.M.; Flegal, K.M.; Mei, Z.; Wei, R.; Curtin, L.R.; Roche, A.F.; Johnson, C.L. 2000 CDC Growth Charts for the United States: Methods and development. *Vital Health Stat.* **2002**, *11*, 1–190.
11. Wang, Y.; Wang, J.Q. A comparison of international references for the assessment of child and adolescent overweight and obesity in different populations. *Eur. J. Clin. Nutr.* **2002**, *56*, 973–982. [CrossRef]
12. Zimmermann, M.B.; Gübeli, C.; Püntener, C.; Molinari, L. Detection of overweight and obesity in a national sample of 6–12-y-old Swiss children: Accuracy and validity of reference values for body mass index from the US Centers for Disease Control and Prevention and the International Obesity Task Force123. *Am. J. Clin. Nutr.* **2004**, *79*, 838–843. [CrossRef] [PubMed]
13. Jagiełło, W. Differentiation of the body composition in taekwondo-ITF competitors of the men's Polish national team and direct based athletes. *Arch. Budo* **2015**, *11*, 329–338.
14. Baya Botti, A.; Pérez-Cueto, F.J.A.; Vasquez Monllor, P.A.; Kolsteren, P.W. International BMI-for-age references underestimate thinness and overestimate overweight and obesity in Bolivian adolescents. *Nutr. Hosp.* **2010**, *25*, 428–436. [PubMed]
15. Khadilkar, V.V.; Khadilkar, A.V.; Chiplonkar, S.A. Growth performance of affluent Indian preschool children: A comparison with the new WHO growth standard. *Indian Pediatr.* **2010**, *47*, 869–872. [CrossRef] [PubMed]
16. Karki, S.; Päkkilä, J.; Laitala, M.-L.; Ojaniemi, M.; Anttonen, V. National reference centiles of anthropometric indices and BMI cut-off values in a child population in Nepal. *Ann. Hum. Biol.* **2018**, *45*, 447–452. [CrossRef] [PubMed]
17. Saha, B.K.; Hoque, M.A.; Dhar, S.K.; Sharmin, M.; Rabbany, M.A.; Ahmad, F.; Nahid, K.L. Comparison of Growth of School Children in Mymensingh City Area, Bangladesh Using the 2000 CDC Standards and 2007 WHO Standards. *Mymensingh Med. J.* **2022**, *31*, 983–991. [PubMed]
18. Asif, M.; Aslam, M.; Wyszyńska, J.; Altaf, S. Establishing Body Mass Index growth charts for Pakistani children and adolescents using the lambda-mu-sigma (LMS) and quantile regression method. *Minerva Pediatr.* **2023**, *75*, 866–875. [CrossRef] [PubMed]
19. Asif, M.; Aslam, M.; Qasim, M.; Altaf, S.; Ismail, A.; Ali, H. A dataset about anthropometric measurements of the Pakistani children and adolescents using a cross-sectional multi-ethnic anthropometric survey. *Data Br.* **2021**, *34*, 106642. [CrossRef]
20. Asif, M.; Aslam, M.; Altaf, S.; Mustafa, S. Developing waist circumference, waist-to-height ratio percentile curves for Pakistani children and adolescents aged 2–18 years using Lambda-Mu-Sigma (LMS) method. *J. Pediatr. Endocrinol. Metab.* **2020**, *33*, 983–993. [CrossRef]
21. Asif, M.; Aslam, M.; Khan, S.; Altaf, S.; Ahmad, S.; Qasim, M.; Ali, H.; Wyszyńska, J. Developing neck circumference growth reference charts for Pakistani children and adolescents using the lambda–mu–sigma and quantile regression method. *Public Health Nutr.* **2021**, *24*, 5641–5649. [CrossRef]
22. McHugh, M.L. Interrater reliability: The kappa statistic. *Biochem. Medica* **2012**, *22*, 276–282. [CrossRef]

23. Wang, Y.; Monteiro, C.; Popkin, B.M. Trends of obesity and underweight in older children and adolescents in the United States, Brazil, China, and Russia. *Am. J. Clin. Nutr.* **2002**, *75*, 971–977. [CrossRef] [PubMed]
24. Qaisar, R.; Karim, A. BMI status relative to international and national growth references among Pakistani school-age girls. *BMC Pediatr.* **2021**, *21*, 535. [CrossRef] [PubMed]
25. Oulamara, H.; Allam, O.; Tebbani, F.; Agli, A.-N. Prevalence of overweight and underweight in schoolchildren in Constantine, Algeria: Comparison of four reference cut-off points for body mass index. *East. Mediterr. Health J.* **2020**, *26*, 349–355. [CrossRef] [PubMed]
26. Partap, U.; Young, E.H.; Allotey, P.; Sandhu, M.S.; Reidpath, D.D. The Use of Different International References to Assess Child Anthropometric Status in a Malaysian Population. *J. Pediatr.* **2017**, *190*, 63–68.e1. [CrossRef]
27. Al-Hazzaa, H.M.; Alrasheedi, A.A.; Alsulaimani, R.A.; Jabri, L.; Alhowikan, A.M.; Alhussain, M.H.; Bawaked, R.A.; Alqahtani, S.A. Prevalence of overweight and obesity among saudi children: A comparison of two widely used international standards and the national growth references. *Front. Endocrinol.* **2022**, *13*, 954755. [CrossRef] [PubMed]
28. Mushtaq, M.U.; Gull, S.; Mushtaq, K.; Abdullah, H.M.; Khurshid, U.; Shahid, U.; Shad, M.A.; Akram, J. Height, weight and BMI percentiles and nutritional status relative to the international growth references among Pakistani school-aged children. *BMC Pediatr.* **2012**, *12*, 31. [CrossRef]
29. Warraich, H.J.; Javed, F.; Faraz-ul-Haq, M.; Khawaja, F.B.; Saleem, S. Prevalence of Obesity in School-Going Children of Karachi. *PLoS ONE* **2009**, *4*, e4816. [CrossRef] [PubMed]
30. Mushtaq, M.U.; Gull, S.; Abdullah, H.M.; Shahid, U.; Shad, M.A.; Akram, J. Prevalence and socioeconomic correlates of overweight and obesity among Pakistani primary school children. *BMC Public Health* **2011**, *11*, 724. [CrossRef] [PubMed]
31. Khan, S.; Abbas, A.; Ali, I.; Arshad, R.; Tareen, M.B.K.; Shah, M.I. Prevalence of overweight and obesity and lifestyle assessment among school–going children of Multan, Pakistan. *Isra Med. J.* **2019**, *11*, 230–233.
32. Tanveer, M.; Hohmann, A.; Roy, N.; Zeba, A.; Tanveer, U.; Siener, M. The Current Prevalence of Underweight, Overweight, and Obesity Associated with Demographic Factors among Pakistan School-Aged Children and Adolescents—An Empirical Cross-Sectional Study. *Int. J. Environ. Res. Public Health* **2022**, *19*, 11619. [CrossRef]

Disclaimer/Publisher's Note: The statements, opinions and data contained in all publications are solely those of the individual author(s) and contributor(s) and not of MDPI and/or the editor(s). MDPI and/or the editor(s) disclaim responsibility for any injury to people or property resulting from any ideas, methods, instructions or products referred to in the content.

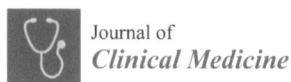

Article

Overweight, Obesity, and Age Are the Main Determinants of Cardiovascular Risk Aggregation in the Current Mexican Population: The FRIMEX III Study

Eduardo Meaney [1], Enrique Pérez-Robles [1], Miguel Ortiz-Flores [1], Guillermo Perez-Ishiwara [2], Alejandra Meaney [3], Levy Munguía [4], Gisele Roman [5] on behalf of the Coalición por el Corazón de México, Nayelli Nájera [1,*] and Guillermo Ceballos [1,*]

1. Laboratorio de Investigación Cardiometabólica Integral, Sección de Estudios de Posgrado e Investigación, Escuela Superior de Medicina, Instituto Politécnico Nacional, Mexico City 11340, Mexico; eperezrobles@gmail.com (E.P.-R.); maortizfl@ipn.mx (M.O.-F.)
2. Escuela Nacional de Medicina y Homeopatía, Instituto Politécnico Nacional, Mexico City 07320, Mexico; dperez@ipn.mx
3. Cardiovascular Unit, Hospital Regional "1° de Octubre", Instituto de Seguridad Social y Servicios para los Trabajadores del Estado, Mexico City 07760, Mexico
4. Dirección Normativa de Salud, Instituto de Seguridad y Servicios Sociales para los Trabajadores del Estado, Mexico City 06030, Mexico
5. Coalición por el Corazón de México, Mexico City 01090, Mexico
* Correspondence: nnajerag@ipn.mx (N.N.); gceballosr@ipn.mx (G.C.)

Abstract: Background: The Mexican population exhibits several cardiovascular risk factors (CVRF) including high blood pressure (HBP), dysglycemia, dyslipidemia, overweight, and obesity. This study is an extensive observation of the most important CVRFs in six of the most populated cities in Mexico. **Methods**: In a cohort of 297,370 participants (54% female, mean age 43 ± 12.6 years), anthropometric (body mass index (BMI)), metabolic (glycemia and total cholesterol (TC)), and blood pressure (BP) data were obtained. **Results**: From age 40, 40% and 30% of the cohort's participants were overweight or obese, respectively. HBP was found in 27% of participants. However, only 8% of all hypertensive patients were controlled. Fifty percent of the subjects 50 years and older were hypercholesterolemic. Glycemia had a constant linear relation with age. BMI had a linear correlation with SBP, glycemia, and TC, with elevated coefficients in all cases and genders. The β1 coefficient for BMI was more significant in all equations than the other β, indicating that it greatly influences the other CVRFs. **Conclusions**: TC, glycemia, and SBP, the most critical atherogenic factors, are directly related to BMI.

Keywords: total cholesterol; glycemia; systolic blood pressure; body mass index; multiple linear regression

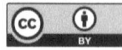

1. Introduction

Contemporary cardiovascular (CV) and cardiometabolic medicines are strongly oriented to fundamental, primary, secondary, and tertiary phases of prevention, basing the prophylaxis and treatment of CV and cardiometabolic diseases on therapeutic modifications of lifestyle, altogether with proven pharmacological and interventional therapies [1–3]. In this context, determining and characterizing the risk profiles of a given population are essential for developing proper public policies and therapeutic and preventive guidelines to mitigate the prevalence and lethality of the epidemic flagella that assail contemporary society.

Cardiac diseases (76.3% are ischemic heart disease) and diabetes mellitus (DM) are the leading causes of total mortality in Mexico, provoking 200,535 deaths in 2022 [4]. Several governmental and academic studies have revealed the high-risk profile affecting the contemporary Mexican population [5–10]. The FRIMEX study [11], an RF survey in six of the most populated cities in Mexico, including more than 140,000 persons of both genders, with an average age of 44 ± 13 years, revealed a population with very high cardiovascular risk, where overweight or obesity (O/O) affected 71.9% of participants, in straight correlation with high blood pressure (HBP), hypercholesterolemia, and elevated glucose serum concentrations. This study and many others indicate that Mexico's leading CV and cardiometabolic risk factor (RF) is O/O, as in many other countries and regions worldwide. However, despite the evident tragic current Mexican epidemiologic panorama, informative and preventive programs have not been established nor have solid public policies that mitigate the prevalence of O/O and their consequences been implemented.

Obesity is a chronic, heterogeneous, relapsing, and progressing structural disease [12] due to the loss of balance between caloric intake and energy expenditure. It is characterized by the excessive accumulation and abnormal distribution of body fat. It is frequently associated with structural and functional alterations of adipocytes as well as hypertrophy, hyperplasia, ischemia, necrosis, apoptosis, and autophagy of fatty tissue. At the same time, it is often accompanied by resistance to insulin and secondary hyperinsulinism, inflammation, oxidative stress, and endothelial dysfunction. The last triad leads to the development of morbid conditions that affect multiple organs and systems [13]. According to the World Health Organization (WHO), obesity is classified, using the body mass index (BMI, kg/m^2), into the following three categories: class 1 (BMI of 30 to <35), class 2 (BMI of 35 to <40), and class 3 (BMI of 40 or higher) [14,15]. In many studies, a strong linear relationship between the degree of obesity and the occurrence of HBP, stroke, and myocardial infarction has been demonstrated [16].

Numerous mechanisms link O/O to the development of multiple cardiovascular diseases, mainly atherosclerotic cardiovascular diseases (ASCVD), but also to heart failure, chronic kidney disease, and obstructive sleep apnea, among many others. Amid several complex mechanisms stand out the already mentioned vascular pathogenic triad. This includes the inflamed ectopic pericardial fat tissue; the binomial insulin resistance/hyperinsulinism; obesity-related comorbidities such as high blood pressure (HBP), dyslipidemia, and diabetes; and systemic inflammation and adverse cytokines, as well as a prothrombotic milieu and the overexpression of renin–angiotensin–aldosterone axis, among others [17,18].

The present report does not aim to show our population's already known pattern of high risk but to highlight the importance of the close interrelationship among the most crucial CVRFs. Moreover, the analysis of this large cohort should show the hierarchical importance of the different CVRFs studied in this survey to profile the risk pattern of the contemporary Mexican population. Likewise, this complex tangle of CV disease-promoting agents imposes therapeutic and preventive strategies that must consider these interrelationships to establish a holistic treatment, better reducing the severity of all CVRFs and metabolic risks.

2. Materials and Methods

The methodology of this study has already been published [11]. The study was conducted following the guidance of Good Clinical Practices [19], the norms from the Declaration of Helsinki, [20] and the Mexican Federal regulations established in the General Law of Health [21]. Mobile units, served by trained health personnel, were placed in commercial malls or civic centers and squares in six of the most populated cities in the country, some located in Central Mexico (the capital Mexico City, Puebla, and León), others in the central western geographic area (Guadalajara), and two in the northernmost regions (Monterrey and Tijuana). The participants, aged 18 years or older, of any gender, were recruited by invitation. The design of this survey allowed the recruitment of any adult who accepted the invitation. Therefore, there were no inclusion criteria. The cohort comprised a non-probabilistic sample of 300,000 participants of both genders (recruited in the last 10 years). Body mass index (BMI, kg/m^2) was obtained in all subjects through weight and height and was classified, according to the WHO, [15] as underweight (BMI < 18.5), healthy weight (BMI 18.5–24.9), overweight (BMI 25.0–29.9), and obesity (BMI ≥ 30.0). Blood pressure (BP) was measured with calibrated mercurial sphygmomanometers following standard recommendations [22]. HBP was considered when systolic blood pressure (SBP) was ≥140 mm Hg associated or not to a diastolic blood pressure (DBP) ≥90 mm Hg, in concordance with the cut-offs accepted by the official Mexican norm on hypertension [23]. The proportions known as the "law of the halves" [24] were estimated from the data collected in the survey which includes the rates of awareness, treatment, and control (treatment type was not recorded). Glucose was measured in capillary blood with a "dry chemistry" apparatus (Accutrend, Roche Diagnostics, Basel, Switzerland) and participants fasted for at least five hours. Dysglycemia was classified as fasting plasma glucose (FPG) between 100 and 125 mg/dL and overt DM with ciphers of ≥126 mg/dL or ≥200 mg/dL, regardless of fasting time, following recommendations of the American Diabetes Association [25]. Total cholesterol (TC) was measured with the same technique. Its concentrations, according to the Adult Treatment Panel III (ATP III), [26] were classified as adequate when TC was <200 mg/dL, borderline hypercholesterolemia when it was between 200 and 239 mg/dL, and definitive hypercholesterolemia with TC ≥ 240 mg/dL (due to logistic and economic restrictions, triglycerides, HDL, or LDL concentrations were not obtained). Finally, smoking status was established as regular consumers if the participants had smoked any amount of tobacco habitually within the last trimester or a longer time and non-smokers if they had never smoked or only occasionally. However, in this first analysis, we omitted tobacco's contribution to CV risk because the number of cigarettes consumed was not registered.

Statistics

Data were presented as mean ± SD; the analysis included year-by-year (20–70 years of age) changes in risk marker levels, an analysis of age-related changes by gender with linear or quadratic correlation between variables when applied. A multilinear regression analysis was performed to generate equations exploring the influence of each variable on body mass index, systolic blood pressure, and cholesterol. This study was conducted using Prism software, 10.1.1 version (www.graphpad.com). Statistical significance was considered when $p < 0.05$.

3. Results

Of the 300,000 participants recruited, those with incomplete data or records showing markedly out-of-range values were excluded, leaving just 297,370 for analysis. This small number, representing 0.87% of all surveyed subjects, cannot influence the analysis results. Most participants (29%) were from Mexico City, while in the rest of the cities, the proportion between them was very similar, between 11% and 15%. Regarding gender, 54% were female, and 46% were male. The mean age was 43 ± 12.6 years (men were 41 ± 11.7 years and women were 44 ± 12.7 years), the mode was 32.3 years, and the 31–40 decade was the most frequent. Concerning educational status, 54.5% of the cohort's participants had elementary education, 21.1% had middle-high or technical subprofessional levels, and 24.4% had college or higher degrees. Considering genders, women obtained 61.5%, 19%, and 19.5% of the three academic mentioned categories, while men obtained 46.2%, 23.4%, and 30.3%, respectively. Table 1 shows the cohort's anthropometric, metabolic, and BP data, as well as the totals and those corresponding to each gender. Although men were more overweight than women, no significant differences were observed between genders in the metabolic or BP data.

Figure 1 reveals that a healthy BMI, starting at age 20, decreases, giving rise to a progressively higher frequency of overweight and obesity (O-O). From the age of 40, O/O affects 75–80% of the study population (overweight was observed in about 40% of the participants and obesity in 30%).

Table 1. Anthropometric, metabolic, and blood pressure data.

Weight, kg Mean ± SD	BMI, kg/m^2 Mean ± SD	TC, mg/dL Mean ± SD	Glycemia, mg/dL Mean ± SD	SBP, mm Hg Mean ± SD	DBP, mm Hg Mean ± SD
All, N = 297,370					
72.64 ± 14.28	27.8 ± 4.76	192.5 ± 35.62	95.33 ± 43.81	118.4 ± 16.19	78.17 ± 18.53
Women, n = 161,264					
67.64 ± 13.1	27.99 ± 5.25	193.6 ± 36.2	94.84 ± 45.52	117.1 ± 17.22	77.06 ± 22.91
Men, n = 136,106					
78.56 ± 13.2	27.57 ± 4.05	191.2 ± 34.86	95.91 ± 41.68	119.9 ± 14.74	79.49 ± 11.19

SD, standard deviation; BMI, body mass index; TC, total cholesterol; SBP, systolic blood pressure; DBP, diastolic blood pressure. See text for details.

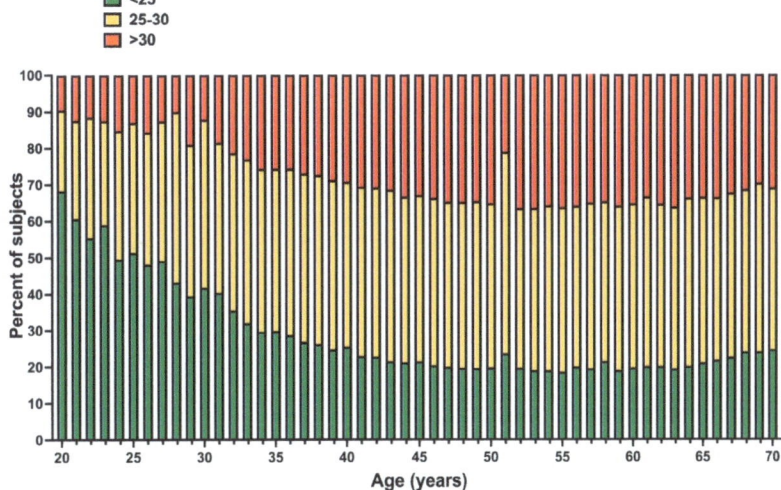

Figure 1. Percentage of normal body mass index (green), overweight (yellow), and obesity (red) by age. An apparent age-related decrease in the percentage of subjects having a normal BMI (<25) was found. An age-related increase in the percentage of subjects with overweight or obesity was also seen.

In Figure 2, the relationship between BMI and age is shown. A straight linear relation exists between both variables from 20 to 40–45 years (with high linear correlation coefficients; r = 0.98 and 0.95 in women and men, respectively), from which the line horizontalizes, and, when reaching 60 or more years, it curves downwards. Men are more overweight than women up to 35 years of age, but from that age to 40, the BMI is similar in both genders. From age 45 years and older, women have a greater body mass than men.

On the contrary, Figure 3 reveals that systolic blood pressure (SBP) rises directly and constantly through all the age stages, with the slope being more significant in women than men. As expected, women showed lower SBP levels until 50–55 years old; there is no difference between genders after that age. The slopes (0.6081 and 0.3525 for women and men, respectively) suggested a higher increase in SBP in women over time.

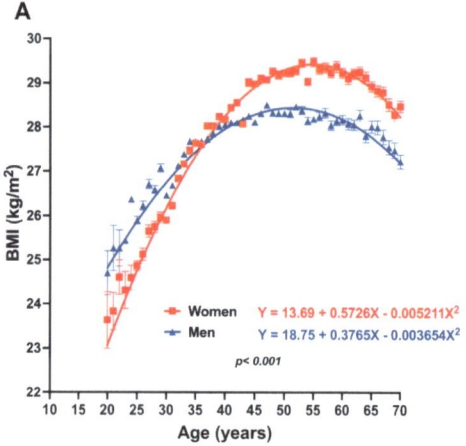

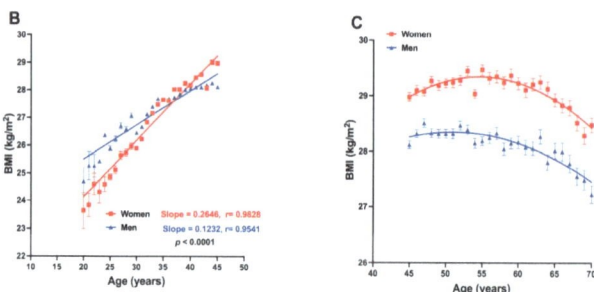

Figure 2. (**A**) Differential age-related BMI changes between women and men; a second-order behavior is appreciated. (**B**) A linear relation between age and BMI is found in the range of 20 to 45 years in both genders. (**C**) A plateau or decreased BMI was found as age advanced, from 45 to 70 years. Data are presented as mean ± SD.

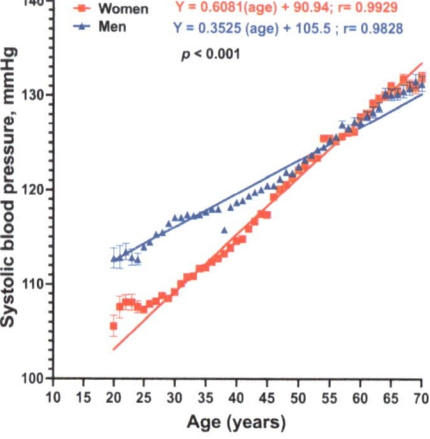

Figure 3. Mean and standard deviation are used to present data on age-related increases in systolic blood pressure.

Figure 4 shows how the concentration of TC changes across age groups. Only 10 to 15% of participants had hypercholesterolemia at younger ages; however, from age 26, the proportion of subjects with hypercholesterolemia (CT greater than 200 mg/dL) increased progressively until age 50, when half of the study population was hypercholesterolemic.

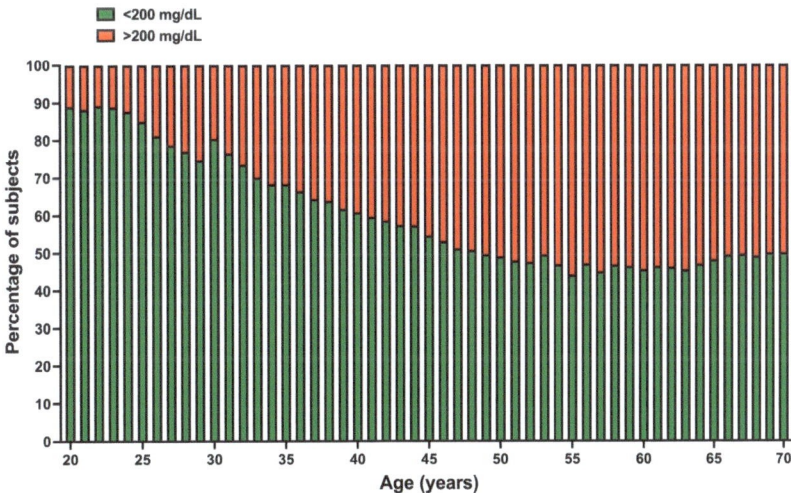

Figure 4. Percentage of normal cholesterol levels (green) and hypercholesterolemia (red) by age. An apparent age-related decrease in the percentage of subjects having normal cholesterol (<200) was found. An age-related increase in the percentage of subjects with hypercholesterolemia was also seen.

Figure 5 shows the same peculiarity between CT and age observed with the BMI. There is a positive and linear relationship between cholesterol and age up to 45 years, followed by a plateau, and, from 65 years, the correlation line is curved downwards. Women had higher values of CT than men, but the fall of this variable is more pronounced in men.

Interestingly, Figure 6 shows that glycemia is normal in 94% of youngsters at 20. From this age, the proportions of pre-diabetic dysglycemia and diabetes increase until a maximum at age 50, where the combination of both comprises 40% of the study's population. From 60 years of age and older, around 30% of subjects have blood glucose levels greater than 126 mg/dL.

Figure 7 reveals that, contrary to what happens with BMI and TC, the correlation between glycemia and age is straightly linear (with very high correlation coefficients) from youth to old age.

On the other hand, Figure 8 shows the proportions of awareness, treatment, and control of the hypertensive population. Of the total cohort universe, 27% of the participants were hypertensives. Less than half were aware of their diagnosis (46.5%). About one-third (36%) of those treated had controlled BP, but the overall proportion of controlled hypertensive subjects was only 8%.

The analysis of the relationship between BMI and SBP, glycemia, and TC is shown in Figure 9. A straight linear correlation between SBP and body mass index was found; however, the linear correlation was lost after a BMI of 28 kg/m^2 when the line curves back and down. The correlation coefficients for women and men are relatively high (0.80 and 0.62, respectively). A more complex relationship between BMI and serum glucose was found. Even though an initial direct correlation was evident up to a BMI of 28–29 kg/m^2, the correlation line also curves back and down later. In this case, the correlation coefficients are less striking (0.68 and 0.46 in women and men). On the other hand, there was a more consistent linear relationship between BMI and TC, with a correlation coefficient greater than 0.9 in both genders.

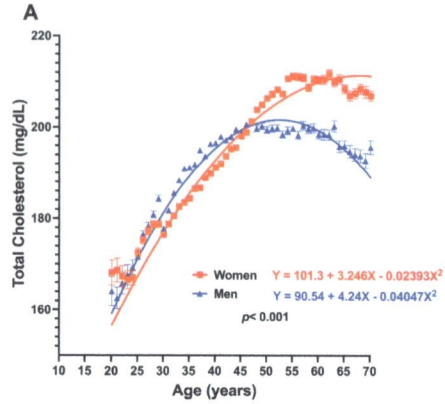

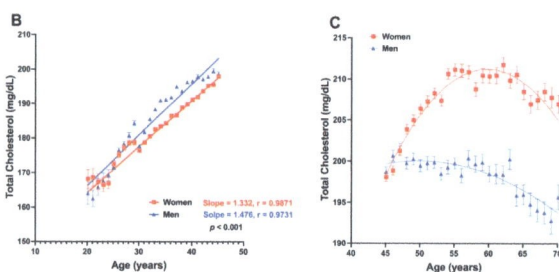

Figure 5. (**A**) Differential age-related cholesterol levels change between women and men; a second-order behavior is appreciated. (**B**) A linear relation between age and cholesterol was found in the range of 20 to 45 years in both genders. (**C**) A plateau or decreased cholesterol levels was found as age advanced, from 45 to 70 years. Data are presented as mean ± SD.

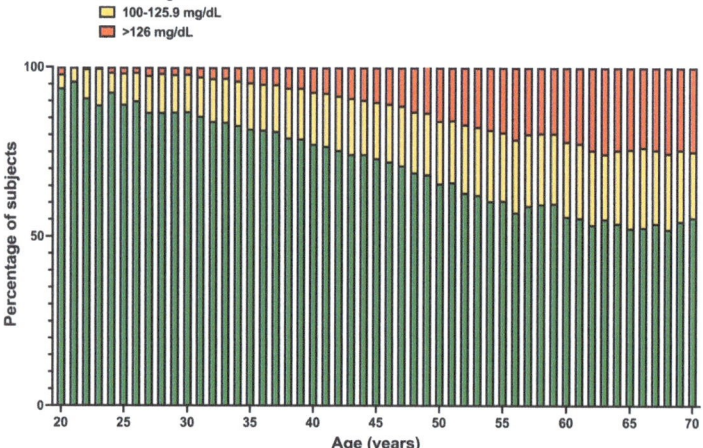

Figure 6. Percentage of normal glucose (green), hyperglycemia (yellow), and DM (red) glucose levels by age. An apparent age-related decrease in the percentage of subjects having normal glycemia (<100 mg/dL) was found. An age-related increase in the percentage of subjects with hyperglycemia and DM was also seen.

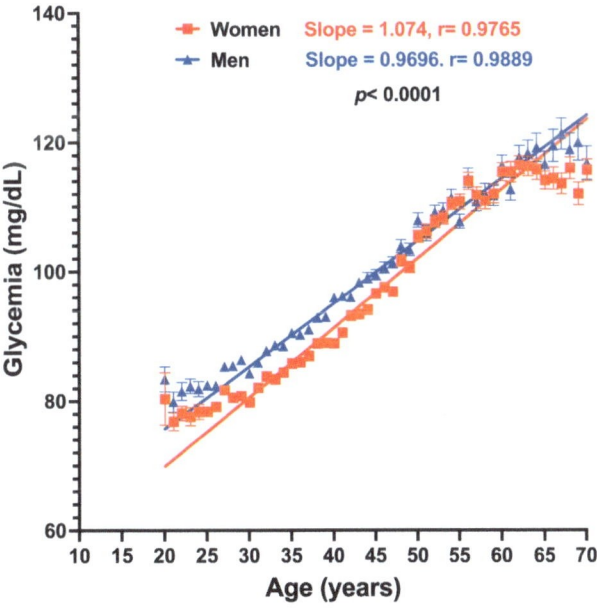

Figure 7. Differential age-related glycemia levels change between women and men; a linear behavior is appreciated in both genders (r ≥ 0.97). Data are presented as mean ± SD.

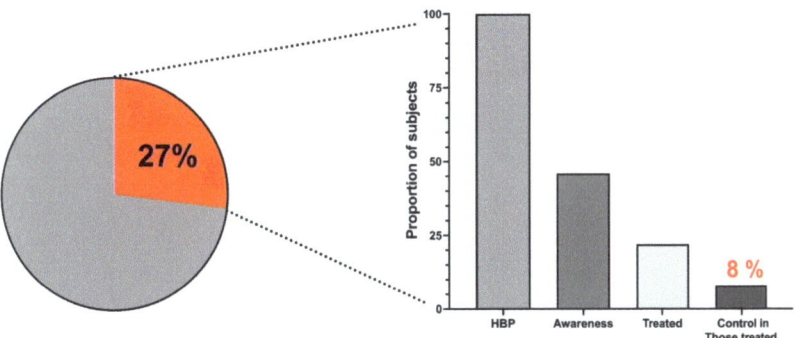

Figure 8. Of the entire cohort universe, 27% (the segment in red) had HBP. The rates of awareness, treatment, and hypertension control are displayed. This represents the "law of the halves" in the hypertensive study's population.

Due to these striking behaviors, we performed a multiple regression analysis. We used multiple regression analyses with the obtained variables to search for a model equation with the highest influence over the other variables. The following approaches were used: (1) the influence of BMI, age, and glycemia in the cholesterol levels; (2) the influence of BMI, cholesterol, and glycemia in SBP; and (3) the influence of age, cholesterol, and glycemia in BMI. The generated equations for both genders are described in Table 2.

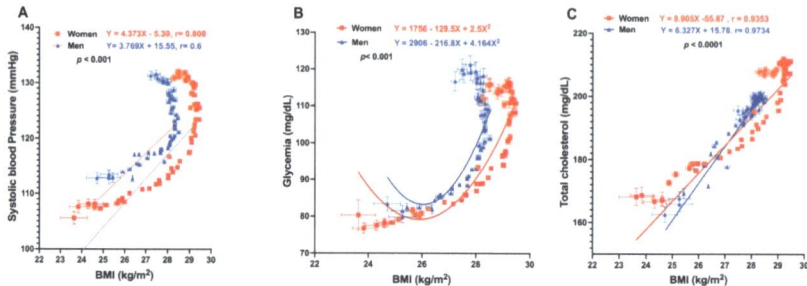

Figure 9. (**A**) shows a linear correlation between SBP and body mass up to a BMI of 28–29 kg/m², from which the linear correlation is lost, and the line curves back and down; this behavior is similar in both genders. (**B**) A more complex relationship between BMI and serum glucose is shown. Even though an initial direct correlation was evident up to a BMI of 28–29 kg/m², the correlation line also curves back and down later. In this case, the correlation coefficients are less striking. (**C**) Shows a more consistent linear relationship between TC and BMI, with a correlation coefficient greater than 0.9 in both genders.

Table 2. Multiple regression equations of total cholesterol, systolic blood pressure, and serum glucose vs. body mass index.

Gender	Risk Factor	Equation
Women	Total cholesterol, mg/dL	TC = 18.21 + 3.936 (BMI) − 0.1087 (age) + 0.7374 (glucose)
	Systolic blood pressure, mm Hg	SBP = 67.64 + 0.4703 (BMI) − 0.1544 (cholesterol) + 0.6989 (glucose)
	Body mass index, kg/m²	BMI = −0.4008 + 0.03528 (age) + 0.2141 (cholesterol) − 0.1543 (glucose)
Men	Total cholesterol, mg/dL	TC = −80.70 + 10.13 (BMI) + 0.2935 (age) + 0.2012 (glucose)
	Systolic blood pressure, mm Hg	SBP = 100.8 − 1.593 (BMI) + 0.1072 (cholesterol) + 0.4391 (glucose)
	Body mass index, kg/m²	BMI = 9.297 − 0.02189 (age) + 0.0912 (cholesterol) + 0.1612 (glucose)

4. Discussion

The results reported here highlight the importance of risk aggregation, which sums the individual components of a set of risks, signals their interrelation, and suggests that overweight/obesity (BMI) is the most relevant risk factor in this population.

Public health policies entail all the modern state's actions to attain some general health goals of social and medical interest applicable in the short, medium, and long range [27,28]. The solidity and transcendence of a public policy depend, on the one hand, on its scientific and epidemiological foundation and, on the other hand, on how it is presented to the community so that the majority of the social segments involved accept it well.

In Mexico, the O/O has reached epidemic proportions and is well documented by the national surveys called ENSANUTs [29–31]. In ENSANUT 2022, O/O was found in 75.2% of the surveyed adult population, in 37.3% of school children, and in 41.1% of teenagers [29,31]. This first epidemic surge supports the secondary waves of DM2 and coronary syndromes [32,33]. Therefore, a pending duty requiring urgent fulfillment is the task of reducing the incidence and prevalence of O/O against powerful economic and political interests and the prejudices and erroneous decisions in the way of life of a society influenced by medical misinformation, marketing propaganda, and unawareness.

In this sense, preventive measures must be based on the facts that link obesity to cardiovascular disease, mainly to ischemic heart disease, the most important epidemiological scourge of contemporary Mexico. Since dyslipidemia (particularly, atherogenic dyslipidemia), HBP, binomial insulin resistance/hyperinsulinism, DM, and inflammation, some of the most important agents promoting atherosclerosis, depend linearly on the grade of obesity, weight loss alone would have a favorable preventive effect. This means that a single preventative therapeutic intervention will have multiple beneficial consequences, improving the overall aggregate risk.

The data in the present analysis indicate that O/O and age are the more influential independent determinants of other analyzed risk factors. The data signal that BMI, glycemia, TC concentration, and BP levels increase from youth to middle-aged adult life (50 or 55 years).

The so-called "law of the halves" is a valuable tool to measure a community's medical and hygienic education level, the fortress of the political policies addressed to the prevention and clinical management of HBP, and the quality of medical care. In developed countries, the principle has evolved to a level called the "law of the thirds", which means that a third of hypertensive patients are unaware of having the disease, another third is treated and controlled, and another third is uncontrolled even if they are treated [28,34]. In the sample analyzed in this work, less than half of the HBP patients were aware, less than half of those who were aware were treated, and a little more than a third of those treated were controlled, with an overall meager 8% of controlled concerning all the universe of hypertensive patients. As the survey was designed, no type of treatment with antihypertensive and lipid-lowering drugs was inquired about. However, at the time data collection was performed, the most frequent treatment in the institutional family care clinics for hypertension was a relatively selective beta-blocker (metoprolol), an ACEI such as captopril or enalapril, sometimes a calcium channel blocker such as amlodipine, and more frequently an ARB such as losartan. Most general physicians used the lowest possible doses of monotherapy, and combined therapy was rarely prescribed.

On the other hand, the only statin prescribed at that time in the public sector was pravastatin, at a modest dose of 10 mg per day. When hypertriglyceridemia was detected, bezafibrate was used. In the private sector, general practitioners who see the bulk of the population with modest resources, drugs, and therapeutic approaches are like those employed in health institutions. In contrast, medical specialists generally serving the middle and upper middle class utilize a wide range of antihypertensives and lipid-lowering agents influenced by American and European guidelines.

The data shown herein agree with the common Mexican epidemiological picture, where combining multiple risk factors constitutes an important atherogenic and dysmetabolic network. All these aggregated CVRFs are biologically and epidemiologically intertwined and influence each other. The population modifies a healthy profile at relatively young ages and shows a growing incidence of O/O, hypercholesterolemia, rising BP, and dysglycemia. When multiple regression equations were employed, it was evident that BMI significantly influences BP and TC. The value of the β coefficient for BMI ($\beta 1$) in the TC regression equation for SBP was 3.963 in women and still more important in men. This coefficient signals to what extent the dependent variable increases when the independent variable becomes more prominent, while the other explanatory variables remain unchanged. BMI had less influence on SBP, which the regression equation showed $\beta 1$ coefficients of 0.4703 in women and 1.593 in men. The β coefficient for BMI was more significant in all equations than the other β. Of all parameters, TC showed a more consistent linear correlation with BMI, with a regression coefficient of 0.9734 in men and slightly less in women of 0.9353. At the highest part of the regression line in women, it curves backwards, signaling that with a maximum BMI, TC no longer rises. In contrast, in men, both variables have a constant positive correlation.

The linearity of most correlations is affected by a phenomenon we already described above. Comparing BMI and TC against age, the linearity is lost once the age of 45 is reached. It is known that TC and LDL-c (cholesterol of the low-density lipoproteins) reach an equilibrium up to 65 years, and then their concentration decreases in both genders [35]. This phenomenon has many possible single or associated explanations that need to be clarified, such as weight loss, concomitant inflammatory chronic diseases, senescent less cholesterol intestinal absorption, and administration of lipid-lowering drugs, among others [36]. In the same context, it has been proved that BMI is a less reliable index of corpulence in the elderly, because, at this stage of life, some changes occur, like less appetite, sarcopenia, osteopenia, loss of height, and concomitant debilitating diseases, among others [37].

On the other hand, we observed the rise of SBP through the age scale explained by senescent changes in elastic arteries, like extracellular matrix dystrophy, calcification, and the development of atherosclerotic plaques [38].

Interestingly, a bizarre curving is observed in both genders in the multiple regression lines of glycemia and BP. In contrast to the behavior of the TC data, the regression line curves backwards and downwards. A theoretical explanation could be that in some aged subjects, there is a loss of weight explained for a handful of reasons, such as sarcopenia, uncontrolled diabetes, better medical care, patient awareness, intercurrent debilitating diseases, and the like. It is known that losing weight improves insulin sensitivity and intra- and extra-renal compression, which are significant mechanisms in dysglycemia and hypertension [39,40].

However, linearity is imperfect in SBP and glycemia multiple regression lines. Still, the correlation coefficient is high in SBP in both women ($r = 0.808$) and men ($r = 0.625$) and is less remarkable, but it is significant in glycemia ($r = 0.68$ in women and 0.46 in men).

5. Conclusions

Obesity (BMI) and age are the more prominent CVRFs, influencing the expression of each other, whose magnitude is aggravated by aging and adiposity. Cholesterol is the most important atherogenic CVRF. The data presented here demonstrate that its serum value is directly related to BMI. From the point of view of public policies, preventive programs directed at lessening coronary atherosclerotic disease must focus primarily on O/O. To this day, considerable efforts are devoted to reducing atherogenic lipids with statins, arterial hypertension with various antihypertensive drugs, and dysglycemia with a set of antidiabetic medications. However, health authorities and individual physicians pay less attention to the primal, basic condition of O/O. Therefore, it is essential to universalize in health institutions, in the therapeutic and preventive practices of health providers, and in the social imagination the importance of a healthy diet and the frequent practice of physical exercise, starting from childhood, to prevent the surge of the entire cluster of diseases and cardiometabolic syndromes, which are nowadays the leading public health threats. Additionally, the dietary and exercise approach reduces, primarily, cardiometabolic and CV risks and improves patients' prognosis and quality of life in secondary prevention. Altogether, the therapeutic modifications of lifestyle, with pharmacological and bariatric treatments and procedures, can benefit society and individual patients [13,35,41]. We need, in addition, a national crusade, powerful and persistent, against obesity to influence the social imagination positively. Only in this way will we subdue or at least diminish the scourge of secondary epidemics of diabetes and ASCVD.

Despite its social lags, Mexico, now considered a middle-income country, is not far from achieving the status of an industrialized nation. But from now on, we suffer from what we have called the "Mexican paradox", meaning that it is a slightly prosperous nation but with an impoverished population affected by the burden of disease typical of developed countries [42]. If this condition prevails and is accentuated with the subsequent expected economic growth, cardiovascular and cardiometabolic epidemics can significantly compromise the well-being of the nation and its public health, making the achieved progress useless. To this day, there are epidemiological differences between Mexico and the developed nations of Europe and North America [43,44]. While in most European nations, CV and coronary incidence and mortality have decreased, in Mexico, they have increased [8]. The median, age-standardized prevalence of HBP varies from 23.8% to 15.7% in middle- and high-income countries. Hypercholesterolemia affects more than 50% of many European nations. Obesity and overweight prevalence have an average value of 53%, while DM affects about 10% of the population.

On the other hand, comparing data with the USA, when the ACC/AHAS cut-off values are used, the rates of HBP are comparable. Obesity and overweight in both countries affect more than four-fifths of the adult populations, and DM is still a little bit higher in Mexico. As can be seen, the epidemiological situation in Mexico is worse. As it happens in Europe, more vascular events occur in the elderly population after many years of negligent diagnosis and insufficient treatment of CV risk factors [43,45–47].

As a perspective, trials exploring the TG/HDL ratio and LDL/HDL ratio to determine their role in cardiovascular risks in Mexicans are initiated.

This study has several limitations, such as the inability to measure triglycerides and HDL concentrations and the lack of a record of specific treatments. We believe that the data's relevance is that, whatever the treatment, only half of the hypertensive subjects are aware of their disease and only half of these are under treatment (any antihypertensives). Only 8% of all subjects with hypertension are under control.

Data showed low treatment compliance and/or efficacy; we do not know who is responsible (patient? physician? economy? medication?). More work is necessary to understand this phenomenon.

Author Contributions: All authors participated in the study's conception and experimental design. E.M., A.M., N.N., E.P.-R., M.O.-F, G.P.-I., L.M., G.R. (Coalición por el Corazón de México) participated in patient and data recruitment and analysis. A.M., E.M., N.N. and G.C. wrote the first draft. All authors revised and edited the manuscript. All authors have read and agreed to the published version of the manuscript.

Funding: This work was supported by Instituto Politécnico Nacional gift #SIP20220789 to G.C. and # SIP20220812 to N.N., and an unrestricted gift from Novartis for publication expenses.

Institutional Review Board Statement: This study was conducted according to the guidelines of the Declaration of Helsinki and approved by the Institutional Ethics Committees (ISSSTE Ethics committee) of participating institutions 250.2022 approved on 1 May 2022.

Informed Consent Statement: Informed consent was obtained from all subjects involved in the study.

Data Availability Statement: Data sharing is available under request.

Acknowledgments: We thank all the societies, institutions, and participants in the Coalición por el Corazón de México for their uninterested participation and advice, Agustin Lara, and Pfizer, for helping in the obtaining of the data, and Novartis Co. for the support.

Conflicts of Interest: G.C. is a stockholder of Epirium, and G.R. is an employee of Novartis Co.; the rest of the authors declare no conflicts of interest.

References

1. Leong, D.P.; Joseph, P.G.; McKee, M.; Anand, S.S.; Teo, K.K.; Schwalm, J.-D.; Yusuf, S. Reducing the global burden of cardiovascular disease, part 2. Prevention and treatment of cardiovascular disease. *Circ. Res.* **2017**, *121*, 695–710. [CrossRef] [PubMed]
2. Rippe, J.M. Lifestyle strategies for risk factor reduction, prevention, and treatment of cardiovascular disease. *Am. J. Lifestyle Med.* **2019**, *13*, 204–212. [CrossRef] [PubMed]
3. Reiner, Ž.; Laufs, U.; Cosentino, F.; Landmesser, U. The year in cardiology 2018: Prevention. *Eur. Heart J.* **2019**, *40*, 336–344. [CrossRef] [PubMed]
4. INEGI. Estadísticas de Defunciones Registradas (EDR) 2022 (Preliminar). Available online: https://www.inegi.org.mx/contenidos/saladeprensa/boletines/2023/EDR/EDR2022.pdf (accessed on 14 November 2023).
5. Aguilar-Salinas, C.A.; Gómez-Pérez, F.J.; Rull, J.; Villalpando, S.; Barquera, S.; Rojas, R. Prevalence of dyslipidemias in the Mexican National Health and Nutrition Survey 2006. *Salud Pública México* **2010**, *52* (Suppl. S1), 44–53. [CrossRef]
6. Campos-Nonato, I.; Oviedo-Solís, C.; Vargas-Meza, J.; Ramírez-Villalobos, D.; Medina-García, C.; Gómez Álvarez, E.; Hernández-Barrera, L.; Barquera, S. Prevalence, treatment, and control of hypertension in Mexican adults: Results of the Ensanut 2022. *Salud Pública México* **2023**, *65* (Suppl. S1), S169–S180. [CrossRef]
7. Basto-Abreu, A.; López-Olmedo, N.; Rojas-Martínez, R.; Aguilar-Salinas, C.A.; Moreno-Banda, G.L.; Carnalla, M.; Rivera, J.A.; Romero-Martinez, M.; Barquera, S.; Barrientos-Gutiérrez, T. Prevalencia de prediabetes y diabetes en México: Ensanut 2022. *Salud Pública México* **2023**, *65*, s163–s168. [CrossRef] [PubMed]

8. Arroyo-Quiroz, C.; Barrientos-Gutierrez, T.; O'Flaherty, M.; Guzman-Castillo, M.; Palacio-Mejia, L.; Osorio-Saldarriaga, E.; Rodriguez-Rodriguez, A.Y. Coronary heart disease mortality is decreasing in Argentina, and Colombia, but keeps increasing in Mexico: A time trend study. *BMC Public Health* **2020**, *20*, 162. [CrossRef] [PubMed]
9. Fanghänel-Salmón, G.; Gutiérrez-Salmeán, G.; Samaniego, V.; Meaney, A.; Sánchez-Reyes, L.; Navarrete, U.; Alcocer, L.; Olivares-Corichi, I.; Najera, N.; Ceballos, G.; et al. Obesity phenotypes in urban middle-class cohorts; the PRIT-Lindavista merging evidence in Mexico: The OPUS PRIME study. *Nutr. Hosp.* **2015**, *32*, 182–188. [CrossRef]
10. Meaney, A.; Ceballos-Reyes, G.; Gutierrez-Salmean, G.; Samaniego-Méndez, V.; Vela-Huerta, A.; Alcocer, L.; Zárate-Chavarría, E.; Mendoza-Castelán, E.; Olivares-Corichi, I.; García-Sánchez, R.; et al. Cardiovascular risk factors in a Mexican middle-class urban population. The Lindavista Study. Baseline Data. *Arch. Cardiol. Mex.* **2013**, *83*, 249–256. [CrossRef] [PubMed]
11. Meaney, E.; Lara-Esqueda, A.; Ceballos-Reyes, G.M.; Asbun, J.; Vela, A.; Martínez-Marroquín, Y.; López, V.; Meaney, A.; de la Cabada-Tamez, E.; Velázquez-Monroy, O.; et al. Cardiovascular risk factors in the urban Mexican population: The Frimex study. *Public Health* **2007**, *121*, 378–384. [CrossRef]
12. Bray, G.A.; Kim, K.K.; Wilding, J.P.H. World Obesity Federation Obesity: A chronic relapsing progressive disease process. A position statement of the World Obesity Federation. *Obes. Rev.* **2017**, *18*, 715–723. [CrossRef] [PubMed]
13. Velázquez Moreno, H.; Gaxiola Cáceres, S.; Alcocer Chauvet, A.; González Coronado, V.J.; Zárate Chavarría, E.; Meaney, E. Obesidad y síndrome metabólico. In *Medicina Cardiovascular*; Navarro Robles, J., Ed.; Elsevier/Asociación Nacional de Cardiólogos de México: Ciudad de México, México, 2012; pp. 124–141.
14. WHO Expert Committee. *Physical Status: The Use and Interpretation of Anthropometry*; WHO Technical Report Series No. 854; WHO: Geneva, Switzerland, 1995.
15. Perone, F.; Pingitore, A.S.; Conte, E.; Halasz, G.; Ambrosetti, M.; Peruzzi, M.; Cavarretta, E. Obesity and cardiovascular risk: Systematic intervention is the key for prevention. *Healthcare* **2023**, *11*, 902. [CrossRef] [PubMed]
16. Akil, L.; Ahmad, H.A. Relationships between obesity and cardiovascular diseases in four southern states and Colorado. *J. Health Care Poor Underserved.* **2011**, *22* (Suppl. S4), 61–72. [CrossRef] [PubMed]
17. Powell-Wiley, T.M.; Poirier, P.; Burke, L.E.; Després, J.-P.; Gordon-Larsen, P.; Lavie, C.J.; Lear, S.A.; Ndumele, C.E.; Neeland, I.J.; Sanders, P.; et al. Obesity and cardiovascular disease: A Scientific Statement From the American Heart Association. *Circulation* **2021**, *143*, e984–e1010. [CrossRef]
18. Lopez-Jimenez, F.; Almahmeed, W.; Bays, H.; Cuevas, A.; Di Angelantonio, E.; le Roux, C.W.; Sattar, N.; Sun, M.C.; Wittert, G.; Pinto, F.J.; et al. Obesity and cardiovascular disease: Mechanistic insights and management strategies. A joint position paper by the World Heart Federation and World Obesity Federation. *Eur. J. Prev. Cardiol.* **2022**, *29*, 2218–2237. [CrossRef] [PubMed]
19. International Conference on Harmonisation. Guidelines on Good Clinical Practice. *Int. Dig. Health Legis.* **1997**, *48*, 231–234. [CrossRef]
20. World Medical Association. Declaration of Helsinki: Ethical principles for medical research involving human subjects. *JAMA* **2013**, *310*, 2191–2194. [CrossRef] [PubMed]
21. Diario de la Federación. Available online: http://www.salud.gob.mx/cnts/pdfs/LEY_GENERAL_DE_SALUD.pdf (accessed on 30 October 2023).
22. Pickering, T.G.; Hall, J.E.; Appel, L.J.; Falkner, B.E.; Graves, J.; Hill, M.N.; Jones, D.W.; Kurtz, T.; Sheps, S.G.; Roccella, E.J. Recommendations for blood pressure measurement in humans and experimental animals: Part 1: Blood pressure measurement in humans: A statement for professionals from the Subcommittee of Professional and Public Education of the American Heart Association Council on High Blood Pressure Research. *Circulation* **2005**, *111*, 697–716. [CrossRef] [PubMed]
23. Proyecto de Norma Oficial Mexicana PROY-NOM030-SSA2-2017, Para la Prevención, Detección, Diagnóstico, Tratamiento y Control de la Hipertensión Arterial Sistémica. Diario Oficial de la Federación 19/04/2017. Available online: https://dof.gob.mx/nota_detalle.php?codigo=5480159&fecha=19/04/2017#gsc.tab=0 (accessed on 30 October 2023).
24. Hadaye, R.; Kale, V.; Manapurath, R.M. Strategic implications of changing rule of halves in hypertension: A cross-sectional observational study. *J. Fam. Med. Prim. Care* **2019**, *8*, 1049–1053. [CrossRef]
25. ElSayed, N.A.; Aleppo, G.; Aroda, V.R.; Bannuru, R.P.; Brown, F.M.; Bruemmer, D.; Collins, B.S.; Gaglia, J.L.; Hilliard, M.E.; Isaacs, D.; et al. Classification and diagnosis of diabetes: Standards of care in Diabetes—2023. *Diabetes Care* **2023**, *46* (Suppl. S1), S19–S40. [CrossRef] [PubMed]
26. Expert Panel on Detection, Evaluation, and Treatment of High Blood Cholesterol in Adults. Executive summary of the third report of the National Cholesterol Education Program (NCEP) expert panel on detection, evaluation, and treatment of high blood cholesterol in adults (Adult Treatment Panel III). *JAMA* **2001**, *285*, 2486–2497. [CrossRef] [PubMed]
27. CDC. Office of Policy, Performance, and Evaluation. Definition of Policy. Available online: https://www.cdc.gov/policy/paeo/process/definition.html (accessed on 19 November 2023).
28. Milio, N. Glossary: Healthy public policy. *J. Epidemiol. Community Health* **2001**, *55*, 622–623. [CrossRef]
29. Shamah-Levy, T.; Villalpando-Hernández, S.; Rivera-Dommarco, J.A. Resultados de Nutrición de la ENSANUT 2006. Cuernavaca, México: Instituto Nacional de Salud Pública, 2007. Available online: https://ensanut.insp.mx/encuestas/ensanut2006/doctos/informes/resultados_ensanut2006.pdf. (accessed on 21 November 2023).

30. Gutiérrez, J.P.; Rivera-Dommarco, J.; Shamah-Levy, T.; Villalpando-Hernández, S.; Franco, A.; Cuevas-Nasu, L.; Romero-Martínez, M. Encuesta Na-Cional de Salud y Nutrición 2012. Resultados Nacionales. Instituto Nacional de Salud Pública (MX): Cuernavaca, México, 2012. Available online: https://ensanut.insp.mx/encuestas/ensanut2012/doctos/informes/ENSANUT2012ResultadosNacionales.pdf (accessed on 21 November 2023).
31. Campos-Nonato, I.; Galván-Valencia, O.; Hernández-Barrera, L.; Oviedo-Solís, C.; Barquera, S. Prevalence of obesity and associated risk factors in Mexican adults: Results of the Ensanut 2022. *Salud Pública México* **2023**, *65* (Suppl. S1), S238–S247. [CrossRef]
32. Al-Goblan, A.S.; Al-Alfi, M.A.; Khan, M.Z. Mechanism linking diabetes mellitus and obesity. *Diabetes Metab. Syndr. Obes.* **2014**, *7*, 587–591. [CrossRef] [PubMed]
33. Piché, M.E.; Poirier, P.; Lemieux, I.; Després, J.P. Overview of epidemiology and contribution of obesity and body fat distribution to cardiovascular disease: An update. *Prog. Cardiovasc. Dis.* **2018**, *61*, 103–113. [CrossRef] [PubMed]
34. Lindblad, U.; Ek, J.; Eckner, J.; Larsson, C.A.; Shan, G.; Råstam, L. Prevalence, awareness, treatment, and control of hypertension: Rule of thirds in the Skaraborg project. *Scand. J. Prim. Health Care* **2012**, *30*, 88–94. [CrossRef]
35. Beckett, N.; Nunes, M.; Bulpitt, C. Is it advantageous to lower cholesterol in the elderly hypertensive? *Cardiovasc. Drugs Ther.* **2000**, *14*, 397–405. [CrossRef] [PubMed]
36. Ferrara, A.; Barrett-Connor, E.; Shan, J. Total, LDL, and HDL Cholesterol decrease with age in older men and women. The Rancho Bernardo Study 1984–1994. *Circulation* **1997**, *96*, 37–43. [CrossRef] [PubMed]
37. Estrella-Castillo, D.F.; Gómez-de-Regil, L. Comparison of body mass index range criteria and their association with cognition, functioning and depression: A cross-sectional study in Mexican older adults. *BMC Geriatr.* **2019**, *19*, 339. [CrossRef]
38. Meaney, E.; Soltero, E.; Samaniego, V.; Alva, F.; Moguel, R.; Vela, A.; Gonzalez, V. Vascular dynamics in isolated systolic arterial hypertension. *Clin. Cardiol.* **1995**, *18*, 721–725. [CrossRef]
39. Clamp, L.D.; Hume, D.J.; Lambert, E.V.; Kroff, J. Enhanced insulin sensitivity in successful, long-term weight loss maintainers compared with matched controls with no weight loss history. *Nutr. Diabetes* **2017**, *7*, e282. [CrossRef] [PubMed]
40. Hall, J.E.; Brands, M.W.; Henegar, J.R. Mechanisms of hypertension and kidney disease in obesity. *Ann. N. Y. Acad. Sci.* **1999**, *892*, 91–107. [CrossRef]
41. Dietz, W.H.; Baur, L.A.; Hall, K.; Puhl, R.M.; Taveras, E.M.; Uauy, R. Management of obesity: Improvement of health-care training and systems for prevention and care. *Lancet* **2015**, *385*, 2521–2533. [CrossRef]
42. Meaney, E.; Munguía, L.; Nájera, N.; Ceballos, G. Mexican epidemiological paradox: A developing country with a burden of "richness" diseases. In *An Update. Encyclopedia of Environmental Health*, 2nd ed.; Elsevier: Amsterdam, The Netherlands, 2011; pp. 738–748. [CrossRef]
43. He, J.; Zhu, Z.; Bundy, J.D.; Dorans, K.S.; Chen, J.; Hamm, L.L. Trends in cardiovascular risk factors in US adults by race and ethnicity and socioeconomic status, 1999–2018. *JAMA* **2021**, *326*, 1286–1298. [CrossRef] [PubMed]
44. Amini, M.; Zayeri, F.; Salehi, M. Trend analysis of cardiovascular disease mortality, incidence, and mortality-to-incidence ratio: Results from global burden of disease study 2017. *BMC Public Health* **2021**, *21*, 401. [CrossRef] [PubMed]
45. European Society of Cardiology: Cardiovascular Disease Statistics 2019. Available online: https://iris.unibocconi.it/retrieve/handle/11565/4023471/115818/Torbica%20EHJ%202019.pdf (accessed on 1 April 2024).
46. Anonymous. Overweight and Obesity—BMI Statistics. Available online: https://ec.europa.eu/eurostat/statistics (accessed on 1 April 2024).
47. Piechocki, M.; Przewłocki, T.; Pieniążek, P.; Trystuła, M.; Podolec, J.; Kabłak-Ziembicka, A. A non-coronary, peripheral arterial atherosclerotic disease (carotid, renal, lower limb) in elderly patients—A review: Part I—Epidemiology, risk factors, and atherosclerosis-related diversities in elderly patients. *J. Clin. Med.* **2024**, *13*, 1471. [CrossRef] [PubMed]

Disclaimer/Publisher's Note: The statements, opinions and data contained in all publications are solely those of the individual author(s) and contributor(s) and not of MDPI and/or the editor(s). MDPI and/or the editor(s) disclaim responsibility for any injury to people or property resulting from any ideas, methods, instructions or products referred to in the content.

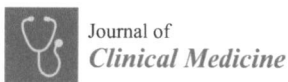

Article

Erectile Dysfunction as an Obesity-Related Condition in Elderly Men with Coronary Artery Disease

Małgorzata Biernikiewicz [1], Małgorzata Sobieszczańska [2], Ewa Szuster [3], Anna Pawlikowska-Gorzelańczyk [4], Anna Janocha [5], Krystyna Rożek-Piechura [6], Agnieszka Rusiecka [7], Jana Gebala [1], Paulina Okrzymowska [6] and Dariusz Kałka [1,6,*]

1 Men's Health Centre in Wroclaw, 53-151 Wroclaw, Poland
2 Clinical Department of Geriatrics, Wroclaw Medical University, 50-369 Wroclaw, Poland
3 Obstetrics and Gynecology Department, Wroclaw Medical University, 50-556 Wroclaw, Poland
4 Cardiosexology Students Club, Wroclaw Medical University, 50-368 Wroclaw, Poland
5 Faculty of Medicine, Wrocław University of Science and Technology, 50-370 Wroclaw, Poland
6 Faculty of Physiotherapy, Wroclaw University of Health and Sport Sciences, 51-612 Wroclaw, Poland
7 Statistical Analysis Centre, Wroclaw Medical University, 50-367 Wroclaw, Poland
* Correspondence: dariusz.kalka@gmail.com

Citation: Biernikiewicz, M.; Sobieszczańska, M.; Szuster, E.; Pawlikowska-Gorzelańczyk, A.; Janocha, A.; Rożek-Piechura, K.; Rusiecka, A.; Gebala, J.; Okrzymowska, P.; Kałka, D. Erectile Dysfunction as an Obesity-Related Condition in Elderly Men with Coronary Artery Disease. *J. Clin. Med.* 2024, 13, 2087. https://doi.org/10.3390/jcm13072087

Academic Editors: Justyna Wyszyńska and Piotr Matłosz

Received: 29 February 2024
Revised: 28 March 2024
Accepted: 2 April 2024
Published: 3 April 2024

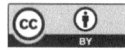

Copyright: © 2024 by the authors. Licensee MDPI, Basel, Switzerland. This article is an open access article distributed under the terms and conditions of the Creative Commons Attribution (CC BY) license (https://creativecommons.org/licenses/by/4.0/).

Abstract: Background: This cross-sectional study aimed to investigate the prevalence of erectile dysfunction (ED) in elderly men with overweight or obesity and coronary artery disease. **Methods**: Patients recruited in cardiac rehabilitation centers post-myocardial infarction provided demographic and anthropomorphic data. ED was assessed using the abbreviated International Index of Erectile Function 5 (IIEF-5) Questionnaire. **Results**: The study included 661 men with a mean age of 67.3 ± 5.57 years, a mean BMI of 27.9 ± 3.6 m/kg^2, and a mean waist circumference of 98.9 ± 10.23 cm. Over 90% of men experienced ED, with similar proportions across BMI categories. The development of ED in men with a waist circumference of ≥ 100 cm had 3.74 times higher odds (OR 3.74; 95% CI: 1.0–13.7; $p = 0.04$) than in men with a waist circumference of <100 cm. Men with obesity and moderate-to-severe and severe ED were older compared to those without these disorders (67.1 ± 5.29 vs. 65.3 ± 4.35; $p = 0.23$). **Conclusions**: The prevalence of ED in men with coronary artery disease surpasses 90%. An increased body weight raises the risk of ED, with waist circumference proving to be a more reliable predictor of this risk compared to BMI. Physicians are encouraged to screen elderly patients with cardiovascular disease for ED and address obesity to enhance overall health.

Keywords: obesity; overweight; erectile dysfunction; sexual dysfunction; prevalence; testosterone; androgens

1. Introduction

Obesity has been deemed an epidemic due to the rapid increase in the percentage of people with abnormally increased body weight. The rise in obesity began in the US between 1976 and 1980 and subsequently spread across Westernized countries [1,2]. Obesity is a complex condition with a significant impact on mortality and morbidity. The Global Burden of Disease Study reported that 4.7 million deaths were directly linked to obesity in 2017 [3], leading to increased societal costs and a decreased health-related quality of life. The burden of obesity results in adverse consequences not only on health. It also contributes to psychological problems, depression, stigmatization, disability, and productivity loss at work [4–6].

Body mass index (BMI) has been widely used for screening increased body weight. This index is a numerical value calculated from a person's weight, in kilograms, and height, in meters. BMI values over 25 kg/m^2 indicate that an individual's weight is higher than what is considered healthy for his/her height. This condition raises the risk of various health issues associated with excess body weight [2,7]. Obesity and being overweight, similarly to other chronic diseases, are considered lifestyle diseases. Furthermore, obesity is a widely recognized independent predictor of cardiovascular disease, which is strongly related to organic erectile dysfunction (ED) [8,9]. Obesity and ED also share common risk factors such as diabetes, hypertension, physical inactivity, smoking, dyslipidemia, and poor diet [8,9]. Data from the literature confirms that men with abnormally increased body weight complain about health issues associated with their sexual health more often. The meta-analysis conducted by Pizzol et al. [10] investigated the link between BMI, waist circumference, and ED. Based on 45 articles involving 42,489 men, the chance of experiencing ED was significantly higher in overweight men (odds ratio [OR] 1.31; 95% confidence interval [CI]: 1.13–1.51) and even higher in men with obesity (OR 1.60; 95% CI: 1.29–1.98). The occurrence of ED was also linked to a higher BMI (mean difference [MD] 0.77; 95% CI: 0.57–0.97 kg/m^2) and a larger waist circumference (MD 5.25; 95% CI: 1.3–9.21) [10]. In another meta-analysis, Li et al. [11] studied how losing weight affects erectile function in men who are overweight or obese. The analysis of 5 studies involving 619 participants revealed a significant weight loss in men undergoing the weight loss intervention, compared to the control group (MD -18.07 kg; $p < 0.01$). A significant BMI difference of -9.6 kg/m^2 ($p < 0.01$) was also reported. Moreover, the improvement in the International Index of Erectile Function (IIEF) was noteworthy at 1.99 ($p < 0.01$), suggesting that weight loss may serve as adjunctive therapy for ED in men who are overweight or obese [11].

Clinical data linking obesity and ED are evident in the biochemical pathways, where testosterone plays a crucial role in mediating this relationship. The definition of hypogonadism in men pertains to testicular failure associated with androgen deficiency in the context of the physiology of the hypothalamus–pituitary–testis axis, which changes across various stages of a man's life [12,13]. The analysis of data from the European Male Aging Study showed that concentrations of testosterone drop progressively by 0.4% for total testosterone and by 1.3% for free testosterone per year. Furthermore, a decrease in free testosterone level was significantly higher in men with obesity (by 5.09 nmol/L; $p < 0.001$), in comparison to normal-weight men [14]. The decreased testosterone levels during aging impact lipid metabolism in cells. Free fatty acids, either released into the bloodstream or obtained from lipoproteins, can be utilized for energy or stored as triglycerides within cells. When testosterone levels are insufficient, there is a reduction in lipolysis, an increase in lipid synthesis, heightened lipid uptake, and enhanced adipocyte differentiation. Additionally, lipids that would typically be broken down during the β-oxidation process are more likely to be stored as triglycerides than utilized for energy. Consequently, hypogonadal men experience a decrease in lean body mass and an increase in fat mass, particularly in the abdominal or central region [15]. Moreover, adipocytes exhibit a high expression of aromatase, an enzyme responsible for converting testosterone to estradiol. This enzymatic process leads to a decrease in circulating androgens. Simultaneously, estrogens, produced as a result of this process, function as part of a negative feedback mechanism on the hypothalamic–pituitary axis. This action suppresses gonadotropin-releasing hormones and, subsequently, luteinizing hormones, ultimately contributing to a decline in gonadal testosterone release [16]. The escalation of body weight fuels a vicious cycle by directly diminishing testosterone levels, thus reinforcing the development of obesity. The interplay of dependencies between the impact of aging on testosterone levels, the development of obesity, and the consequent negative effects on health is illustrated in Figure 1.

While the connection between obesity and ED is evident clinically and pathophysiologically, there are gaps in the current knowledge regarding real-world data on the strength of the relationship between body weight and the occurrence of ED. To fill this gap, we conducted a cross-sectional study to examine the prevalence of ED in elderly men who are overweight or obese and have comorbid coronary artery disease, considering accompanying modifiable risk factors. The evidence regarding the prevalence of ED in men who are obese or overweight is limited. The novelty of this study lies in providing robust data on the prevalence of ED among elderly men with cardiac conditions and elevated body weight.

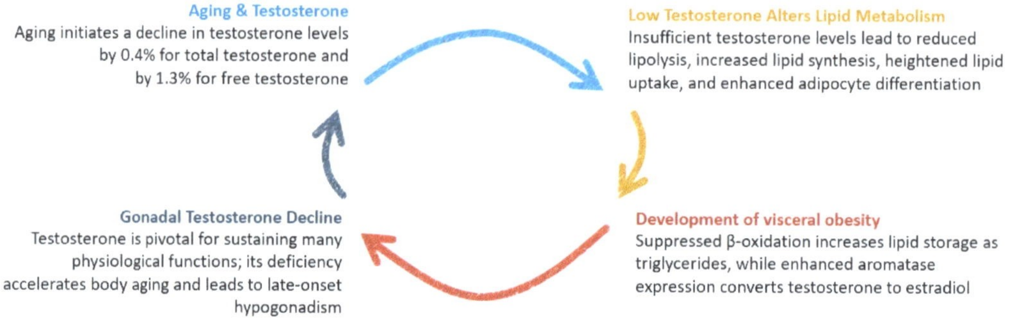

Aging & Testosterone
Aging initiates a decline in testosterone levels by 0.4% for total testosterone and by 1.3% for free testosterone

Low Testosterone Alters Lipid Metabolism
Insufficient testosterone levels lead to reduced lipolysis, increased lipid synthesis, heightened lipid uptake, and enhanced adipocyte differentiation

Gonadal Testosterone Decline
Testosterone is pivotal for sustaining many physiological functions; its deficiency accelerates body aging and leads to late-onset hypogonadism

Development of visceral obesity
Suppressed β-oxidation increases lipid storage as triglycerides, while enhanced aromatase expression converts testosterone to estradiol

Figure 1. Domino effect of testosterone decline.

2. Materials and Methods

Patients were recruited from cardiac rehabilitation centers while undergoing rehabilitation following an event of myocardial infarction. All were diagnosed with coronary artery disease. Demographic data and details regarding modifiable risk factors were gathered through questionnaires. Clinical data were obtained from medical records. The intensity of physical activity was assessed using a form modeled on the Framingham questionnaire, following the instructions of the original questionnaire [17]. A standard of 1000 kcal per week was established as the minimum intensity for leisure-time physical activity, aligning with efforts to prevent cardiovascular diseases as a primary intervention [18]. To assess the occurrence of ED, we utilized an abbreviated International Index of Erectile Function 5 (IIEF-5) Questionnaire [19]. This questionnaire consists of five questions, each scored from 0 to 5. ED was diagnosed when the overall score was 21 or lower.

We included men diagnosed with coronary artery disease who were 60 years old or above, despite the common use of a 65 year threshold and above to define the elderly population. The age of 65 is based on the traditional retirement age in many countries; however, the United Nations consider adults between the ages of 20 and 60 years to be fully productive [20]. Furthermore, individuals with chronic diseases, particularly cardiovascular disease, may be considered elderly at an earlier age of 60 years.

Additional inclusion criteria required participants to have a recorded BMI value and to complete the IIEF-5 questionnaire. Exclusion criteria included previous surgery for prostatic hyperplasia or prostate cancer, repair of the abdominal aorta or iliac arteries, treatment for any vascular event in the central nervous system, injuries to the spine or pelvis, psychiatric disorders, hormonal disorders other than testosterone deficiency, and undergoing dialysis. None of the patients were undergoing a weight reduction intervention.

All patients provided written informed consent to participate in the study. The study received approval from the local Bioethics Committee at Wroclaw Medical University. It was conducted within the framework of the PREVANDRO project, serving as an introduction to targeted cardiosexology education. Initiated in 2011, the project is ongoing, consistently reporting outcomes on ED in cardiac patients.

Data were statistically analyzed using Statistica software version 13.3 (StatSoft, Tulsa, OK, USA) and were presented as means ± standard deviation (SD) for continuous variables, and numbers (%) for categorical variables. The distribution of values was assessed using the Shapiro–Wilk test. Depending on the group characteristics and the number of groups selected for a single comparison, we employed the Mann–Whitney U test, Chi-square test, or the Kruskal–Wallis test with the post hoc median test. Relationships were examined using Spearman's rank correlation coefficient. The OR and 95% CI were calculated to compare the risks of ED. Statistical significance was interpreted at $p < 0.05$.

3. Results

3.1. Characteristics of the Study Group

The study included 661 men with a mean age of 67.3 ± 5.57 years, a mean BMI of 27.9 ± 3.6 m/kg², and a mean waist circumference of 98.9 ± 10.23 cm. None of the patients had a BMI below 18.5, so, to facilitate comparison, they were stratified into three BMI groups, as follows: men with normal weight or with weight within a normal range (*n* = 143; 21.6%), men who were overweight (*n* = 344; 52.0%), and men with obesity (*n* = 174; 26.3%). Regarding the occurrence of risk factors and comorbidities, the groups stratified by BMI category did not significantly differ in terms of age, education, severity of ED, dyslipidemia, smoking, and leading a sedentary lifestyle. However, hypertension and type 2 diabetes were more frequent in men with an increased BMI. All patients were on pharmacotherapy, with 95.2% taking statins, 93.2% taking beta-blockers, 81.6% acetylsalicylic acid, 72.2% taking angiotensin-converting-enzyme inhibitors, 42.9% clopidogrel, 41.8% diuretics, 20.7% calcium channel blockers, 10.4% angiotensin receptor blockers, and 6.8% beta-adrenergic blockers. Table 1 presents the characteristics of the study group.

Table 1. Characteristics of the study group.

Variable	Total	18.5 ≤ BMI < 25	25 ≤ BMI < 30	BMI ≥ 30	*p* Value
No of patients, *n* (%)	661	143 (21.6%)	344 (52.0%)	174 (26.3%)	
Age, years					
Mean ± SD	67.3 ± 5.57	68.7 ± 5.52	67.1 ± 5.20	67.6 ± 5.26	0.32
Median	66.0	67.0	66.0	66.00	
IQR	63.0–71.0	64.0–73.0	63.0–70.0	62.0–70.0	
Range	60.0–90.0	60.0–90.0	60.0–85.0	60.0–84.0	
Education, *n* (%)					
Higher	127 (19.2%)	118 (19.6%)	68 (19.8%)	31 (17.8%)	0.05
Secondary	211 (31.9%)	46 (32.2%)	120 (34.9%)	45 (25.9%)	
Vocational	191 (28.9%)	32 (22.4%)	96 (27.9%)	63 (36.2%)	
Primary	46 (7.0%)	12 (8.4%)	17 (4.9%)	17 (9.8%)	
Missing data	86 (13.0)	25 (17.5%)	43 (12.5%)	18 (10.3%)	
Erectile dysfunction *, *n* (%)					
Severe	142 (21.5%)	29 (20.3%)	75 (21.8%)	38 (21.8%)	0.96
Moderate-to-severe	95 (14.4%)	21 (14.7%)	44 (12.8%)	30 (17.2%)	
Moderate	208 (31.5%)	46 (32.2%)	112 (32.6%)	50 (28.7%)	
Mild	154 (23.3%)	34 (23.8%)	81 (23.5%)	39 (22.4%)	
No dysfunction	62 (9.4%)	13 (9.1%)	32 (9.3%)	17 (9.8%)	
Hypertension, *n* (%)					
Yes	382 (57.8%)	66 (46.2%)	194 (56.4%)	122 (70.1%)	0.004
No	89 (13.5%)	29 (20.3%)	39 (11.3%)	21 (12.1%)	
Missing data	190 (28.7%)	48 (33.6%)	111 (32.3%)	31 (17.8%)	
Type 2 diabetes, *n* (%)					
Yes	157 (23.8%)	21 (14.7%)	75 (21.8%)	61 (35.1%)	0.003
No	281 (42.5%)	68 (47.6%)	141 (41.0%)	72 (41.4%)	
Missing data	223 (33.7%)	54 (37.8%)	128 (37.2%)	41 (23.6%)	
Dyslipidemia, *n* (%)					
Yes	273 (41.3%)	58 (40.6%)	125 (36.3%)	90 (51.7%)	0.15
No	165 (25.0%)	31 (21.7%)	91 (26.5%)	43 (24.7%)	
Missing data	223 (33.7%)	54 (37.8%)	128 (37.2%)	41 (23.6%)	

Table 1. Cont.

Variable	Total	18.5 ≤ BMI < 25	25 ≤ BMI < 30	BMI ≥ 30	p Value
		Smoking, n (%)			
Yes	336 (50.8%)	69 (48.3%)	165 (48.0%)	102 (58.6%)	0.97
No	103 (15.6%)	20 (14.0%)	51 (14.8%)	32 (18.4%)	
Missing data	222 (33.6%)	54 (37.8%)	128 (37.2%)	40 (23.0%)	
		Sedentary lifestyle **			
Yes	539 (81.5%)	115 (80.4%)	280 (81.45%)	144 (82.8%)	0.81
No	85 (12.9%)	19 (13.3%)	41 (11.9%)	25 (14.4%0	
Missing data	37 (5.6%)	9 (6.3%)	23 (6.7%)	5 (2.9%)	
		Waist circumference			
Mean ± SD	98.9 ± 10.23	92.1 ± 8.60	97.6 ± 7.83	107.0 ± 10.42	<0.001
Median	98.0	90.0	97.0	105.0	
IQR	92.0–104.0	86.0–98.0	93.0–102.0	100.0–104.0	
Range	70.0–160.0	70.0–116.0	76.0–160.0	85.0–154.0	

BMI, body mass index; IQR, interquartile range; SD, standard deviation; * Erectile dysfunction was classified using an abbreviated International Index of Erectile Function 5 (IIEF-5) Questionnaire, as follows: severe (5–7 scores), moderate-to-severe (8–11 scores), moderate (12–16 scores), mild (17–21 scores), and no dysfunction (>21 scores); ** A threshold of <1000 kcal/week was established to identify men who are leading a sedentary lifestyle.

3.2. Association between BMI and ED

The correlation between BMI and IIEF-5 score was weak and not significant (r = −0.02; $p = 0.60$). Additionally, no numerical increase in the IIEF-5 score was observed when patients were stratified by BMI categories and five degrees of ED severity. However, there was a slight numerical increase in the percentage of patients classified as having moderate to severe ED; nevertheless, this increase was not statistically significant with $p = 0.987$ (Table 2).

Table 2. Study group stratified by BMI categories and erectile dysfunction severity.

	18.5 ≤ BMI < 25	25 ≤ BMI < 30	BMI ≥ 30
Moderate-to-severe ED	96 (67.1%)	231 (67.2%)	118 (67.8%)
No ED and mild ED	47 (32.9%)	113 (32.8%)	56 (32.2%)

BMI, body mass index; ED, erectile dysfunction.

3.3. Association between Waist Circumference and ED

The correlation between waist circumference and IIEF-5 score was weak but significant (r = −0.20; $p < 0.0001$). The distribution of waist circumference values across BMI categories is illustrated in Figure 2.

A significant numerical rise in the percentage of patients classified as having moderate to severe ED was observed across quartiles of waist circumference ($p = 0.02$) (Table 3).

Table 3. Study group stratified by waist circumference quartiles and erectile dysfunction severity.

	WC Q1	WC Q2	WC Q3	WC Q4
Moderate-to-severe ED	89 (69.5%)	96 (64.4%)	117 (66.1%)	141 (75.8%)
No ED and mild ED	58 (39.5%)	53 (35.6%)	60 (33.9%)	45 (24.2%)

Q, quartile; WC, waist circumference.

Additionally, when considering a threshold of 100 cm (75% percentile) for waist circumference, in relation to the occurrence of ED, the OR was 3.74 (95% CI: 1.0–13.7; $p = 0.04$). This means that the odds for the development of ED were 3.74 times higher for men with a waist circumference of 100 cm and above, compared to men with a waist circumference below 100 cm.

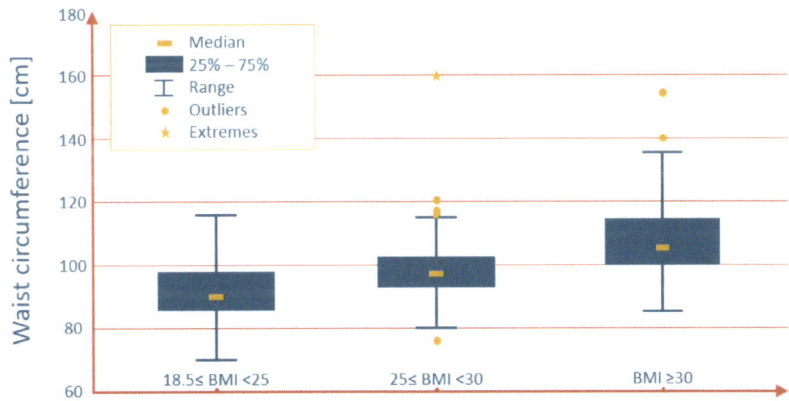

Figure 2. Distribution of waist circumference values by BMI categories.

3.4. Characteristics of Obese Men with ED

To characterize men with obesity and erectile dysfunction, we compared men with a normal weight, who did not report having ED, to men with obesity and who are overweight, with an IIEF-5 score of 21 and below. Although numerical differences were observed in some variables, only the difference in waist circumference reached statistical significance. A detailed comparison of both groups is presented in Table 4.

Table 4. Comparison between normal-weight men without ED and obese and overweight men with ED.

Variable	Normal Weight, No ED (BMI < 25 and IIEF-5 * > 21)	Obesity, Overweight, ED (BMI ≥ 25 and IIEF-5 * ≤ 21)	p Value
Number of patients, n	13 (2.7%)	469 (97.3%)	
Age, years			
Mean ± SD	65.3 ± 4.35	67.1 ± 5.29	0.23
Median (IQR)	65.0 (62.0–67.0)	66.0 (63.0–70.0)	
Range	60.0–75.0	60.0–84.0	
Education, n (%)			
Higher	3 (25.0%)	81 (19.8%)	0.77
Secondary	5 (41.7%)	154 (37.7%)	
Vocational	4 (33.3%)	144 (35.2%)	
Primary	0 (0.0%)	30 (7.3%)	
Hypertension, n (%)			
Yes	9 (90.0%)	285 (96.9%)	0.62
No	1 (22.0%)	53 (15.7%)	
Type 2 diabetes, n (%)			
Yes	4 (44.4%)	126 (40.3%)	0.80
No	5 (55.6%)	187 (97.4%)	
Dyslipidemia, n (%)			
Yes	6 (66.7%)	192 (61.3%)	0.75
No	3 (33.3%)	121 (38.7%)	
Smoking, n (%)			
Yes	6 (66.7%)	243 (77.4%)	0.45
No	3 (33.3%)	71 (22.6%)	

Table 4. *Cont.*

Variable	Normal Weight, No ED (BMI < 25 and IIEF-5 * > 21)	Obesity, Overweight, ED (BMI ≥ 25 and IIEF-5 * ≤ 21)	*p* Value
Sedentary lifestyle **			
Yes	9 (75.00%)	381 (86.2%)	0.27
No	3 (25.00%)	61 (13.8%)	
Waist circumference			
Mean ± SD	91.6 ± 8.88	101.1 ± 9.91	<0.001
Median (IQR)	89.0 (86.0–95.0)	100.0 (95.0–105.0)	
Range	83.0–112.0	76.0–160.0	

BMI, body mass index; ED, erectile dysfunction; IQR, interquartile range; SD, standard deviation. * Erectile dysfunction was classified using an abbreviated International Index of Erectile Function 5 (IIEF-5) Questionnaire, as follows: severe (5–7 scores), moderate-to-severe (8–11 scores), moderate (12–16 scores), mild (17–21 scores), and no dysfunction (>21 scores); ** A threshold of <1000 kcal/week was established to identify men who are leading a sedentary lifestyle.

4. Discussion

Our study found that the prevalence of ED is over 90% in elderly men with coronary artery disease, with similar proportions across BMI categories. The correlation between BMI and IIEF-5 score was weak and not significant ($r = -0.02$; $p = 0.60$), while the correlation between waist circumference and IIEF-5 score was significant ($r = -0.20$; $p < 0.0001$). Both an elevated BMI and a waist circumference of <100 cm (75% percentile) increased the risk of developing ED. No important differences were found between typical-weight men without ED and men with ED who were obese or overweight, including age; however, the group of men with increased body weight and ED was numerically older by almost 2 years.

In our study, we employed two methods to assess increased body weight, namely BMI and waist circumference. Both are recommended by the European Association of Urology Guidelines on Sexual and Reproductive Health to be taken during the physical examination of all individuals suspected of late-onset hypogonadism [21]. In the literature, there are few publications on how common ED is in men with a high BMI. We found only one study that looked at ED in elderly men based on their BMI. Cho et al. [22] conducted a study with 208 elderly Koreans in a suburban area, all aged 65 or older (average age 67.4 ± 8.2 years). ED was diagnosed using the IIEF-5 questionnaire; however, the cutoff value for ED was a score of 18, in contrast to Rosen et al.'s [19] cutoff value of ≤21 for diagnosing ED. As a result, some men with mild ED were categorized as not having ED, potentially leading to underestimated percentages of men experiencing ED. After excluding sexually inactive men and using the second quintile of BMI (23.2–24.4) as a reference, the authors observed an increased risk of ED in both the first BMI quintile (23.1 and below), with an OR of 14.09 (95% CI: 2.35–84.60) and the fifth BMI quintile (27.1 and above), with an OR of 4.92 (95% CI: 0.96–25.34) [22]. We added a similar threshold of a score of 18 in the IIEF-5 questionnaire in our analysis. It showed a numerical increase in the percentage of men affected by ED across BMI categories, but this increase was not significant.

Other measures of obesity, particularly focused on visceral fat, involve measuring waist circumference and indices derived from waist circumference measurements. The WHO regards waist circumference as a measure of metabolic risk. A waist circumference above 94 cm indicates an increased risk for metabolic complications, while a waist circumference above 102 cm signifies a substantially increased risk of metabolic complications, when taking into account the male population [23]. The experts from the European Group for the Study of Insulin Resistance (EGIR) [24] included central obesity, defined as a waist circumference of 94 cm and over, as part of metabolic syndrome. According to the National Cholesterol Education Program (NCEP), the Expert Panel on Detection, Evaluation, and Treatment of High Blood Cholesterol in Adults [25] provided one threshold for the determination of abdominal obesity as part of metabolic syndrome (>102 cm); however, with the caveat that metabolic syndrome can also develop in patients burdened with multiple risk factors and marginally increased waist circumference (94–102 cm). Our study did not specifically address metabolic syndrome, but the threshold of 100 cm (75% percentile) indicated a significant increase in the risk of ED. In a study on the general population, Cao et al. [26] explored the relationship between the weight-adjusted waist index (WWI) and ED. The WWI was calculated by dividing waist circumference, in centimeters, by the square root of weight, in kilograms. Data for this analysis were obtained from the National Health and Nutrition Examination Survey (NHANES) 2001–2004, comprising 3884 participants, of whom 1056 (27.19%) had a history of ED. This cohort was regarded as a representative sample of noninstitutionalized civilian residents in the US. The study population, with a mean age of 60.62 ± 0.48 years (range: 20 to 85 years) was younger compared to our sample and reflected the characteristics of the general population. While the prevalence of ED was low, their study demonstrated an increase in ED prevalence with rising body weight, 22.98% for a BMI below 25, 26.77% for a BMI of 25 and above but below 30, and 31.95% for a BMI of 30 and higher. The WWI was significantly higher in men with ED compared to those without ED (11.22 ± 0.03 cm/$\sqrt{kg}$ vs. 10.59 ± 0.02 cm/$\sqrt{kg}$, $p < 0.001$). Additionally, the WWI exhibited a stronger predictive value for ED than BMI and waist circumference. It is worth noting that NHANES used a self-reported single-item Massachusetts Male Aging Study (MMAS) question to classify men with ED, while we employed the IIEF-5 questionnaire, indicating another difference between our studies [26]. Kessler et al. pointed out that the prevalence of ED measured using MMAS tends to produce slightly different levels in comparison to those measured using IIEF questionnaires [27]. To relate to this study, we investigated the correlation between waist circumference and the IIEF-5 score. Waist circumference appeared to be more tightly connected with the IIEF-5 score than BMI, which may indicate that it could serve as a more reliable predictor of ED risk than BMI. Nevertheless, a direct comparison between these studies is not possible due to using different questionnaires for ED.

There is a growing body of evidence that suggests that BMI is not an ideal indicator of excess body weight in the elderly, as confirmed by our analysis. The International Atherosclerosis Society (IAS) and International Chair on Cardiometabolic Risk (ICCR) Working Group on Visceral Obesity underscored that abdominal obesity serves as a risk factor for premature atherosclerosis and cardiovascular disease. The consensus among experts in the group meeting was that relying solely on BMI is insufficient for accurately assessing and managing the cardiometabolic risk linked to higher levels of body fat. This is because BMI does not distinguish between fat distribution patterns and may underestimate the risk associated with central adiposity. Thus, experts advocate for incorporating waist circumference as a routine measurement in clinical practice alongside BMI to more effectively classify obesity [28]. Another significant factor is age-related changes, which encompass the loss of muscle mass, the redistribution of fat, and frailty, all of which are common in older adults [29]. In older people, BMI can either underestimate or overestimate body fat mass. Given that fat deposition in the elderly tends to accumulate intra-abdominally, measuring waist circumference provided a more accurate assessment of obesity, as waist circumference provides a more direct measure of adiposity and can better capture changes in body composition that occur with aging. Sarcopenic obesity is characterized by poor quality and an insufficient amount of muscle mass, leading to functional limitations and disability [30]. BMI alone cannot accurately determine sarcopenic obesity because it does not differentiate between fat mass and lean muscle mass. In elderly people, measuring waist circumference provides a better assessment; however, other methods such as hydrostatic densitometry, bioelectrical impedance, or dual-energy x-ray absorptiometry would more accurately assess the degree of obesity. Despite the limitations of BMI, it remains widely utilized in clinical studies involving elderly populations.

Diabetes is widely recognized as a risk factor for both ED and cardiovascular diseases. In our study, we investigated diabetes as one of the risk factors. Al-Hunayan et al. [31] conducted a study involving 323 men newly diagnosed with type 2 diabetes from primary care centers in Kuwait. The mean age was 41.7 ± 0.6 years, ranging from 21 to 65 years. To diagnose ED, the IIEF-5 questionnaire was used. The study reported that the percentage of men experiencing ED increased with BMI, 21.5% in normal-weight men, 40% in overweight men, and 59.3% in men with obesity [31]. In our study, 23.8% of the study population were diagnosed with diabetes. Furthermore, the percentage of men with diabetes was 14.7% among those with a normal weight and 35.1% among those with obesity. The same trend pertains to the cardiovascular system's link with obesity. Visceral obesity adversely affects endothelial function and testosterone levels [32]. In our study, the percentage of men with hypertension was 46.2% among those with a normal weight and 70.1% among those with obesity. Finally, an interesting finding considered the fact that obese and overweight men experienced ED at an equivalent age compared to normal-weight men without ED, 65.3 ± 4.35 years vs. 67.1 ± 5.29 years; $p = 0.23$. This finding indicates that an excess of body weight accelerated the development of ED. We did not identify any other study that investigated whether obesity could accelerate the onset of ED. Nevertheless, these findings highlight an escalating burden of risk factors with increasing body weight in our senior population with coronary artery disease.

Several limitations should be kept in mind while interpreting our results. The study cohort comprised older men with coronary artery disease undergoing cardiac rehabilitation. Patients with cardiovascular diseases have an increased risk of developing ED due to shared risk factors for both conditions. For example, in a similar cohort without age limitation having coronary heart disease with a mean age of 60.73 ± 9.20 age, ED was reported in 79.23% of the men [33]. The global prevalence of ED, as reported by Kessler et al. [27], spans a wide range, starting from 13.1% and reaching 71.2%. The summary of IIEF data obtained from men aged 60 to 69 indicates that a range of 18.1% to 94.1% experience some degree of ED. Another limitation is the use of BMI to define obesity. Although it fails to differentiate between body fat and lean mass and does not provide information about the distribution of body mass, it remains very popular among patients and physicians. For this reason, we recommend increasing awareness about the use of waist circumference for determining central obesity, so this measure can be used alongside BMI. Waist circumference has been proven to be useful and is associated with ED [10,34]. Furthermore, this is a cross-sectional study, which means it cannot establish causality, while ED is self-reported by survey participants and is susceptible to bias. Finally, this study pertains to a Polish population of patients with chronic cardiovascular disease. The association between BMI and IIEF-5 scores, as identified in this study, requires further research in different populations before generalization can be considered.

5. Conclusions

The prevalence of ED in men with coronary artery disease surpasses 90%. Men with obesity and who are overweight face an increased risk of developing ED; however, it appears that waist circumference is a more reliable predictor of this risk than BMI. Notably, obese and overweight men experienced ED at a similar age. As a proactive measure, physicians are advised to screen all elderly patients with cardiovascular disease for the occurrence of ED and address obesity to enhance their overall health.

Author Contributions: Conceptualization, M.B., M.S., P.O. and D.K.; methodology, M.B., M.S., D.K., E.S., K.R.-P., A.R. and J.G.; formal analysis, M.B., A.R. and D.K.; investigation, D.K., A.P.-G. and A.J.; resources, D.K.; data curation, M.B., M.S., E.S., A.P.-G., A.J., K.R.-P., A.R., J.G. and D.K.; writing—original draft preparation, M.B., M.S., D.K., E.S., A.P.-G., A.J., K.R.-P., A.R. and J.G.; writing—review and editing, M.B., M.S., D.K., K.R.-P., P.O. and A.R.; visualization, M.B.; supervision, D.K. All authors have read and agreed to the published version of the manuscript.

Funding: This research received no external funding.

Institutional Review Board Statement: This study was conducted in accordance with the Declaration of Helsinki, and was approved by the Bioethics Committee at Wroclaw Medical University (KB 3/2019 dated on 11 January 2019).

Informed Consent Statement: Informed consent was obtained from all subjects involved in the study.

Data Availability Statement: The data that support the findings of this study are available on request from the corresponding author.

Conflicts of Interest: The authors declare no conflicts of interest.

References

1. Temple, N.J. The Origins of the Obesity Epidemic in the USA-Lessons for Today. *Nutrients* **2022**, *14*, 4253. [CrossRef] [PubMed]
2. Obesity. World Health Organization (WHO). Available online: https://www.who.int/health-topics/obesity (accessed on 25 September 2023).
3. Dai, H.; Alsalhe, T.A.; Chalghaf, N.; Riccò, M.; Bragazzi, N.L.; Wu, J. The global burden of disease attributable to high body mass index in 195 countries and territories, 1990-2017: An analysis of the Global Burden of Disease Study. *PLoS Med.* **2020**, *17*, e1003198. [CrossRef] [PubMed]
4. Plackett, B. The vicious cycle of depression and obesity. *Nature* **2022**, *608*, S42–S43. [CrossRef] [PubMed]
5. Cawley, J.; Biener, A.; Meyerhoefer, C.; Ding, Y.; Zvenyach, T.; Smolarz, B.G.; Ramasamy, A. Job Absenteeism Costs of Obesity in the United States: National and State-Level Estimates. *J. Occup. Environ. Med.* **2021**, *63*, 565–573. [CrossRef] [PubMed]
6. Hecker, J.; Freijer, K.; Hiligsmann, M.; Evers, S. Burden of disease study of overweight and obesity; the societal impact in terms of cost-of-illness and health-related quality of life. *BMC Public Health* **2022**, *22*, 46. [CrossRef] [PubMed]
7. What Is the Body Mass Index (BMI)? National Health Servise (NHS). Available online: https://www.nhs.uk/common-health-questions/lifestyle/what-is-the-body-mass-index-bmi/ (accessed on 25 September 2023).
8. Powell-Wiley, T.M.; Poirier, P.; Burke, L.E.; Després, J.P.; Gordon-Larsen, P.; Lavie, C.J.; Lear, S.A.; Ndumele, C.E.; Neeland, I.J.; Sanders, P.; et al. Obesity and Cardiovascular Disease: A Scientific Statement From the American Heart Association. *Circulation* **2021**, *143*, e984–e1010. [CrossRef] [PubMed]
9. Kałka, D.; Domagała, Z.; Rakowska, A.; Womperski, K.; Franke, R.; Sylwina-Krauz, E.; Stanisz, J.; Piłot, M.; Gebala, J.; Rusiecki, L.; et al. Modifiable risk factors for erectile dysfunction: An assessment of the awareness of such factors in patients suffering from ischaemic heart disease. *Int. J. Impot. Res.* **2016**, *28*, 14–19. [CrossRef] [PubMed]
10. Pizzol, D.; Smith, L.; Fontana, L.; Caruso, M.G.; Bertoldo, A.; Demurtas, J.; McDermott, D.; Garolla, A.; Grabovac, I.; Veronese, N. Associations between body mass index, waist circumference and erectile dysfunction: A systematic review and META-analysis. *Rev. Endocr. Metab. Disord.* **2020**, *21*, 657–666. [CrossRef] [PubMed]
11. Li, H.; Xu, W.; Wang, T.; Wang, S.; Liu, J.; Jiang, H. Effect of weight loss on erectile function in men with overweight or obesity: A meta-analysis of randomised controlled trials. *Andrologia* **2022**, *54*, e14250. [CrossRef]
12. Rey, R.A.; Grinspon, R.P.; Gottlieb, S.; Pasqualini, T.; Knoblovits, P.; Aszpis, S.; Pacenza, N.; Stewart Usher, J.; Bergadá, I.; Campo, S.M. Male hypogonadism: An extended classification based on a developmental, endocrine physiology-based approach. *Andrology* **2013**, *1*, 3–16. [CrossRef]
13. Kałka, D.; Biernikiewicz, M.; Gebala, J.; Sobieszczańska, M.; Jakima, S.; Pilecki, W.; Rusiecki, L. Diagnosis of hypogonadism in patients treated with low energy shock wave therapy for erectile dysfunction: A narrative review. *Transl. Androl. Urol.* **2020**, *9*, 2786–2796. [CrossRef] [PubMed]
14. Wu, F.C.; Tajar, A.; Pye, S.R.; Silman, A.J.; Finn, J.D.; O'Neill, T.W.; Bartfai, G.; Casanueva, F.; Forti, G.; Giwercman, A.; et al. Hypothalamic-pituitary-testicular axis disruptions in older men are differentially linked to age and modifiable risk factors: The European Male Aging Study. *J. Clin. Endocrinol. Metab.* **2008**, *93*, 2737–2745. [CrossRef]
15. Kelly, D.M.; Jones, T.H. Testosterone and obesity. *Obes. Rev.* **2015**, *16*, 581–606. [CrossRef] [PubMed]
16. Cohen, P.G. The hypogonadal–obesity cycle: Role of aromatase in modulating the testosterone–estradiol shunt—A major factor in the genesis of morbid obesity. *Med. Hypotheses* **1999**, *52*, 49–51. [CrossRef]
17. Drygas, W.; Kostka, T.; Jegier, A.; Kuński, H. Long-term effects of different physical activity levels on coronary heart disease risk factors in middle-aged men. *Int. J. Sports Med.* **2000**, *21*, 235–241. [CrossRef]
18. Arsenault, B.J.; Rana, J.S.; Lemieux, I.; Després, J.P.; Wareham, N.J.; Kastelein, J.J.; Boekholdt, S.M.; Khaw, K.T. Physical activity, the Framingham risk score and risk of coronary heart disease in men and women of the EPIC-Norfolk study. *Atherosclerosis* **2010**, *209*, 261–265. [CrossRef] [PubMed]
19. Rosen, R.C.; Cappelleri, J.C.; Smith, M.D.; Lipsky, J.; Peña, B.M. Development and evaluation of an abridged, 5-item version of the International Index of Erectile Function (IIEF-5) as a diagnostic tool for erectile dysfunction. *Int. J. Impot. Res.* **1999**, *11*, 319–326. [CrossRef]
20. World Population Ageing 2019. United Nations: Department of Economic and Social Affairs. Available online: https://www.un.org/en/development/desa/population/publications/pdf/ageing/WorldPopulationAgeing2019-Report.pdf (accessed on 15 November 2023).
21. Salonia, A.; Bettocchi, C.; Capogrosso, P.; Carvalho, J.; Corona, G.; Hatzichristodoulou, G.; Jones, T.H.; Kadioglu, A.; Martinez-Salamanca, J.I.; Minhas, S.; et al. EAU Guidelines on Sexual and Reproductive Health. European Association of Urology. Available online: https://d56bochluxqnz.cloudfront.net/documents/full-guideline/EAU-Guidelines-on-Sexual-and-Reproductive-Health-2023.pdf (accessed on 25 October 2023).

22. Cho, Y.G.; Song, H.J.; Lee, S.K.; Jang, S.N.; Jeong, J.Y.; Choi, Y.H.; Hong, K.S.; Choi, M.G.; Kang, S.H.; Kang, J.H.; et al. The relationship between body fat mass and erectile dysfunction in Korean men: Hallym Aging Study. *Int. J. Impot. Res.* **2009**, *21*, 179–186. [CrossRef]
23. Waist Circumference and Waist-Hip Ratio—Report of a WHO Expert Consultation. World Health Organization. Available online: https://iris.who.int/bitstream/handle/10665/44583/9789241501491_eng.pdf?sequence=1 (accessed on 26 March 2024).
24. Balkau, B.; Charles, M.A. Comment on the provisional report from the WHO consultation. European Group for the Study of Insulin Resistance (EGIR). *Diabet. Med.* **1999**, *16*, 442–443. [CrossRef]
25. Expert Panel on Detection, Evaluation, and Treatment of High Blood Cholesterol in Adults. Executive Summary of the Third Report of the National Cholesterol Education Program (NCEP) Expert Panel on Detection, Evaluation, and Treatment of High Blood Cholesterol in Adults (Adult Treatment Panel III). *JAMA* **2001**, *285*, 2486–2497. [CrossRef]
26. Cao, S.; Hu, X.; Shao, Y.; Wang, Y.; Tang, Y.; Ren, S.; Li, X. Relationship between weight-adjusted-waist index and erectile dysfunction in the United State: Results from NHANES 2001–2004. *Front. Endocrinol.* **2023**, *14*, 1128076. [CrossRef]
27. Kessler, A.; Sollie, S.; Challacombe, B.; Briggs, K.; Van Hemelrijck, M. The global prevalence of erectile dysfunction: A review. *BJU Int.* **2019**, *124*, 587–599. [CrossRef] [PubMed]
28. Ross, R.; Neeland, I.J.; Yamashita, S.; Shai, I.; Seidell, J.; Magni, P.; Santos, R.D.; Arsenault, B.; Cuevas, A.; Hu, F.B.; et al. Waist circumference as a vital sign in clinical practice: A Consensus Statement from the IAS and ICCR Working Group on Visceral Obesity. *Nat. Rev. Endocrinol.* **2020**, *16*, 177–189. [CrossRef] [PubMed]
29. Buch, A.; Marcus, Y.; Shefer, G.; Zimmet, P.; Stern, N. Approach to Obesity in the Older Population. *J. Clin. Endocrinol. Metab.* **2021**, *106*, 2788–2805. [CrossRef]
30. McKee, A.M.; Morley, J.E. Obesity in the Elderly. Available online: https://www.ncbi.nlm.nih.gov/books/NBK532533/ (accessed on 29 February 2024).
31. Al-Hunayan, A.; Al-Mutar, M.; Kehinde, E.O.; Thalib, L.; Al-Ghorory, M. The prevalence and predictors of erectile dysfunction in men with newly diagnosed with type 2 diabetes mellitus. *BJU Int.* **2007**, *99*, 130–134. [CrossRef] [PubMed]
32. Traish, A.M.; Feeley, R.J.; Guay, A. Mechanisms of obesity and related pathologies: Androgen deficiency and endothelial dysfunction may be the link between obesity and erectile dysfunction. *FEBS J.* **2009**, *276*, 5755–5767. [CrossRef] [PubMed]
33. Kałka, D.; Karpiński, Ł.; Gebala, J.; Rusiecki, L.; Biełous-Wilk, A.; Krauz, E.S.; Piłot, M.; Womperski, K.; Rusiecka, M.; Pilecki, W. Sexual health of male cardiac patients—Present status and expectations of patients with coronary heart disease. *Arch. Med. Sci.* **2017**, *13*, 302–310. [CrossRef] [PubMed]
34. Yassin, A.A.; Nettleship, J.E.; Salman, M.; Almehmadi, Y. Waist circumference is superior to weight and BMI in predicting sexual symptoms, voiding symptoms and psychosomatic symptoms in men with hypogonadism and erectile dysfunction. *Andrologia* **2017**, *49*, e12634. [CrossRef]

Disclaimer/Publisher's Note: The statements, opinions and data contained in all publications are solely those of the individual author(s) and contributor(s) and not of MDPI and/or the editor(s). MDPI and/or the editor(s) disclaim responsibility for any injury to people or property resulting from any ideas, methods, instructions or products referred to in the content.

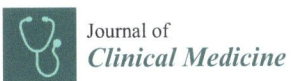

Article

Time Trend Analysis of Comorbidities in Ankylosing Spondylitis: A Population-Based Study from 53,142 Hospitalizations in Poland

Katarzyna Helon [1,*], Małgorzata Wisłowska [1], Krzysztof Kanecki [2], Paweł Goryński [2], Aneta Nitsch-Osuch [2] and Krzysztof Bonek [1]

1. Department of Rheumatology, National Institute of Geriatrics, Rheumatology and Rehabilitation, 02-637 Warsaw, Poland; mwislowska@wp.pl (M.W.); krzysztof.bonek@spartanska.pl (K.B.)
2. National Institute of Public Health—National Institute of Hygiene, 00791 Warsaw, Poland; kanecki@mp.pl (K.K.); pawel@pzh.gov.pl (P.G.); aneta.nitsch-osuch@wum.edu.pl (A.N.-O.)
* Correspondence: katarzyna.helon@spartanska.pl

Abstract: Background: (1) Influence of comorbidities on life expectancy and treatment outcomes is one of the main concerns of modern rheumatology, due to their rising prevalence and increasing impact on mortality and disability. The main objective of our study was to analyze the time trends and shifts in the comorbidity profile and mortality over 10 years in the Polish population with ankylosing spondylitis (AS). (2) Data from 2011–2020 years were acquired from the General Hospital Morbidity Study in the National Institute of Public Health—National Institute of Hygiene (NIH-PIB) as ICD-10 codes. Based on ICD10 codes, we calculated the percentage shares for comorbidities, with the relative risk ratios and odds ratios. We analyzed the hospitalization rates and mortality from the overlapping conditions. Also, we analyzed age and sex related differences in the clinical manifestations of AS patients. (3) Results: From 53,142 hospitalizations of patients with AS, we found that the male population presented higher rates of cardiovascular (2.7% vs. 1.3% $p < 0.001$) and pulmonary conditions (1.2% vs. 0.8% $p < 0.025$). Inflammatory bowel diseases were more common in the female population than in males (2.3% vs. 1.7%, $p < 0.001$). In the years 2011–2020, we observed a decline in the number of hospitalized patients due to cardiovascular ($p < 0.001$) and respiratory system conditions ($p < 0.001$), yet the relative risk and odd ratios remained high. In the years 2011–2020, 4056 patients received biological treatment (7%). The number of initiated biological therapies correlated negatively with the number of reported hospitalizations due to ischemic heart diseases (IHD) ($p < 0.031$, $r = -0.8$). Furthermore, in the logistic regression model, we found strong collinearity between cardiovascular and pulmonary comorbidities (VIF = 14; tolerance = 0.1); also, the number of reported IHD's correlated positively with the number of pulmonary infections ($p < 0.031$, $r = 0.7$) (4). Conclusions: Cardiopulmonary comorbidities are a main factor associated with increased mortality in patients with AS, especially in hospitalized patients. The mortality rates among patients with AS admitted to hospital due to other conditions other than movement disorders exceed the populational risk. The number of biologically treated patients correlated negatively with hospital admissions due to IHD.

Keywords: ankylosing spondylitis; cardiovascular risk; epidemiology; atherosclerosis

1. Introduction

Ankylosing spondylitis (AS) is an autoinflammatory disease affecting the spine and sacroiliac joints that is also associated with increased occurrence of comorbidities [1]. Comorbidities in spondyloarthritis (SpA) add to the burden of disease by contributing to disease activity, functional and work disability, and a higher risk for depression [2]. This leads to lower life quality [2] and higher overall mortality rates [3]. Thus, awareness of comorbidities in SpA is crucial to improve their screening and management of SpA [3].

Yet, due to rapid development of medical knowledge and implementation of new treatment methods, a shift in comorbidities and mortality in the general population has been observed [4], which also affects patients with autoinflammatory diseases [5]. Additionally, a rapid increase of socioeconomic costs of health care systems has been observed [6]; therefore, big-data, population-based research is required for clinicians and health care providers to focus their efforts to balance the cost-effectiveness. Cardiovascular diseases (CVD) were identified as the leading cause of death in patients with AS. Several studies showed that systemic inflammation as well as secondary lipid profile alterations lead to increased CV incidents [7]. Research on CVD and CVD-related death in SpA suggests a cause-and-effect relationship. Cohort and populational studies suggest that the prevalence of ischemic heart disease and cardiac failure is higher among patients with AS in comparison to the general population [7]. Moreover, despite a world trend of decrease in CVD-related mortality and disability, prognosis for AS patients is still less favorable. Gastrointestinal tract involvement is considered as one of the major comorbidities in AS. Occurrence of peptic ulcers, infection of Helicobacter pylori, and post-NSAID enteropathy have been widely described in AS. Inflammatory bowel diseases (IBD) are a group of chronic autoinflammatory diseases sharing their pathophysiology and pathogenesis with Spondyloarthropaties [8]. The clinical manifestations of ulcerative colitis (UC) mainly involve abdominal pain, diarrhea, and hematochezia [9]. According to available studies, in about 6% of patients with AS, IBD is being reported [10]. Also, several studies on comorbidities in AS have reported subclinical IBDs [11]. Interestingly, the occurrence of radiological signs of AS, without inflammatory back pain among patients with IBDs has been reportedly approximately in 3–5% of patients [11]. Occurrence of eye inflammatory diseases is considered as one of the major health problems because sight deterioration or loss of vision leads to the major disability and lower quality of life. Ocular involvement is frequently encountered in SpA, of which uveitis is the most common manifestation. Acute anterior uveitis (AAV) is reported in almost 40% of the patients with SpA [12]. Ocular manifestations in AS were widely addressed in population studies. As novel research has suggested, the occurrence of AAV, episcleritis, and scleritis is associated with unfavorable disease progression [12]. Also, some researchers suggest that the occurrence of AAV is associated with a higher CVD risk, yet this is still under research [13]. Constant inflammatory state and gene changes that lead to ankylosing spondylitis could also play a role in cancer development. The results from national registers [14–17] revealed that the overall incidence of cancer seems to be elevated in patients with AS, yet the outcomes between populations seem to differ. In patients from Hong Kong, Chang et al. [14] reported an increased risk of hematological malignancy in both sexes, colon cancer in females, and bone and prostate cancer in males. On the contrary, Feltelius et al. [15], in their retrospective analysis, reported only increased prevalence of kidney neoplasm, which was not observed by Bittar et al. [16]. Research by Bitter stated that among patients with AS, skin cancers (squamous cell, malignant melanoma, and basal cell) and head and neck cancers were reported as significantly increased [16]. Similar observations were made by Kagan et al. [17], who reported increased risk for solid tumors in AS.

Accurate estimates of treatment trends and populational comorbidities drifts are important in planning health policy [18,19]. Data obtained from outpatient clinics are often lacking due to the requirement of reporting a single ICD-10 number. We decided to analyze data acquired from the General Hospital Morbidity Study conducted by the Institute of Public Health—National Institute of Hygiene (NIH-PIB), as health care providers, except psychiatric facilities, are required to send data to the NIH-PIB. Because AS affects less than 0.5% of the global population, observational or single-center studies on small groups do not provide enough data for estimating population drifts or trends in comorbidities or mortality. There is a need for studies performed on large populations. Yet, due to COVID-19 epidemics, data from years 2021–2023 are burdened with the influence of a strong single factor dominating general mortality rates. This also includes populational studies on mortality and comorbidities in AS. Therefore, we decided to analyze pre-pandemic data from the years 2011–2020 involving over 53,000 hospitalizations. In our study, we wanted to present trends and changes of comorbidities with concomitant mortality in patients with ankylosing spondylitis in Poland.

2. Materials and Methods

Raw data were acquired from National Institute of Public Health—National Institute of Hygiene (NIH-PIB) as anonymized numerical data from the 2011–2020 period. Data consisted of up to four ICD-10 codes with patients' unique number, age, and additional procedures presented with ICD-9 codes. Each study procedure complied with the Declaration of Helsinki or similar standards of ethics. All patients' data were searched for relevant diagnosis codes for AS.

2.1. Study Population

The study was approved by the local ethical committee (KBT-2/3/2022). Data were obtained from the NIH-PIB database, regarding patients diagnosed with AS (M45) from 1 January 2011 to 31 December 2020 covering 95% of the Polish population. The NIH-PIB collects information on patients including sociodemographic data, ICD-10 coded diagnoses, procedures patients underwent as ICD-9 codes, dates of admission and discharge, sex, and cause of death. The authors excluded repeated hospitalizations from analysis.

We used the following criteria for inclusion in this analysis: (1) diagnosis of M45, and (2) age above 18 years (3). We excluded patients who (1) did not meet these criteria and (2) were diagnosed with other autoinflammatory disease or autoimmune disease including M00, M05, M06, M46, M31, M32, M33, M35, and M31. Patients diagnosed with L40 (psoriasis), sarcoidosis (D86), reactive arthritis (M02), gout (M10), and infective arthritis (M00) were excluded from the study. Patients diagnosed with overlapping inflammatory bowel diseases (K50) were included in the analysis if they were also diagnosed with M45. Patients reported with an ICD-9 code of 00.181 or 00.18 (Introduction of Therapeutic Monoclonal Antibody) were considered as biologically treated. In the study group, we defined and analyzed a group with ischemic heart disease (IHD)—patients with the presence of diseases identified by the ICD 10 I20.0–ICD 25.9

2.2. Statistical Analysis

Statistical analysis was performed with the PS IMAGO v 26 SPSS module. Data were expressed as mean (±SD) for normal distribution and as interquartile ranges (IQR) for non-normal distribution. A Shapiro–Wilk test for normality for all measured parameters was performed. Pearson's test for normal ranges and Spearman's correlation test for not normal ranges were performed. For comparing non-paired nominal data, we used the Chi2 and Wilcoxon tests. A McNemar test was used for paired numerical data. A 2-sided $p < 0.05$ or an IRR whose 95% CI excluded 1.0 was considered statistically significant.

3. Results

Into our analysis, we included N = 53,142 hospitalizations (males N = 38,974 vs. females N = 14,168 $p < 0.001$), with a median age of 46.6 ± 13.7 for males and 48.5 ± 13.5 for females ($p = 0.001$) (Table 1). Statistically significant differences in reported comorbidities were found predominantly in the male population in comparison to female patients in cardiovascular diseases (n = 6546 patients) (2.7% vs. 1.3% $p < 0.001$) and pulmonary conditions (1.2% vs. 0.8% $p < 0.023$) ratios. After analysis of the correlation matrix, we found positive correlations between CVD and pulmonary conditions ($p < 0.031$ tau = 0.5). After regression analysis, we concluded that they are secondary to the "suppressor effect" based on collinearity (VIF = 14; tolerance = 0.1) between pulmonary diseases, such as COPD, pulmonary infections, and cardiovascular diseases in male patients. In the other groups, no statistically significant differences were found. Among CVD diseases, the most common was hypertension (HT) affecting 15% of patients, yet after an adjustment for age above 40 years, the percentage rose up to 25%. In hospitalized patients, group CVD was present in 45% of inpatients.

Similarly, among the pulmonary comorbidities of hospitalized patients, the most common were infections (22%) and COPD/Asthma (32%). There were no significant differences in the occurrence of neoplasmatic or hematological diseases, traumas, and kidney diseases. The general mortality was 2.5%, yet analysis of subgroups of patients admitted to hospital due to conditions other than AS revealed a higher mortality of 13%. In Table 1, we present the typical clinical features of AS reported by medical services providers. In the statistical analysis, occurrences of acute anterior uveitis were not statistically significant between the male and female patients (1.7% vs. 1.6% $p < 0.34$). In the female group, we observed a tendency toward a higher occurrence of inflammatory bowel diseases (2.3% vs. 1.7 $p < 0.031$) despite a similar ratio of ICD10-ths codes reported involving ICD-10:K symbol (gastrointestinal conditions). There were no significant differences in skin conditions other than psoriasis and osteoporosis.

Table 1. Clinical and demographic data comparing male and female groups. Data are presented as means ± SD or in percentages.

	All Patients	Males	Females	p
Age (years)	47.1 ± 13.7	46.6 ± 13.7	48.5 ± 13.5	<0.001
Gender(Male/Female)	53,142	38,974	14,168	<0.001
Median length of hospitalization (Days)	2 [0–10]	2 [0–10]	2 [0–9]	0.071
Psoriasis [%]	710	325 (45%)	389 (55%)	0.4
Eye inflammation [%]	882 (1.7%)	658 (1.7%)	224 (1.6%)	0.392
Inflammatory bowel diseases [%]	996 (1.9%)	675 (1.7%)	321 (2.3%)	<0.001
Crohns disease [%]	295 (0.6%)	157 (0.4%)	138 (1.0%)	<0.001
Colitis Ulcerosa [%]	702 (1.3%)	519 (1.8%)	183 (1.3%)	0.721

In the further analysis, we included patients admitted to the hospital with a reported code for AS (M45) between the years 2011–2020. Data were divided by categories following the ICD-10 codes, as shown in Table 2. Groups of ICD-10 including P00–P96 (certain conditions originating in the perinatal period), Q00–Q99 (congenital malformations, deformations, and chromosomal abnormalities), V01–Y98 (external causes of morbidity and mortality), H60–H95 (diseases of the ear and mastoid process) were excluded from analysis because their frequency was too low for the requirements of the statistical analysis.

Table 2. Hospital admissions divided by year of admission and ICD-10 codes.

	ICD-Code	2011	2012	2013	2014	2015	2016	2017	2018	2019	2020
Certain infectious and parasitic diseases	A00–B99	40	52	40	51	57	52	47	49	49	39
Neoplasms	C00–D49	42	54	55	84	73	102	104	117	113	95
Diseases of the blood and blood-forming organs and certain disorders involving the immune mechanism	D50–D89	93	83	91	73	99	83	72	130	82	102
Endocrine, nutritional, and metabolic diseases	E00–E90	389	395	461	454	595	615	498	604	604	470
Mental and behavioral disorders	F00–F99	41	41	27	29	33	27	19	50	41	31
Diseases of the nervous system	G00–G99	81	73	88	92	129	111	157	80	94	81
Diseases of the eye and adnexa	H00–H59	76	164	220	220	223	209	92	110	108	88
Diseases of the circulatory system	I00–I99	999	1155	1102	1254	1317	1294	1118	1100	1128	802
Diseases of the respiratory system	J00–J99	188	231	216	205	230	267	206	227	226	140
Diseases of the digestive system	K00–K93	232	284	363	355	388	387	322	441	413	384
Diseases of the skin and subcutaneous tissue	L00–L99	51	67	61	66	59	75	62	110	105	54

Table 2. Cont.

	ICD-Code	2011	2012	2013	2014	2015	2016	2017	2018	2019	2020
Diseases of the musculoskeletal system and connective tissue other than ankylosing spondylitis	M00–M99 without M45	927	1050	1199	570	3186	1307	1403	1230	1362	970
Diseases of the genitourinary system	N00–N99	165	156	206	177	184	203	208	189	207	110
Pregnancy, childbirth, and the puerperium	O00–O99	121	116	101	138	135	138	170	170	177	153
Symptoms, signs, and abnormal clinical and laboratory findings, not elsewhere classified	R00–R99	41	53	32	68	56	59	84	88	95	77
Injury, poisoning, and certain other consequences of external cause	S00–T98	92	80	68	86	83	85	100	85	90	93
Factors influencing health status and contact with health services	Z00–Z99	87	75	96	119	122	169	215	150	154	137

3.1. Hospitalisations Due to AS

In the analysis of all hospitalizations, a decrease in number of hospitalizations in patients due to AS was observed. Also, a decline in the total number of hospitalizations ($p < 0.031$), hospitalizations due to cardiovascular diseases (ICD-10: I; $p < 0.041$), and movement disorders (ICD-10: M; $p < 0.051$) were observed. There were no statistically significant differences in hospital admissions due to neoplastic processes (ICD-10: C, D and Z), kidney diseases (ICD-10 N), infections (ICD-10: A, B, J and U), or trauma (ICD-10: T, S). Interestingly, despite a numerical decline, differences in the proportions presented in the percentages between the analyzed conditions remained similar and statistically insignificant, as shown in Table 2.

3.2. Overall Hospitalization and Comorbidities Risk Analysis

On the trend analysis, we calculated relative risk (RR) ratios of the mortality for statistically significant ($p < 0.05$) factors based on Table 2. In Figure 1, we present the changes in RR with the time trends for CVD (Figure 1) and for pulmonary conditions. As shown on Figure 1, there is a tendency toward increased mortality among patients with AS who were hospitalized (RR median: 1.6 OR median: 7). Despite, the observed lowering in occurrence of CVD, the relative risk ratios remained on a stable level. Similarly, the CVD pulmonary conditions presented similar tendencies with increased mortality rates (RR median: 2 OR median: 5) and similar mortality risks despite the observed trends.

In the further analysis, we included only patients with AS admitted to hospitals due to conditions other than M45. In the analysis, we included n = 1562 patients and among them 156 deaths were reported. We analyzed direct, secondary, and underlying causes of death. Ambiguous codes such as R09.2 (lack of breath) that didn't refer to a direct cause of death were excluded unless an unambiguous secondary or underlying cause was given. Cases without secondary or underlying or other following conditions were excluded from our analysis. In the statistical analysis, we used the Chi2 test and multivariate logistic regression analysis. In the logistic regression, we created a statistically significant model including two covariates (chi-square $p < 0.001$, Hosner–Lewershaw test $p = 0.31$, Nagerkelke R Square = 0.38) with two covariates: cardiovascular diseases (B – 5.7 $p < 0.01$) and pulmonary conditions (B = 3.0, $p < 0.031$), as presented in Figure 2 (ICD-10: J and I). Further analysis suggests a strong collinearity (VIF > 4; tolerance < 0.25; condition index > 30) between those two variables. No statistical significance was observed for the other analyzed factors.

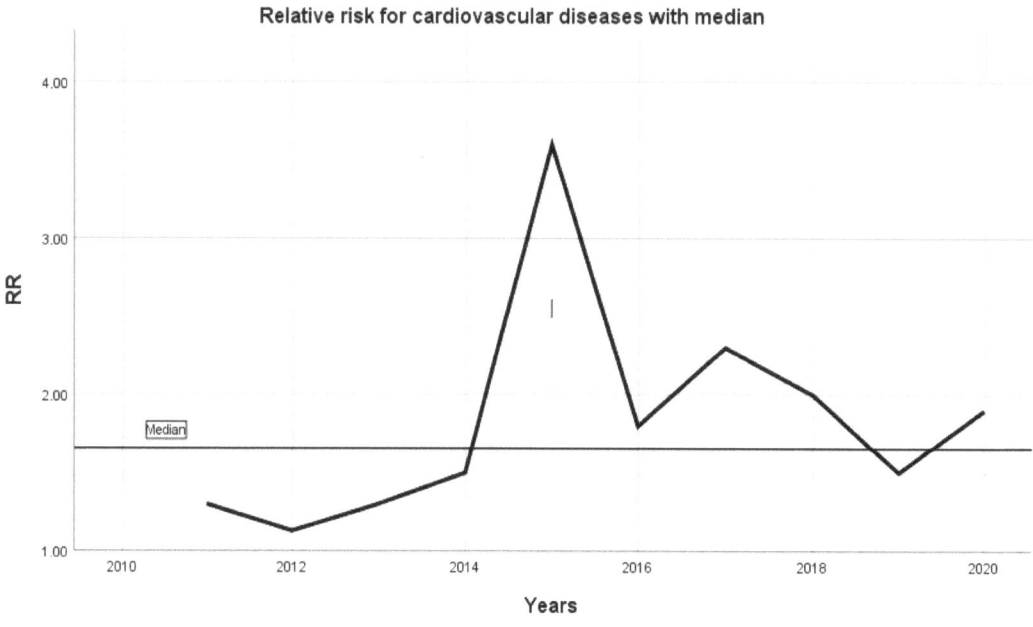

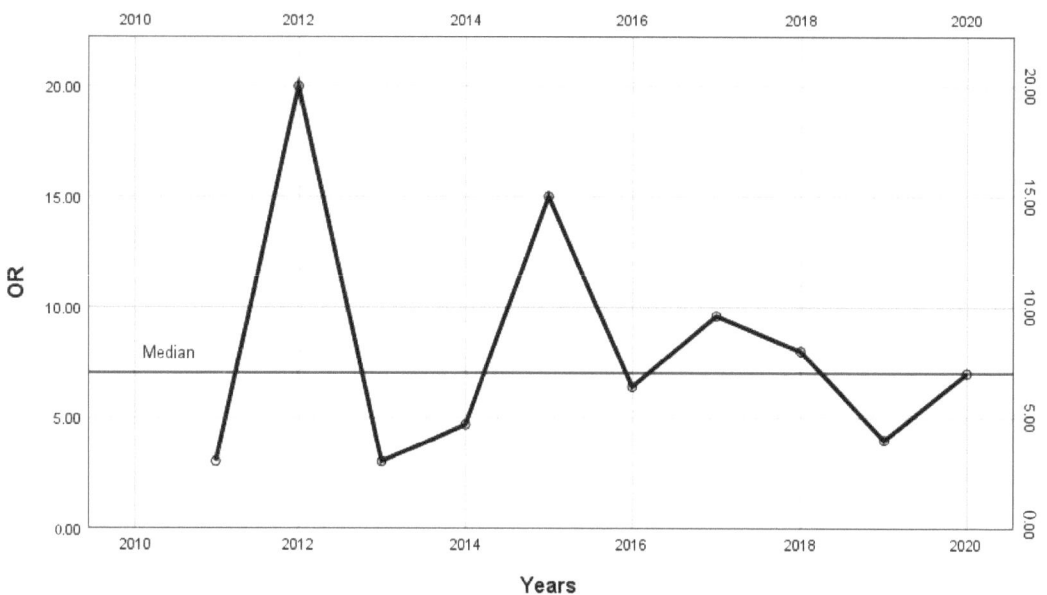

Figure 1. Relative risk (RR) ratios and odds ratio (OR) changes for cardiovascular conditions in patients with AS with medians.

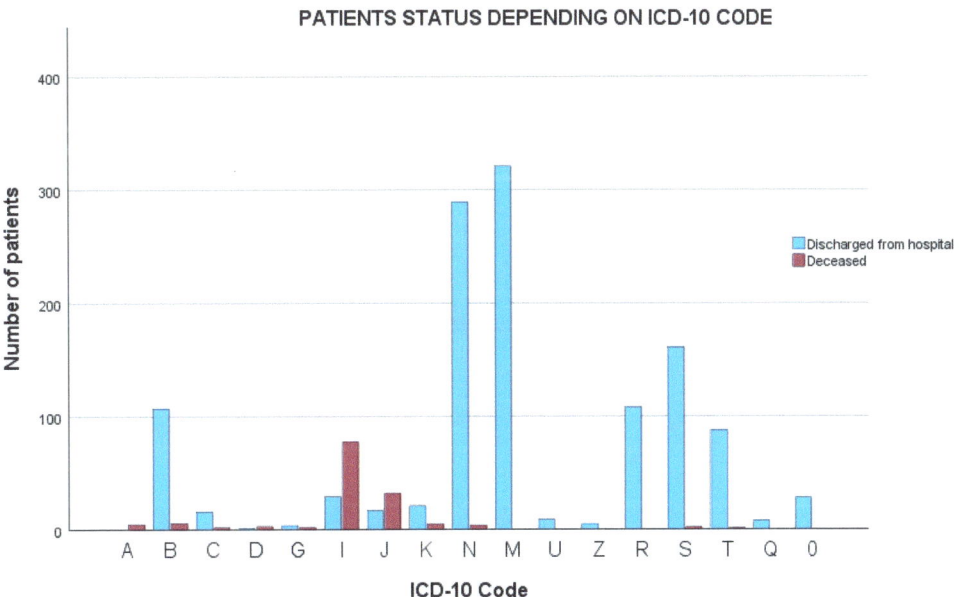

Figure 2. Percentage share of ICD-10 related deaths.

3.3. Associations between Initiation of Biological Treatment and Comorbidities

A total number of 4056 patients (7%) were hospitalized to administer the dosage of biological treatment (ICD-9 code 00.181). Demographic data are given in Table 3. In Poland, biological treatment is carried out in accordance with the EULAR standards [19], taking into account the recommendations of the Polish Society of Rheumatology and Polish law regulations. Patients with severe infection and pregnant were omitted from the analysis. Patients who qualified for biological therapy had lower rates of comorbidities, which can be explained partially by contradictions to anticytokine treatment, and so this that analysis was limited. Occurrence of uveitis was higher in the biologically treated group in comparison to the remaining patients with AS (10% vs. 3%). Since 2016, we observed a significant rise in the number of patients qualified for the biological treatment, namely from 2% in 2011 to 16% in 2020. We further analyzed the associations between comorbidities and hospital admission between 2011 and 2020, and significant correlations between the measured parameters, shown in Figure 3A–D. The total number of n = 256 patients were admitted to the hospital due to IHD. We found a statistically significant negative correlation between the number of patients with IHD per year and the number of patients initiating biological treatment ($p < 0.031$, $r = -0.8$), shown in Figure 3A. Also, the number of hospital admissions due to IHD correlated strongly and positively with the number of patients with pulmonary infections ($p < 0.021$ $r = 0.8$), given in Figure 3B. There was also a significant positive correlation between the total hospitalization count and pulmonary infections ($r = 0.65$; $p < 0.01$), as shown in Figure 3C. Finally, we observed a strong negative correlation between the number of IHD-based hospitalizations and the number of newly biologically treated patients per year ($r = -0.8$; $p < 0.008$), Figure 3D. There were no statistically significant correlations between the number of biologically treated patients and the number of newly diagnosed patients with neoplasms, hematological malignancies, and skin conditions, other than AS movement disorders, endocrinological disorders, eye disorders, neuropsychiatric conditions, or other conditions during pregnancy. There was only a statistically significant decline in the occurrence of CVD ($p < 0.001$) and pulmonary conditions ($p < 0.001$), but changes in the remaining comorbidities were statistically nonsignificant. There were also no correlations between the number of patients initiating biological treatment and hospital admissions or with overall hospital mortality.

Table 3. Comparison of comorbidities in patients treated with biologics in comparison to non-biological treatment group.

	ICD-Code	Biological Treatment (n = 4056)	Non-Biological Treatment (n = 49,086)
Endocrine, nutritional, and metabolic diseases	E00–E90	15 (0.3%)	4481 (0.8%)
Mental and behavioral disorders	F00–F99	10 (0.2%)	298 (0.5%)
Diseases of the nervous system	G00–G99	5 (0.1%)	906 (2%)
Diseases of the eye and adnexa	H00–H59	400 (10%)	1400 (3%)
Diseases of the circulatory system	I00–I99	52 (1,2%)	10,169 (19%)
Diseases of the respiratory system	J00–J99	4 (0.1%)	1909 (4%)
Diseases of the digestive system	K00–K93	123 (3%)	3128 (6%)
Diseases of the skin and subcutaneous tissue	L00–L99	3 (0.007%)	600 (1%)
Diseases of the genitourinary system	N00–N99	10 (0.02%)	1616 (3%)

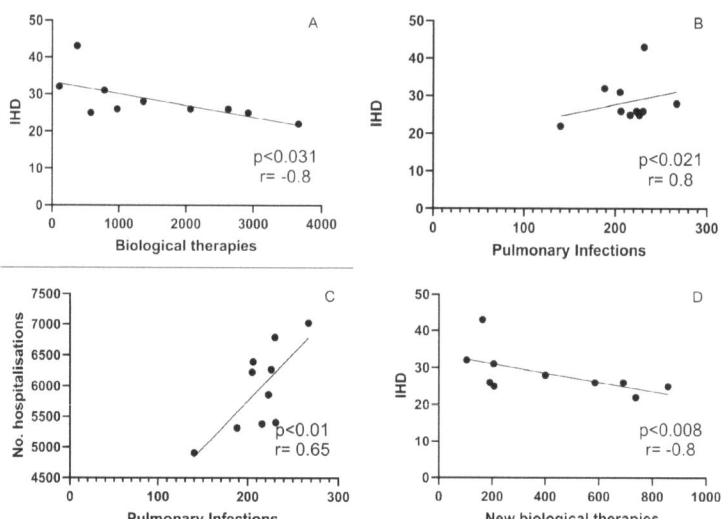

Figure 3. Correlations between (**A**)-cardiovascular diseases and number of biologically treated patients (**B**)-Correlations between IHD and pulmonary infections (**C**)-orrelation between hospitalization and pulmonary infections (**D**)-Correlations between IHD and new biological treatment programs.

4. Discussion

Increasing comorbidity, mortality, and associated socioeconomic costs position AS as a major public health problem. Patients with AS are burdened with higher cardiovascular risk as compared to the general population [20,21]. Following Gökşenoğlu et al. [22], the population with AS is burdened with more comorbidities that also seem to affect predicted pharmacological and surgical treatment outcomes [23]. Interestingly, despite differences between the enrolled populations in terms of chronic kidney disease or diabetes [22,24], our data are consistent with other research showing that AS is not associated with an increased risk of cancer or hematological malignancies [24,25]. Our first and key finding is that, despite the decline in hospitalization rates, relative mortality ratios from cardiovascular (CV) and pulmonary conditions remain higher among patients with AS compared to the observed for the general population admitted to the hospital. This is especially highlighted in male patients with AS. According to population studies, cardiovascular and circulatory system involvement is the main cause of an increased risk of stroke, myocardial infarct, and sudden cardiac death [21]. The increase in the general death ratio in the AS population is estimated from 1.36-fold up to 2.3 times [3,26] with a 50% higher cardiovascular risk (CVR) [26] in comparison to the general population. This phenomenon seems to originate from two main sources. First are the populational factors from INTERHEART [27] study such as smoking, gender, genetic factors, and lipid profile. Second are the factors that are secondary to chronic inflammation, typical for SpA [28–30]. So far, several studies have investigated factors suspected of being associated with an increased cardiovascular risk and with disease activity in patients with AS [31–33]. Also, there were data suggesting that clinical symptoms such as uveitis were associated with increased CVR [12,13]. Despite the high percentage of patients treated for uveitis in our study, we did not observe significantly higher mortality nor CV conditions in this group of patients. Also, in our study, there was no significant correlation between the occurrence of uveitis and the risk for mortality or other comorbidities. On the contrary, populational studies from Hong Kong by Feng et al. [34] had shown that uveitis is associated with a higher risk for mortality and risk for developing IHD. There are several differences between our study and the one conducted by Feng et al., as our study was based on the ICD codes, while the work by those authors was based on clinical data. Although there were more patients with AS included in our research, the group treated due to uveitis was relatively smaller (1400/53,145 vs. 1111/5555). Also, due to the retrospective nature of this study, our observations should be treated with caution.

Despite the limitations of our study, overall cardiovascular mortality in our research group was a total of 2.5% for all AS patients and 13% for patients with AS who were hospitalized for comorbidities other than movement disorders. Although the general mortality of the AS patients enrolled into our study surpassed 0.5% of the mortality described for the European population [35], our data were acquired from hospitals and are not comparable with those for the general population. Therefore, they should be addressed in a separate study. Yet, despite the limitations of this study, mortality due to comorbidities among in-hospitalized patients with AS(13%) was higher than one described by Walicka et al. for average mortality (4.1%), as well as for short term (5–7 days long) hospitalizations (2.63%) in Poland [36]. Also, in our cohort, CVD-related mortality (13% vs. 11.4%) as well as mortality related to pulmonary diseases (13% vs. 7.4%) was higher than the estimates for the general Polish population [37]. Yet, again due to the selective nature of our study, such observations should be verified in a separate study.

The EUROASPIRE III and EUROASPIRE IV (European Action on Secondary Prevention by Intervention to Reduce Events) survey showed that hypertension (HT) is the main cardiovascular risk factor [38,39], which translates to 40.6% of deaths from cardiovascular disease globally [40]. Our research shows that HT affected 15% of patients diagnosed with AS, which was compatible with populational studies [40–43] and similar to the research in the general Polish population by Liput-Sikora [44]. Yet, in our research after adjustment for age above 40 years, this percentage rose up to 25% in hospitalized patients. Such a discrepancy matches the populational data from the general population studies such as the NATPOL 2011 Survey (22%) and WOBASZ I and WOBASZ II (33%) [43]. Also, similar trends were described for the general Polish population [43]. Yet, despite positive trends for HT, mortality ratios and relative risk remain high despite the general trend for lowering of cardiovascular mortality in Poland [45]. This observation suggests discrepancies between patients with AS and the general population, supposedly delivering from chronic inflammation and disease activity. Yet, our data represent trends for the mainly male, high-CV risk population. Because of typical for AS imbalance in the male/female ratio, the presented data do not fully relate to the general population and should be interpreted within the context of studies focusing on AS.

Consequently, our findings show associations between a risk of hospitalization and cardiopulmonary comorbidities. Our outcomes stay in line with other research such as the study by Bittnar et al., which was obtained from the US population [16] and other studies [46]. In the analysis of hospitalized patients, we found that 45% of patients were diagnosed during hospitalization for CV condition, but also that 32% of AS patients were hospitalized due to obstructive airways diseases. Also, among inpatients, 22% were admitted to the hospital due to respiratory tract infections. This observation seems to originate from multiple overlapping factors. Lung diseases are associated with environmental factors such as air pollution [47,48], cigarette smoking, and several other risk factors. In recent years, research has focused on phenotypes of lung changes observed in the course of ankylosing spondylitis. Despite the fact that UIP/NSIP is not commonly associated with AS [49], several researchers had reported higher rates of pleural thickening, fibrotic changes, emphysema, and non-specific interstitial changes compared to the healthy controls [47]. Impairment in lung function leads to increased vulnerability for infections and development of COPD/emphysema, especially in actively smoking patients [48]. Also, the aforementioned conditions tend to share similar risk factors with secondary pulmonary hypertension, heart valvular diseases, arrhythmias, and chronic heart failure [49], further increasing the overall CV risk and general mortality rates. This issue has been addressed by Shrikrishina et al. in the European Heart Journal [43], where the authors suggested a new term, namely a cardiopulmonary risk. The above observations stand in line with the others available, supporting our findings considering the collinearity between CVD and pulmonary conditions [43]. Also, the rapidly increasing number of biologically treated patients seem to correlate negatively with the number of patients with AS admitted to the hospital with IHD. Yet, despite the promising results, due to the retrospective nature of this register analysis and the lack of clinical data (such as traditional CV risk factors) on biological treatment, we cannot directly associate the initiation of biological treatment with a decrease in IHDs, and so this should be addressed in further studies. Due to the small number of patients diagnosed with AS (below 0.5% of population) and overlapping multiple factors, the research on the populational scale is difficult in AS. Considering the limitations of our study, the most efficient further approach would be combining populational and clinical data in the form of a register, such as the British Society for Rheumatology Biologics Register in Ankylosing Spondylitis (BSRBR-AS) [50] or the Framingham Heart Study [51].

Our second finding concerns the different disease phenotype in female patients with AS. Our study revealed a higher occurrence of inflammatory bowel diseases in female patients. Several other researchers [50–52] had reported similar clinical differences in the SpA's disease progression, but also higher rates of subclinical bowel inflammation in female patients with AS [8,53,54]. In other studies, higher ratios of insidious back pain, worse responses to anti-TNF treatment, and higher rates of peripheral joint inflammation [52] were described in females with AS. Therefore, a personalized clinical approach should be advised, considering other than axial symptoms of SpA in female patietns.

Finally, our study has several limitations. First, our analysis was retrospectively based on reported ICD-10 codes and in-hospital procedures and not on real life data. This analytic approach limits our outcomes because we were unable to analyze clinical data, biochemical parameters, or potential differences between biological drugs used in treatment of AS. Secondly, due to our retrospective approach, we were not able to verify the diagnosis of AS/M45 or obtain additional data on disease progression nor clinical data such as occurrence of dactylitis, spondylitis, or other comorbidities such as dyslipidemia or obesity. Also, we encountered difficulties during analysis that are typical for register-based studies, mainly the lack of data and necessity to exclude missing valuables from analysis. Finally, we were unable to perform a direct cause–effect analysis of multiple overlapping factors such as biological treatments on CV risk or comorbidities due to the lack of clinical data.

5. Conclusions

A decrease in hospitalizations of patients with AS was observed, yet overall mortality in the AS population seems to be higher than in the general Polish population. Despite a decrease in hospitalization rates and morbidity remaining at a stable 2.5% level, in-hospital mortality exceeded the indices for the general population in patients with AS when they were hospitalized due to comorbidities. Cardiopulmonary comorbidities seem to be a main factor associated with increased mortality rates and higher than populational mortality. Our research shows that biological treatment might be associated with lower risk of IHD, yet due to the limitations of our study it should be approached with caution and addressed in further research. Male patients with AS seem to be at a higher risk of overall mortality; thus, prevention and health programs should focused on patients with AS.

Author Contributions: Conceptualization, K.B., K.H., M.W., K.K., A.N.-O. and P.G.; data curation; K.B., K.H., M.W., K.K., A.N.-O. and P.G.; formal analysis; K.B., K.H., and K.K.; investigation, K.H.; methodology, M.W., K.K., A.N.-O., and P.G.; Resources, M.W.; validation, M.W., K.K., A.N.-O., and P.G.; visualization, K.B. and K.H.; writing—original; draft preparation, K.B., K.H., M.W., K.K., A.N.-O., and P.G.; writing—review and editing, K.B., K.H., M.W., K.K., A.N.-O., and P.G.; supervision M.W., P.G., A.N.-O., and P.G.; funding acquisition, M.W. All authors have read and agreed to the published version of the manuscript.

Funding: This research received no external funding.

Institutional Review Board Statement: The study was conducted in accordance with the Declaration of Helsinki and approved by the Ethics Committee of the National Institute of Geriatrics, Rheumatology, and Rehabilitation, Warsaw, Poland (approval N KBT-2 March 2022) for studies involving raw data.

Informed Consent Statement: Not applicable.

Data Availability Statement: Data are available upon reasonable request according to ICMJE requirements: Data shared: All the individual participant data were collected during the trial, after deidentification. Available documents: study protocol, statistical analysis, analytic code. When will data be available: beginning three months and ending two years following the article's publication. With whom: Researchers who provide a methodologically sound proposal. For what type of analyses: to achieve the aim of the approved proposal. By what mechanism will data be made available: The proposal should be directed to katarzyna.helon@spartanska.pl.

Conflicts of Interest: The authors declare no conflicts of interest.

References

1. Moltó, A.; Nikiphorou, E. Comorbidities in Spondyloarthritis. *Front. Med.* **2018**, *5*, 62. [CrossRef] [PubMed]
2. Webers, C.; Vanhoof, L.; Leue, C.; Boonen, A.; Köhler, S. Depression in ankylosing spondylitis and the role of disease-related and contextual factors: A cross-sectional study. *Arthritis Res. Ther.* **2019**, *21*, 215. [CrossRef] [PubMed]
3. Kelty, E.; Ognjenovic, M.; Raymond, W.D.; Inderjeeth, C.A.; Keen, H.I.; Preen, D.B.; Nossent, J.C. Mortality Rates in Patients with Ankylosing Spondylitis with and without Extraarticular Manifestations and Comorbidities: A Retrospective Cohort Study. *J. Rheumatol.* **2022**, *49*, 688–693. [CrossRef] [PubMed]
4. Deng, P.; Fu, Y.; Chen, M.; Wang, D.; Si, L. Temporal trends in inequalities of the burden of cardiovascular disease across 186 countries and territories. *Int. J. Equity Health* **2023**, *22*, 164. [CrossRef] [PubMed]
5. Nikiphorou, E.; Nurmohamed, M.T.; Szekanecz, Z. Editorial: Comorbidity Burden in Rheumatic Diseases. *Front. Med.* **2018**, *5*, 197. [CrossRef] [PubMed]
6. Kim, T.E.; Lee, R.G.; Park, S.Y.; Oh, I.H. Measuring Trends in the Socioeconomic Burden of Disease in Korea, 2007–2015. *J. Prev. Med. Public Health* **2022**, *55*, 19–27. [CrossRef]
7. Toussirot, E. The Risk of Cardiovascular Diseases in Axial Spondyloarthritis. Current Insights. *Front. Med.* **2021**, *8*, 782150. [CrossRef]
8. Fragoulis, G.E.; Liava, C.; Daoussis, D.; Akriviadis, E.; Garyfallos, A.; Dimitroulas, T. Inflammatory bowel diseases and spondyloarthropathies: From pathogenesis to treatment. *World J. Gastroenterol.* **2019**, *25*, 2162–2176. [CrossRef]
9. Rosen, M.J.; Dhawan, A.; Saeed, S.A. Inflammatory bowel disease in children and adolescents. *JAMA Pediatr.* **2015**, *169*, 1053–1060. [CrossRef]
10. Ranganathan, V.; Gracey, E.; Brown, M.A.; Inman, R.D.; Haroon, N. Pathogenesis of ankylosing spondylitis—Recent advances and future directions. *Nat. Rev. Rheumatol.* **2017**, *13*, 359–367. [CrossRef]

11. Lin, A.; Tan, Y.; Chen, J.; Liu, X.; Wu, J. Development of ankylosing spondylitis in patients with ulcerative colitis: A systematic meta-analysis. *PLoS ONE.* **2023**, *18*, e0289021. [CrossRef] [PubMed]
12. Pandey, A.; Ravindran, V. Ocular Manifestations of Spondyloarthritis. *Mediterr. J. Rheumatol.* **2023**, *34*, 24–29. [CrossRef] [PubMed]
13. Lai, Y.F.; Lin, T.Y.; Chien, W.C.; Sun, C.A.; Chung, C.H.; Chen, Y.H.; Chen, J.T.; Chen, C.L. Uveitis as a Risk Factor for Developing Acute Myocardial Infarction in Ankylosing Spondylitis: A National Population-Based Longitudinal Cohort Study. *Front. Immunol.* **2022**, *12*, 811664. [CrossRef] [PubMed]
14. Chang, C.C.; Chang, C.W.; Nguyen, P.A.; Chang, T.H.; Shih, Y.L.; Chang, W.Y.; Horng, J.T.; Lee, O.K.; Ho, J.H. Ankylosing spondylitis and the risk of cancer. *Oncol. Lett.* **2017**, *14*, 1315–1322. [CrossRef] [PubMed]
15. Feltelius, N.; Ekbom, A.; Blomqvist, P. Cancer incidence among patients with ankylosing spondylitis in Sweden 1965–95: A population based cohort study. *Ann. Rheum. Dis.* **2003**, *62*, 1185–1188. [CrossRef] [PubMed]
16. Bittar, M.; Merjanah, S.; Alkilany, R.; Magrey, M. Malignancy in ankylosing spondylitis: A cross-sectional analysis of a large population database. *BMC Rheumatol.* **2022**, *6*, 44. [CrossRef] [PubMed]
17. Kagan, P.; Horesh, N.; Amital, H.; Tsur, A.M.; Watad, A.; Cohen, A.D.; Ben-Shabat, N. The Risk and Predictors of Malignancies in Ankylosing Spondylitis Patients in Israel—A Retrospective Electronic Data-Based Study. *J. Clin. Med.* **2023**, *12*, 5153. [CrossRef]
18. Charlson, M.E.; Wells, M.T. Comorbidity: From a Confounder in Longitudinal Clinical Research to the Main Issue in Population Management. *Psychother. Psychosom.* **2022**, *91*, 145–151. [CrossRef]
19. Shrikrishna, D.; Taylor, C.J.; Stonham, C.; Gale, C.P. Exacerbating the burden of cardiovascular disease: How can we address cardiopulmonary risk in individuals with chronic obstructive pulmonary disease? *Eur. Heart J.* **2023**, ehad669. [CrossRef]
20. Kao, C.-M.; Wang, J.-S.; Ho, W.-L.; Ko, T.-M.; Chen, H.-M.; Lin, C.-H.; Huang, W.-N.; Chen, Y.-H.; Chen, H.-H. Factors Associated with the Risk of Major Adverse Cardiovascular Events in Patients with Ankylosing Spondylitis: A Nationwide, Population-Based Case—Control Study. *Int. J. Environ. Res. Public Health* **2022**, *19*, 4098. [CrossRef]
21. Joodi, G.; Maradey, J.A.; Bogle, B.; Mirzaei, M.; Sadaf, M.I.; Pursell, I.; Henderson, C.; Mounsey, J.P.; Simpson, R.J., Jr. Coronary Artery Disease and Atherosclerotic Risk Factors in a Population-Based Study of Sudden Death. *J. Gen. Intern. Med.* **2020**, *35*, 531–537. [CrossRef] [PubMed]
22. Gökşenoğlu, G.; Buğdaycı, D.; Paker, N.; Yıldırım, M.A.; Etli, Ö. The prevalence of comorbidity and predictors in ankylosing spondylitis. *Turk. J. Phys. Med. Rehabil.* **2018**, *65*, 132–138. [CrossRef] [PubMed]
23. Ull, C.; Yilmaz, E.; Hoffmann, M.F.; Reinke, C.; Aach, M.; Schildhauer, T.A.; Kruppa, C. Factors Associated with Major Complications and Mortality During Hospitalization in Patients with Ankylosing Spondylitis Undergoing Surgical Management for a Spine Fracture. *Glob. Spine J.* **2022**, *12*, 1380–1387. [CrossRef] [PubMed]
24. Kelty, E.; Raymond, W.; Inderjeeth, C.; Keen, H.; Nossent, J.; Preen, D.B. Cancer diagnosis and mortality in patients with ankylosing spondylitis: A Western Australian retrospective cohort study. *Int. J. Rheum. Dis.* **2021**, *24*, 216–222. [CrossRef] [PubMed]
25. Ye, W.; Zhuang, J.; Yu, Y.; Li, H.; Leng, X.; Qian, J.; Qin, Y.; Chen, L.; Li, X.M. Gender and chronic kidney disease in ankylosing spondylitis: A single-center retrospectively study. *BMC Nephrol.* **2019**, *20*, 457. [CrossRef]
26. Eriksson, J.K.; Jacobsson, L.; Bengtsson, K.; Askling, J. Is ankylosing spondylitis a risk factor for cardiovascular disease, and how do these risks compare with those in rheumatoid arthritis? *Ann. Rheum. Dis.* **2017**, *76*, 364–370. [CrossRef]
27. Yusuf, S.; Hawken, S.; Ounpuu, S.; Dans, T.; Avezum, A.; Lanas, F.; McQueen, M.; Budaj, A.; Pais, P.; Varigos, J.; et al. Effect of potentially modifiable risk factors associated with myocardial infarction in 52 countries (the INTERHEART study): Case-control study. *Lancet* **2004**, *364*, 937–952. [CrossRef]
28. Berg, I.J.; van der Heijde, D.; Dagfinrud, H.; Seljeflot, I.; Olsen, I.C.; Kvien, T.K.; Semb, A.G.; Provan, S.A. Disease activity in ankylosing spondylitis and associations to markers of vascular pathology and traditional cardiovascular disease risk factors: A cross-sectional study. *J. Rheumatol.* **2015**, *42*, 645–653. [CrossRef]
29. Berger, M.; Fesler, P.; Roubille, C. Arterial stiffness, the hidden face of cardiovascular risk in autoimmune and chronic inflammatory rheumatic diseases. *Autoimmun. Rev.* **2021**, *20*, 102891. [CrossRef]
30. Asenjo-Lobos, C.; González, L.; Bulnes, J.F.; Roque, M.; Muñoz Venturelli, P.; Rodríguez, G.M. Cardiovascular events risk in patients with systemic autoimmune diseases: A prognostic systematic review and meta-analysis. *Clin. Res. Cardiol.* **2023**, ahead of print. [CrossRef]
31. Bengtsson, K.; Forsblad-d'Elia, H.; Lie, E.; Klingberg, E.; Dehlin, M.; Exarchou, S.; Lindström, U.; Askling, J.; Jacobsson, L.T. Are ankylosing spondylitis, psoriatic arthritis and undifferentiated spondyloarthritis associated with an increased risk of cardiovascular events? A prospective nationwide population-based cohort study. *Arthritis Res. Ther.* **2017**, *19*, 102. [CrossRef] [PubMed]
32. Brembilla, N.C.; Senra, L.; Boehncke, W.H. The IL-17 family of cytokines in psoriasis: IL-17A and beyond. *Front. Immunol.* **2018**, *9*, 1682. [CrossRef] [PubMed]
33. Bonek, K.; Kuca-Warnawin, E.; Kornatka, A.; Zielińska, A.; Wisłowska, M.; Kontny, E.; Głuszko, P. Associations of IL-18 with Altered Cardiovascular Risk Profile in Psoriatic Arthritis and Ankylosing Spondylitis. *J. Clin. Med.* **2022**, *11*, 766. [CrossRef] [PubMed]
34. Feng, K.M.; Chien, W.-C.; Chen, Y.-H.; Sun, C.-A.; Chung, C.-H.; Chen, J.-T.; Chen, C.-L. Increased Risk of Acute Coronary Syndrome in Ankylosing Spondylitis Patients with Uveitis: A Population-Based Cohort Study. *Front. Immunol.* **2022**, *13*, 890543. [CrossRef] [PubMed]

35. Karmacharya, P.; Shahukhal, R.; Crowson, C.S.; Murad, M.H.; Davis, J.M., 3rd; Shrestha, P.; Bekele, D.; Wright, K.; Chakradhar, R.; Dubreuil, M. Effects of Therapies on Cardiovascular Events in Ankylosing Spondylitis: A Systematic Review and Meta-Analysis. *Rheumatol. Ther.* **2020**, *7*, 993–1009. [CrossRef] [PubMed]
36. Bała, M.M.; Koperny, M.; Stefanoff, P. In-hospital mortality in Poland: What can we learn from administrative data? *Pol. Arch. Intern. Med.* **2020**, *130*, 264–265. [CrossRef] [PubMed]
37. Walicka, M.; Chlebus, M.; Śliwczyński, A.; Brzozowska, M.; Rutkowski, D.; Czech, M.; Tuszyńska, A.; Jacyna, A.; Puzianowska-Kuźnicka, M.; Franek, E. Predictors of in-hospital mortality in nonsurgical departments: A multivariable regression analysis of 2855029 hospitalizations. *Pol. Arch. Intern. Med.* **2020**, *130*, 268–275. [CrossRef]
38. De Smedt, D.; De Bacquer, D.; De Sutter, J.; Dallongeville, J.; Gevaert, S.; De Backer, G.; Bruthans, J.; Kotseva, K.; Reiner, Ž.; Tokgözoğlu, L.; et al. The gender gap in risk factor control: Effects of age and education on the control of cardiovascular risk factors in male and female coronary patients. The EUROASPIRE IV study by the European Society of Cardiology. *Int. J. Cardiol.* **2016**, *209*, 284–290. [CrossRef]
39. Kotseva, K.; Wood, D.; De Bacquer, D.; De Backer, G.; Rydén, L.; Jennings, C.; Gyberg, V.; Amouyel, P.; Bruthans, J.; Castro Conde, A.; et al. EUROASPIRE IV: A European Society of Cardiology survey on the lifestyle, risk factor and therapeutic management of coronary patients from 24 European countries. *Eur. J. Prev. Cardiol.* **2016**, *23*, 636–648. [CrossRef]
40. Go, A.S.; Mozaffarian, D.; Roger, V.L.; Benjamin, E.J.; Berry, J.D.; Blaha, M.J.; Dai, S.; Ford, E.S.; Fox, C.S.; Franco, S.; et al. Executive summary: Heart disease and stroke statistics—2014 update: Report from the American Heart Association. *Circulation* **2014**, *129*, 399–410. [CrossRef]
41. Hung, Y.M.; Chang, W.P.; Wei, J.C.; Chou, P.; Wang, P.Y.P. Midlife ankylosing spondylitis increases the risk of cardiovascular diseases in males 5 years later: A national population-based study. *Medicine* **2016**, *95*, e3596. [CrossRef] [PubMed]
42. Ahmed, N.; Prior, J.A.; Chen, Y.; Hayward, R.; Mallen, C.D.; Hider, S.L. Prevalence of cardiovascular-related comorbidity in ankylosing spondylitis, psoriatic arthritis and psoriasis in primary care: A matched retrospective cohort study. *Clin. Rheumatol.* **2016**, *35*, 3069–3073. [CrossRef] [PubMed]
43. Niklas, A.; Flotyńska, A.; Puch-Walczak, A.; Polakowska, M.; Topór-Mądry, R.; Polak, M.; Piotrowski, W.; Kwaśniewska, M.; Nadrowski, P.; Pająk, A.; et al. Prevalence, awareness, treatment and control of hypertension in the adult Polish population—Multi-center National Population Health Examination Surveys—WOBASZ studies. *Arch. Med. Sci.* **2018**, *14*, 951–961. [CrossRef] [PubMed]
44. Liput-Sikora, A.; Cybulska, A.M.; Fabian, W.; Stanisławska, M.; Kamińska, M.S.; Grochans, E.; Jurczak, A. The Severity of Changes in Cardiovascular Risk Factors in Adults over a Five-Year Interval. *Clin. Interv. Aging* **2020**, *15*, 1979–1990. [CrossRef] [PubMed]
45. Moryson, W.; Kalinowski, P.; Kotecki, P.; Stawińska-Witoszyńska, B. Changes in the Level of Premature Mortality in the Polish Population Due to Selected Groups of Cardiovascular Diseases before and during the Pandemic of COVID-19. *J. Clin. Med.* **2023**, *12*, 2913. [CrossRef] [PubMed]
46. Pond, Z.A.; Hernandez, C.S.; Adams, P.J.; Pandis, S.N.; Garcia, G.R.; Robinson, A.L.; Marshall, J.D.; Burnett, R.; Skyllakou, K.; Garcia Rivera, P.; et al. Cardiopulmonary Mortality and Fine Particulate Air Pollution by Species and Source in a National U.S. Cohort. *Environ. Sci. Technol.* **2022**, *56*, 7214–7223. [CrossRef] [PubMed]
47. Momeni, M.; Taylor, N.; Tehrani, M. Cardiopulmonary manifestations of ankylosing spondylitis. *Int. J. Rheumatol.* **2011**, *2011*, 728471. [CrossRef]
48. Bhat, T.A.; Panzica, L.; Kalathil, S.G.; Thanavala, Y. Immune Dysfunction in Patients with Chronic Obstructive Pulmonary Disease. *Ann. Am. Thorac. Soc.* **2015**, *12* (Suppl. 2), S169–S175. [CrossRef]
49. Oakes, J.M.; Xu, J.; Morris, T.M.; Fried, N.D.; Pearson, C.S.; Lobell, T.D.; Gilpin, N.W.; Lazartigues, E.; Gardner, J.D.; Yue, X. Effects of Chronic Nicotine Inhalation on Systemic and Pulmonary Blood Pressure and Right Ventricular Remodeling in Mice. *Hypertension* **2020**, *75*, 1305–1314. [CrossRef]
50. Available online: https://www.abdn.ac.uk/iahs/research/epidemiology/bsrbras-1438.php (accessed on 11 June 2023).
51. Lungaro, L.; Costanzini, A.; Manza, F.; Barbalinardo, M.; Gentili, D.; Guarino, M.; Caputo, F.; Zoli, G.; De Giorgio, R.; Caio, G. Impact of Female Gender in Inflammatory Bowel Diseases: A Narrative Review. *J. Pers. Med.* **2023**, *13*, 165. [CrossRef]
52. Available online: https://www.framinghamheartstudy.org/ (accessed on 11 June 2023).
53. Laganà, B.; Zullo, A.; Scribano, M.L.; Chimenti, M.S.; Migliore, A.; Picchianti Diamanti, A.; Lorenzetti, R.; Scolieri, P.; Ridola, L.; Ortona, E.; et al. Sex Differences in Response to TNF-Inhibiting Drugs in Patients with Spondyloarthropathies or Inflammatory Bowel Diseases. *Front. Pharmacol.* **2019**, *10*, 47. [CrossRef] [PubMed]
54. Rusman, T.; van Vollenhoven, R.F.; van der Horst-Bruinsma, I.E. Gender Differences in Axial Spondyloarthritis: Women Are Not So Lucky. *Curr. Rheumatol. Rep.* **2018**, *20*, 35. [CrossRef] [PubMed]

Disclaimer/Publisher's Note: The statements, opinions and data contained in all publications are solely those of the individual author(s) and contributor(s) and not of MDPI and/or the editor(s). MDPI and/or the editor(s) disclaim responsibility for any injury to people or property resulting from any ideas, methods, instructions or products referred to in the content.

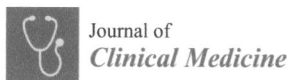

Article

Sex Differences in the Relationship between Personal, Psychological and Biochemical Factors with Blood Pressure in a Healthy Adult Mexican Population: A Cross-Sectional Study

Blanca Estela Ríos-González [1,2], Ana Míriam Saldaña-Cruz [3,*], Sergio Gabriel Gallardo-Moya [4] and Aniel Jessica Leticia Brambila-Tapia [5,*]

1. Unidad Médico Familiar #92, Instituto Mexicano del Seguro Social (IMSS), Guadalajara 44340, Mexico; blanca2282@hotmail.com
2. Especialidad en Medicina Familiar, Centro Universitario de Ciencias de la Salud (CUCS), Universidad de Guadalajara, Guadalajara 44340, Mexico
3. Departamento de Fisiología, Centro Universitario de Ciencias de la Salud (CUCS), Universidad de Guadalajara, Guadalajara 44340, Mexico
4. Programa de Doctorado en Farmacología, Departamento de Fisiología, Centro Universitario de Ciencias de la Salud (CUCS), Universidad de Guadalajara, Guadalajara 44340, Mexico; sergio.gallardo@alumnos.udg.mx
5. Departamento de Psicología Básica, Centro Universitario de Ciencias de la Salud (CUCS), Universidad de Guadalajara, Guadalajara 44340, Mexico
* Correspondence: ana.saldanac@academicos.udg.mx (A.M.S.-C.); aniel.brambila@academicos.udg.mx (A.J.L.B.-T.)

Abstract: Hypertension is one of the main risk factors related to cardiovascular mortality, being the levels of blood pressure (BP) related to a variety of personal, anthropometric, biochemical and psychological variables; however, the study evaluating the association of all these factors in systolic blood pressure (SBP) and diastolic blood pressure (DBP) in a sample of relatively healthy subjects has not been performed. The aim of the study was to determine the main variables associated with SBP and DPB in a sample of relatively healthy subjects. A total of 171 participants were included, in which personal, anthropometric, positive and negative psychological variables and biochemical variables were measured. We observed that men showed higher levels of SBP and DBP than women, with more differences for SBP. Among the biochemical factors and SBP, we found that albumin and monocytes were positively correlated with it, while potassium, phosphorus and eosinophils were negatively correlated with it. Additionally, schooling was a constant variable negatively correlated with SBP in all samples (global, men and women). Among psychological variables, we observed that emotional perception was negatively correlated with SBP in men's and women's samples, while autonomy was positively correlated with SBP in the men's sample; however, their association was less when compared with the personal and biochemical variables included in the multivariate model. With regard to DBP, we observed that the biochemical variables, hemoglobin, sodium, uric acid and glucose, were positively correlated with DBP in the global sample, while chloride and BUN were negatively correlated with it. In addition, many personal and behavioral variables, including BMI, age and smoking consumption frequency, also correlated with DBP in the global sample. In conclusion, BP is affected by different factors, and these affect each sex differently.

Keywords: systolic blood pressure; diastolic blood pressure; biochemical variables; psychological factors; anthropometric factors; sex

Citation: Ríos-González, B.E.; Saldaña-Cruz, A.M.; Gallardo-Moya, S.G.; Brambila-Tapia, A.J.L. Sex Differences in the Relationship between Personal, Psychological and Biochemical Factors with Blood Pressure in a Healthy Adult Mexican Population: A Cross-Sectional Study. *J. Clin. Med.* **2024**, *13*, 378. https://doi.org/10.3390/jcm13020378

Academic Editors: Justyna Wyszyńska and Piotr Matłosz

Received: 22 November 2023
Revised: 4 January 2024
Accepted: 6 January 2024
Published: 10 January 2024

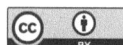

Copyright: © 2024 by the authors. Licensee MDPI, Basel, Switzerland. This article is an open access article distributed under the terms and conditions of the Creative Commons Attribution (CC BY) license (https://creativecommons.org/licenses/by/4.0/).

1. Introduction

High levels of blood pressure (BP) are associated with cardiovascular mortality since high levels are associated with a greater probability of acute myocardial infarction or stroke [1]. BP can be modified by several factors, including personal (age and ethnicity), anthropometric (those related to body adiposity), biochemical (blood count cells, uric acid and serum electrolytes) and psychological ones [1–6]. In the case of psychological factors, this relationship is explained by considering that emotions affect BP by impacting the sympathetic nervous system and the hypothalamic–pituitary–adrenal axis [2]. Norepinephrine is an indirect marker of sympathetic tone, and this is usually elevated in hypertensive patients, both in the sympathetic nerve terminals as well as in the urine. In addition, high levels of noradrenaline and dopamine have also been observed in depression [7]. This shows a link between emotional states and hypertension. In addition, a previous report showed that variations in depression and mental health in people with hypertension and metabolic syndrome produced a modification in BP over time [8]. Another report showed that emotion recognition ability was higher in normotensive people when compared with pre-hypertensives and hypertensives [9]. Furthermore, a recent report showed that anxiety disorders and depression are associated with resistant hypertension [10]. Finally, it was recently demonstrated that trait anger was associated with increases in BP in an experimental group of hypertensive people [11].

On the other hand, it has been shown that serum electrolytes and biochemical parameters influence BP. A study performed in hypertensive and normotensive men showed that hypertensive men had higher levels of glucose, cholesterol and triglycerides, as well as higher levels of sodium, chloride and potassium when compared with normotensive men [12]. Additionally, high salt intake has been related to an increase in BP and arterial stiffness [13], while potassium intake has been associated with BP-lowering effects, mainly in hypertensive people [3]. However, a study searching for the association between personal, biochemical, anthropometric and psychological factors in order to determine their correlation with systolic blood pressure (SBP) and diastolic blood pressure (DBP) in relatively healthy people has not been performed. This study is necessary in order to understand the relationships among all these variables with BP when adjusted with the other ones.

Therefore, our objective was to determine the association between personal, anthropometric, biochemical and psychological variables, including positive (positive emotions, well-being, optimism and emotional intelligence) and negative (negative emotions, depression and anxiety) psychological factors, with BP in a sample of a relatively healthy population.

The hypotheses were: (1) There are sex differences in BP, with men having higher levels of it; (2) Presence of negative psychological factors are associated with higher BP, while positive factors are associated with lower BP, after adjustment for biochemical factors; (3) The association of psychological, personal, anthropometric and biochemical factors in BP impacts differently between sexes.

2. Subjects and Methods

2.1. Ethical Considerations

The study was conducted according to the guidelines of the Declaration of Helsinki and was approved by the ethical committee of the Health Sciences University Center, with the registration number: 19–21, approval date: 14 October 2019. All the participants signed an informed consent.

2.2. Subjects

The inclusion criteria were: (a) to be older than 18 years old, (b) do not have chronic or acute diseases known by the subject (self-reported), (c) subjects who were not consuming illegal drugs, (d) subjects who were not consuming hormonal products to increase muscular mass, (e) subjects who were not pregnant, (f) subjects who were not genetically related to another participant of the study (i.e., brothers, cousins), and (g) subjects who preferably did not smoke. The elimination criterium was: the absence of the measurement of any variable.

2.2.1. Study Design: Cross-Sectional Study

This study consists of the measurement of several variables at the same point in time in order to establish possible relationships between them.

2.2.2. Procedures

The invitation was performed through the distribution of an announcement via social networks (WhatsApp, Facebook); additionally, in order to complete the minimum sample size, we invited university students personally. All the potential participants met the inclusion criteria; if they accepted to participate, they were cited in computer rooms of the University of Guadalajara, where they signed informed consent and filled out Google Forms questionnaires which included personal, behavioral and psychological variables. After filling out the questionnaire, the anthropometric indexes, body mass index (BMI) and waist-to-hip ratio (WHR), were obtained, along with the SBP and DBP measurements.

The blood and samples were obtained by trained personnel who worked for a certified laboratory. All the samples were transported to a certified laboratory, where the biochemical analyses were performed. No payment was offered to participants. As an advantage for participating, their biochemical results were sent to them along with a medical interpretation. In this sense, it is important to clarify that all the surveys were filled on computers and in person, where any doubt could be clarified by the research team.

2.2.3. Sample Size

The sample size was calculated with the formula for bivariate correlations [14], which was estimated to detect a statistical confidence of 95% and a statistical power of 80% for a minimum correlation value of 0.2, which means a very low correlation. This formula yielded a total of 67 subjects. However, the minimum sample size intended was 80 individuals per sex. In this sense, we used this formula in order to detect very low bivariate correlations as significant, and we did not adjust for a specific number of independent variables because no formulas for multivariate analyses were found. However, with this formula, we expected to detect clinically relevant correlations in the bivariate and multivariate analyses.

When multivariate analyses are carried out, a large sample size is desirable in order to avoid false results, with a minimum of 10 participants per variable; nevertheless, when it is not reachable, multivariate analyses can also be performed in order to diminish the confusion bias produced by the influence of multiple variables in a dependent variable, being cautious with the interpretation.

2.3. Personal Variables

The following personal and behavioral variables were measured: age, sex, schooling, whether they had a job, a romantic partner, and children, socioeconomic level, daily hours of physical activity, daily free hours, and monthly extra money. The monthly extra money variable was measured with 5 categories, ranging from nothing to more than USD 180. The frequency of alcohol and smoking consumption was measured with 5 categories: from never to 4 or more times in a week. Sleep satisfaction was measured with the first item of the OVIEDO sleep questionnaire, with the answer options ranging from 1 (very unsatisfied) to 7 (very satisfied); sleep quality was measured with the second item (which included 5 items) of the OVIEDO sleep questionnaire, which ranged from 1–5 (low sleep quality to high sleep quality) [15]. We measured the quality of food intake with the Mini-Ecca scale, which ranged from 1–12 (very low quality to very high quality) [16]. We also measured two questions of eating behavior: (a) the frequency of food consumption in excess and (b) the frequency of food consumption outside the home. Both questions were measured with 7 answer options, ranging from 1 (less than once in a month) to 7 (all the days); these two questions were obtained from the eating behavioral questionnaire [17].

2.4. Measurement of Anthropometric Variables

The height and weight were obtained by trained personnel with a Tanita brand scale (model bc-533) and measuring tape attached to the wall to calculate the BMI. The hips and waist circumferences were also obtained by trained personnel by using a measuring tape. These measurements were used to calculate the waist/hip ratio (WHR).

2.5. Measurement of Blood Pressure

The measurements of SBP and DBP of the participants were performed with the subject sitting with the left arm placed in semiflexion at the level of the hearth. This was performed through an automated procedure by using an upper arm BP monitor brand Omron (model Hem-7320).

2.6. Psychological Variables

We measured the following psychological variables: depressive symptoms, with the 10-items CES-D scale, ranging from 1 (none of the days) to 4 (all the days) [18,19]; anxiety symptoms, with the Generalized Anxiety Disorder test (GAD-7), ranging from 0 (never) to 3 (almost all the days) [20]; the presence of positive and negative emotions, with the positivity-self scale (PSS), ranging from 1 (never) to 5 (almost always) [21]; the 6 subscales of the shortened version of the scale of psychological well-being (PWB) (including self-acceptance, environmental mastery, autonomy, personal growth, purpose in life and positive relations with others), with the scale ranging from 1 (totally disagree) to 6 (totally agree) [22]; optimism was measured with the Life Orientation Test (LOT-R), ranging from 1 (totally disagree) to 5 (totally agree) [23]; additionally, we measured 5–6 items of 4 subscales of the Trait Emotional Intelligence Questionnaire (TEIQUE), which included: emotion perception (5 items), self-motivation (5 items), emotion regulation (6 items) and assertiveness (6 items), which ranged from 1 (totally disagree) to 7 (totally agree). These items are described in the Supplementary file [24].

2.7. Biochemical Variables Measurement

Analyses of biochemical variables were performed in a certificated laboratory. Blood samples were obtained to quantify the following: (1) complete blood count test (including leucocytes and their subpopulations, erythrocytes and hematocrit), (2) complete lipid profile test (total cholesterol, low-density lipoprotein (LDL), high-density lipoprotein (HDL) and triglycerides), (3) liver function tests (gamma-glutamyl transferase (GGT), aspartate aminotransferase (AST), alkaline phosphatase (ALP), alanine aminotransferase (ALT), lactate dehydrogenase (LDH) enzymes and direct and indirect bilirubin, albumin and total proteins), (4) blood chemistry (creatinine, glucose, urea, uric acid and blood urea nitrogen (BUN)), (5) serum electrolytes (including calcium, phosphorus, magnesium, iron, sodium, potassium and chloride) and (6) pancreatic enzymes (amylase and lipase). All the values detected that were out of range were double-checked in order to verify them.

2.8. Statistical Analysis

In order to perform the description of continuous variables, mean and standard deviations were used when the distribution was parametric, and median and ranges when it was non-parametric. In order to compare sociodemographic variables between the sexes, we used the chi-squared test for categorical variables and the Student's *t*-test or Mann–Whitney U test for continuous ones (for parametric or non-parametric distribution, respectively). In order to compare categories of SBP and DBP, as well as WHR and BMI, we used chi-squared and Fisher's exact tests. In order to correlate quantitative variables with SBP and DBP, we used Pearson and Spearman correlation tests, depending on the parametric or non-parametric distribution of the data.

In order to detect the association of independent variables with SBP and DBP, we performed multiple linear regression analysis (using the stepwise method). This analysis was performed by considering that the dependent variables (SBP and DBP) were continuous and normally distributed, and the independent variables were continuous, dichotomic and ordinal. The stepwise method was selected in order to obtain a model with all the included variables being significant. This analysis was performed for all the samples and segmented by sex. The segmented analyses were performed in order to detect specific correlations between independent and dependent variables in each sex. We did not perform interaction analyses between sex and each independent variable in order to better understand the results, analyzing the effect of each variable (without interactions) on the dependent variables in each sex. This decision of doing stratified analyses by sex was performed a priori.

The determination of multicollinearity was performed in order to avoid collinear variables in each multivariate model, and this was confirmed by including only variables with tolerance values above 0.3.

In addition, we performed the Cronbach's alpha test for all the psychological instruments in order to obtain the reliability of each scale and subscale used. All analyses were performed with the software SPSS v.25, and a p-value < 0.05 was considered significant.

3. Results

A total of 171 participants were included, from whom 91 (53.2%) were women; the mean ± SD of the age of the sample was 27.17 ± 10.68. All scales and subscales employed had a Cronbach's alpha test >0.6.

The descriptive data of sociodemographic and psychological variables are described in Table 1, where we observe that all sociodemographic variables were similar between the sexes. We observed some differences in psychological variables between the sexes, where anxiety and negative emotions were significantly higher in women than in men, and assertiveness and autonomy were significantly higher in men than in women (Table 1). In Table 2, we show the descriptive data of SBP and DPB, where we could detect significantly higher levels of both variables in men when compared with women. These differences were corroborated when the values were categorized as normal, pre-hypertension or hypertension, according to the values proposed by the Joint National Committee 7 (JCN-7) [25]. The highest differences between the sexes were observed for SBP, where men showed 10 times more frequency of individuals in the pre-hypertension category when compared with women (Table 2). We also showed the descriptive data of BMI and HWR, where we found a significant difference between the sexes, with higher levels of WHR in men than in women. This was compared with the numeric values and the values categorized as normal or high, according to the desirable WHR values for the Mexican population [26].

Table 1. Descriptive data of sociodemographic and psychological variables and their comparison between the sexes.

Variable	Women (n = 91)	Men (n = 80)	p-Value
Age	27.91 ± 10.99	26.33 ± 10.91	0.334
With romantic partner, n (%)	45 (49.5)	43 (53.8)	0.646
With children, n (%)	24 (26.4)	11 (13.8)	0.057
With job, n (%)	51 (56.0)	38 (47.5)	0.286
Schooling, n (%)			
- Elementary school	1 (1.1)	0 (0.0)	
- Secondary	3 (3.3)	2 (2.5)	
- Preparatory	48 (52.7)	50 (62.5)	0.582
- University (Bachelor's degree)	32 (35.2)	21 (26.3)	
- Master's degree	7 (7.7)	6 (7.5)	
- Ph.D. degree	0 (0.0)	1 (1.2)	

Table 1. *Cont.*

Variable	Women (n = 91)	Men (n = 80)	*p*-Value
Socioeconomic level, n (%)			
- Very low	0 (0.0)	2 (2.5)	
- Low	16 (17.6)	15 (18.7)	
- Average	74 (81.3)	59 (73.8)	0.185
- High	1 (1.1)	4 (5.0)	
- Very high	0 (0.0)	0 (0.0)	
Monthly extra money, n (%)			
- Nothing	6 (6.5)	9 (11.2)	
- Less than USD 60	33 (36.3)	16 (20.0)	
- From USD 61 to USD 120	28 (30.8)	25 (31.3)	0.146
- From USD 121 to USD 180	9 (9.9)	10 (12.5)	
- More than USD 180	15 (16.5)	20 (25.0)	
Smoking frequency, n (%)			
- Never	83 (91.2)	69 (86.2)	
- Two to four times in a year	4 (4.4)	7 (8.8)	
- Once a month or less	1 (1.1)	1 (1.2)	0.371
- Two to three times in a week	2 (2.2)	0 (0.0)	
- Four or more times in a week	1 (1.1)	3 (3.8)	
Alcohol consumption frequency, n (%)			
- Never	14 (15.4)	16 (20.0)	
- Two to four times in a year	28 (30.8)	22 (27.5)	
- Once a month or less	42 (46.2)	33 (41.2)	0.612
- Two to three times in a week	6 (6.5)	9 (11.3)	
- Four or more times in a week	1 (1.1)	0 (0.0)	
Daily free hours, median (range)	4 (0–11)	4 (0–14)	0.012 *
Daily physical activity hours, median (range)	1 (0–5)	1 (0–4)	0.399

Table 1. *Cont.*

Variable	Women (n = 91)	Men (n = 80)	*p*-Value
Sleep satisfaction (OVIEDO scale), mean ± SD			
- Very unsatisfied	7 (7.7)	2 (2.5)	0.385
- Quite unsatisfied	9 (9.9)	9 (11.3)	
- Unsatisfied	14 (15.4)	15 (18.8)	
- Medium	32 (35.1)	25 (31.2)	
- Satisfied	18 (19.8)	12 (15.0)	
- Quite satisfied	8 (8.8)	9 (11.2)	
- Very Satisfied	3 (3.3)	8 (10.0)	
Sleep quality (OVIEDO scale), mean ± SD	3.55 ± 0.96	3.74 ± 0.93	0.185
Frequency of food consumption outside the home, n (%)			
- Less than once a month	8 (8.8)	1 (1.2)	0.024 *
- Once a month	4 (4.4)	1 (1.2)	
- Once every 15 days	12 (13.2)	11 (13.8)	
- 1–2 times a week	43 (47.3)	29 (36.2)	
- 3–4 times a week	14 (15.4)	15 (18.8)	
- 5–6 times a week	6 (6.5)	13 (16.3)	
- Daily	4 (4.4)	10 (12.5)	
Frequency of food consumption in excess, mean, n (%)			
- Less than once a month	14 (15.4)	5 (6.3)	0.115
- Once a month	10 (11.0)	11 (13.8)	
- Once every 15 days	13 (14.3)	17 (21.3)	
- 1–2 times a week	36 (39.6)	29 (36.3)	
- 3–4 times a week	8 (8.8)	14 (17.5)	
- 5–6 times a week	6 (6.5)	1 (1.3)	
- Daily	4 (4.4)	3 (3.5)	

Table 1. Cont.

Variable	Women (n = 91)	Men (n = 80)	p-Value
Quality of food intake (Mini-Ecca scale), mean ± SD	7.70 ± 2.65	7.19 ± 2.39	0.122
Psychological variables			
Anxiety (GAD-7), mean ± SD	1.19 ± 0.74	0.90 ± 0.60	0.019 *
Depression (CES-D), mean ± SD	1.96 ± 0.58	1.78 ± 0.45	0.095
Psychological well-being (PWB), mean ± SD			
- Self-acceptance	4.59 ± 1.23	4.83 ± 1.04	0.237
- Autonomy	3.88 ± 0.99	4.35 ± 0.98	0.002 *
- Purpose in life	4.53 ± 1.22	4.65 ± 1.13	0.568
- Positive relations with others	4.88 ± 1.04	4.72 ± 0.99	0.242
- Personal growth	5.08 ± 0.97	5.01 ± 0.92	0.333
- Environmental mastery	4.37 ± 1.10	4.47 ± 0.98	0.524
Emotional intelligence (TIEQUE), mean ± SD			
- Assertiveness	4.63 ± 0.96	5.13 ± 1.10	0.002 *
- Emotion regulation	4.84 ± 1.17	5.04 ± 1.26	0.290
- Self-motivation	5.16 ± 1.19	4.97 ± 1.20	0.300
- Emotion perception	4.94 ± 1.45	5.06 ± 1.38	0.663
Positive emotions (PSS), mean ± SD	3.65 ± 0.65	3.83 ± 0.52	0.051
Negative emotions (PSS), mean ± SD	2.61 ± 0.65	2.39 ± 0.57	0.018 *
Optimism (LOT-R), mean ± SD	3.66 ± 0.74	3.70 ± 0.67	0.848

* p-value obtained with chi-squared test, Student's t-test and Mann-Whitney U test. Monthly extra money: five categories, from nothing to more than USD 180. Smoking and alcohol consumption frequencies were measured, from 0–4 (never to more than four times in a week); sleep satisfaction (OVIEDO scale), from 1–7 (very unsatisfied to very satisfied); sleep quality (OVIEDO scale), from 1–5 (low quality to high quality); quality of food intake (Mini-Ecca scale) from 1–12 (very low quality to very high quality); frequency of food consumption outside the home and frequency of food consumption in excess, from 1–7 (less than once in a month to all the days); anxiety (GAD-7 scale), from 0–3 (never to almost all the days); depression (CES-D scale), from 1–4 (none of the days to all the days); subscales from psychological well-being (PWB), from 1–6 (totally disagree to totally agree); emotional intelligence (TEIQUE scale), from 1–7 (totally disagree to totally agree), positive and negative emotions (PSS scale), from 1–5 (never to almost always) and optimism (LOT-R), from 1–5 (totally disagree to totally agree).

The descriptive data of biochemical variables are described in Table 3, and the values out of the reference range are also mentioned. The laboratory ranges are according to the desirable values and not the normal values found in the general population; therefore, we included the values out of the reference range in the analyses. In addition, all the values out of range detected in the laboratory tests were double-checked (performed twice) in order to verify them.

Table 2. Comparison between systolic blood pressure, diastolic blood pressure and anthropometric variables between the sexes.

Variable, Mean ± SD	Quantitatively Measured		
	Women (n = 91)	Men (n = 80)	p-Value
Systolic blood pressure (SBP)	103.40 ± 12.11	121.96 ± 14.30	1.35×10^{-16}
Diastolic blood pressure (DBP)	72.93 ± 7.6	78.61 ± 9.88	<0.001 *
Body mass index (BMI)	24.05 ± 3.72	24.80 ± 4.22	0.218
Waist-to-hip ratio (WHR)	0.77 ± 0.05	0.84 ± 0.07	<0.001 *
Categorized BMI and WHR			
Body mass index (BMI)			
Normal < 25 kg/m^2	57 (62.6)	45 (56.2)	0.436
High > 25 kg/m^2	34 (37.4)	35 (43.8)	
Waist-to-hip ratio (WHR)			
Normal: Women < 0.86 and Men < 0.90	86 (94.5)	64 (80.0)	0.005 *
High: Women ≥ 0.86 and Men ≥ 0.90	5 (5.5)	16 (20.0)	
Categorized SBP and DBP			
Systolic blood pressure			
Normal ≤ 120 mmHg	84 (92.3)	35 (43.7)	
Pre-hypertension (121–139 mmHg)	4 (4.4)	38 (47.5)	1.71×10^{-12}
High ≥ 140 mmHg	3 (3.3)	7 (8.8)	
Diastolic blood pressure			
Normal ≤ 80 mmHg	76 (83.5)	47 (58.8)	
Pre-hypertension (81–89 mmHg)	13 (14.3)	24 (30.0)	0.002 *
High ≥ 90 mmHg	2 (2.2)	9 (11.2)	

* Significant values; p-values obtained with Student's t-test and chi-squared test.

Table 3. Descriptive data of the laboratory variables studied and their comparison between the sexes.

Variable	Women (n = 91)	Men (n = 80)	Laboratory Reference Values	Participants Out of Range n (%)
Leukocytes (10^3/μL), mean ± SD	6.80 ± 1.48	6.58 ± 1.81	5.00–10.00	28 (16.4)
- Lymphocytes	2.23 ± 0.53	2.17 ± 0.56	1.00–4.20	1 (0.6)
- Monocytes	0.49 ± 0.14	0.53 ± 0.16	0.10–1.00	1 (0.6)
- Neutrophils	3.88 ± 1.18	3.78 ± 1.44	1.50–7.00	4 (2.3)
- Eosinophils	0.14 ± 0.12	0.13 ± 0.09	0.05–0.40	20 (11.7)
- Basophils	0.04 ± 0.02	0.05 ± 0.02	0.01–0.05	42 (24.6)
Hemoglobin (g/dL), mean ± SD	13.79 ± 1.18	16.32 ± 0.79	W: 12.00–16.00, M: 14.00–17.00	W: 7 (7.7), M: 17 (21.3)
Hematocrit (%)	42.29 ± 3.19	48.48 ± 2.31	W: 36.0–48.0, M: 36.0–52.0	W: 9 (9.9), M: 5 (6.3)
Erythrocytes	4.71 ± 0.35	5.44 ± 0.33	W: 4.0–5.0, M: 4.5–6.2	W: 20 (22.0), M: 0 (0.0)

Table 3. *Cont.*

Variable	Women (n = 91)	Men (n = 80)	Laboratory Reference Values	Participants Out of Range n (%)
Platelets ($10^3/\mu L$), mean ± SD	278.00 ± 53.61	260.18 ± 51.29	141.00–400.00	3 (1.8)
Glucose (g/dL), mean ± SD	87.30 ± 8.59	90.99 ± 14.81	74.00–106.00	11 (6.4)
Urea (mg/dL), mean ± SD	25.56 ± 6.52	28.44 ± 7.06	16.60–48.50	6 (3.5)
Blood urea nitrogen (BUN), mg/dL, mean ± SD	11.95 ± 3.04	13.29 ± 3.30	6.00–20.0	8 (4.6)
Creatinine (mg/dL), mean ± SD	0.74 ± 0.11	0.95 ± 0.13	W: 0.50–0.90	8 (8.8)
			M: 0.70–1.20	4 (5.0)
Uric acid (mg/dL), mean ± SD	4.21 ± 1.00	6.05 ± 1.10	W: 2.40–5.70	7 (7.7)
			M: 3.40–7.00	14 (17.5)
Lipid levels (mg/dL), mean ± SD				
Total cholesterol	166.18 ± 29.18	176.71 ± 36.43	≤200.00	36 (21.10)
High-density lipoprotein (HDL)	51.97 ± 11.72	44.47 ± 10.25	W ≥ 45.00, M ≥ 35.00	31 (34.1), 13 (16.3)
Low-density lipoprotein (LDL)	95.72 ± 24.19	108.96 ± 29.70	≤100.00	82 (48.0)
Triglycerides	92.59 ± 43.84	130.58 ± 97.97	≤150.00	34 (19.9)
Total proteins (g/dL)	7.47 ± 0.38	7.65 ± 0.39	6.4–8.3	5 (2.9)
Albumin (g/dL)	4.71 ± 0.26	5.01 ± 0.27	3.97–4.94	63 (36.8)
Liver enzymes (U/L), mean ± SD				
- AST	19.99 ± 16.10	29.93 ± 39.77	W ≤ 32.00, M ≤ 40.00	4 (4.4), 7 (8.6)
- ALT	17.52 ± 15.45	28.91 ± 21.20	W ≤ 33.00, M ≤ 41.00	6 (6.5), 11 (13.8)
- GGT	16.15 ± 7.62	27.58 ± 22.56	W ≤ 40.00, M ≤ 60.00	2 (2.2), 4 (5.0)
- ALP	78.61 ± 17.59	97.46 ± 26.99	W ≤ 104.00, M ≤ 129.00	5 (5.5), 12 (15.0)
- LDH	169.56 ± 32.03	187.03 ± 100.98	W ≤ 214.00, M ≤ 225.00	4 (4.4), 5 (6.3)
Serum electrolytes				
- Calcium, mg/dL	9.71 ± 0.31	9.97 ± 0.34	8.6–10.0	39 (22.8)
- Phosphorus, mg/dL	3.62 ± 0.50	3.59 ± 0.50	2.5–4.5	6 (3.5)
- Magnesium, mg/dL	2.05 ± 0.11	2.08 ± 0.14	W: 1.7–2.2, M: 1.6–2.6	W: 2 (2.2), M: 0 (0.0)
- Iron, μg/dL	83.53 ± 36.81	116.58 ± 38.76	33.0–193.0	10 (5.8)
- Sodium, meq/L	139.05 ± 1.93	139.60 ± 1.97	136.0–145.0	5 (2.9)

Table 3. Cont.

Variable	Women (n = 91)	Men (n = 80)	Laboratory Reference Values	Participants Out of Range n (%)
- Potassium, meq/L	4.52 ± 0.41	4.45 ± 0.45	3.5–5.10	11 (6.4)
- Chloride, meq/L	103.78 ± 1.76	102.72 ± 1.91	98.0–107.0	4 (2.3)
Pancreatic enzymes				
Amilase, U/L	71.13 ± 25.65	72.24 ± 50.33	28.0–100.0	20 (11.7)
Lipase, U/L	34.52 ± 11.77	32.04 ± 20.12	13.0–60.0	4 (2.3)

AST: aspartate aminotransferase; ALT: alanine aminotransferase; GGT: gamma-glutamyl transferase; ALP: Alkaline phosphatase; LDH: lactate dehydrogenase; W: women; M: men.

3.1. Bivariate Correlations

In the bivariate correlations between the studied variables and SBP/DBP performed in the whole sample (Table 4), we observed that the variable most positively correlated with SBP was male sex (r = 0.607), followed by uric acid (r = 0.522), WHR (r = 0.482) and creatinine levels (r = 0.459); we also observed that all liver enzymes showed low but positive significant correlations with SBP, with the highest correlation value for GGT (r = 0.369). Electrolyte levels also showed significant correlations with SBP, with a low positive correlation between SBP and calcium levels (r = 0.222) and low negative correlations with phosphorus and chloride levels (r = −0.246 and r = −0.217). The psychological variable "autonomy" showed a low positive correlation with SBP (r = 0.221), while "depression" showed a low negative correlation with it (r = −0.164).

Table 4. Significant bivariate correlations between the studied variables and systolic blood pressure and diastolic blood pressure in the global sample.

Variable	SBP (n =171)	DBP (n = 171)
Sex (Female = 1, male = 2)	0.607 **	0.322 **
With children	0.114	0.151 *
Erythrocytes	0.445 **	0.325 **
Hemoglobin	0.424 **	0.346 **
Hematocrit	0.400 **	0.336 **
Glucose	0.248 **	0.262 **
Creatinine	0.459 **	0.238 **
Uric acid	0.522 **	0.347 **
Cholesterol	0.208 **	0.123
Triglycerides	0.229 **	0.219 **
High-density lipoprotein (HDL)	−0.296 **	−0.231 **
Low-density lipoprotein (LDL)	0.275 **	0.175 *
Aspartate aminotransferase (AST)	0.241 **	0.128
Alanine aminotransferase (ALT)	0.288 **	0.215 **
Gamma-glutamyl transferase (GGT)	0.396 **	0.326 **
Alkaline Phosphatase (ALP)	0.304 **	0.178 *
Lactate Dehydrogenase (LDH)	0.193 *	0.135
Total proteins	0.282 **	0.250 **
Albumin	0.294 **	0.185 *
Calcium	0.222 **	0.171 *
Phosphorus	−0.246 **	−0.196 *
Magnesium	0.104	0.228 **
Lipase	−0.169 *	−0.033
Iron	0.158 *	0.102
Sodium	0.123	0.169 *
Chloride	−0.217 **	−0.113

Table 4. Cont.

Variable	SBP (n =171)	DBP (n = 171)
Depression	−0.164 *	−0.104
Autonomy	0.221 **	0.162 *
Body mass index (BMI)	0.340 **	0.289 **
Waist/hip ratio (WHR)	0.482 **	0.341 **
Sleep satisfaction	0.197 **	0.120
Sleep quality	0.174 *	0.163 *

p-values obtained with Pearson and Spearman correlation tests. * p-value < 0.05; ** p-value < 0.01.

In the case of DBP, we observed that the most associated variable was uric acid (r = 0.347), followed by hemoglobin (r = 0.346), erythrocytes (r = 0.325), hematocrit (r = 0.336), WHR (r = 0.341), male sex (r = 0.322), GGT (r = 0.326) and total proteins (r = 0.250). The electrolytes calcium, sodium and magnesium showed low positive correlations with DBP, while phosphorus showed a very low negative correlation with DBP (Table 4). The only psychological variable associated was "autonomy", with a very low positive correlation with DBP (r = 0.162).

3.2. Multivariate Regression Analysis for SBP

In the multivariate regression analysis for SBP in the whole sample (Table 5), we observed that male sex was the most positively associated variable with SBP, followed by BMI and age, while schooling was negatively correlated with SBP. In the case of biochemical variables, we observed that albumin, monocytes, glucose and creatinine were positively correlated with SBP, while phosphorus, potassium and eosinophils were negatively correlated with it, with a robust R of the model: 0.770.

Table 5. Multivariate regression analysis for systolic blood pressure in the global sample.

Variable	B	Beta Coefficient	Significance	Change in R^2	Tolerance
Constant	22.058	-	0.341		-
Male sex	8.870	0.276	0.001	0.334	0.380
Body mass index (BMI)	0.939	0.232	0.000	0.082	0.721
Age	0.347	0.230	0.000	0.026	0.621
Schooling	−4.837	−0.219	0.000	0.033	0.849
Albumin	13.731	0.258	0.000	0.030	0.575
Sleep satisfaction	0.981	0.091	0.085	0.015	0.932
Phosphorus	−5.230	−0.162	0.007	0.012	0.728
Monocytes	15.992	0.149	0.007	0.012	0.866
Eosinophils	−23.278	−0.156	0.005	0.014	0.868
Potassium	−5.483	−0.146	0.006	0.011	0.920
Glucose	0.186	0.139	0.014	0.013	0.824
Creatinine	4.978	0.146	0.048	0.010	0.479

R of the model: 0.770.

In the multivariate regression analysis for SBP performed in women (Table 6), we observed that BMI and age were the most positively associated variables with SBP, while schooling, eosinophils, ALP, emotion perception and having children were variables negatively correlated with SBP, with an R of the model of 0.673.

Table 6. Multivariate regression analysis for systolic blood pressure in women.

Variable	B	Beta Coefficient	Significance	Change in R^2	Tolerance
Constant	67.277	-	0.000	-	-
Body mass index (BMI)	1.015	0.312	0.002	0.129	0.676
Age	0.697	0.604	0.000	0.055	0.282
Schooling	−5.623	−0.341	0.001	0.056	0.743
Monocytes	22.109	0.252	0.005	0.047	0.889
Eosinophils	−24.884	−0.252	0.005	0.049	0.871
Alkaline phosphatase (ALP)	−0.162	−0.235	0.011	0.027	0.840
Glucose	0.318	0.225	0.013	0.034	0.858
Emotion perception	−1.751	−0.209	0.026	0.025	0.794
With children	−8.330	−0.305	0.038	0.030	0.324

R of the model = 0.673.

Finally, in the multivariate regression analysis for SBP in men (Table 7), we observed that total proteins, daily physical activity hours, autonomy, monthly free money and calcium were positively correlated with SBP, while schooling, phosphorus, potassium, iron, frequency of alcohol consumption, socioeconomic level and emotion perception were negatively correlated with it. The R of the model was also robust at 0.757.

Table 7. Multivariate regression analysis for systolic blood pressure in men.

Variable	B	Beta Coefficient	Significance	Change in R^2	Tolerance
Constant	113.988	-	0.004	-	-
Schooling	−8.540	−0.433	0.000	0.062	0.654
Total proteins	10.486	0.284	0.005	0.125	0.665
Daily physical activity hours	6.894	0.434	0.000	0.076	0.828
Phosphorus	−16.906	−0.590	0.000	0.046	0.733
Potassium	−11.893	−0.375	0.000	0.048	0.813
Autonomy	6.228	0.426	0.000	0.038	0.652
Iron	−0.111	−0.300	0.001	0.031	0.817
Socioeconomic level	−11.160	−0.432	0.000	0.029	0.544
Monthly free money	3.256	0.302	0.008	0.024	0.524
Frequency of alcohol consumption	−3.257	−0.214	0.018	0.034	0.816
Calcium	8.317	0.196	0.054	0.026	0.639
Emotion perception	−1.862	−0.180	0.071	0.020	0.665

R of the model = 0.757.

3.3. Multivariate Regression Analysis for DBP

In the multivariate regression analysis for DBP in the global sample, we detected that the positively correlated variables were age, hemoglobin, glucose, LDH, BMI, sodium and magnesium, while the negatively correlated variables with DBP were BUN, schooling, chloride and frequency of smoking consumption. The R of the model was 0.644 (Table 8).

Table 8. Multivariate regression analysis for diastolic blood pressure in the global sample.

Variable	B	Beta Coefficient	Significance	Change in R^2	Tolerance
Constant	−13.916	-	0.737	-	-
Age	0.163	0.190	0.008	0.140	0.736
Hemoglobin	0.956	0.169	0.026	0.054	0.650
Glucose	0.198	0.259	0.000	0.046	0.835
Lactate dehydrogenase (LDH)	0.016	0.126	0.044	0.026	0.951
Blood urea nitrogen	−0.476	−0.168	0.009	0.026	0.921
Schooling	−2.589	−0.205	0.002	0.021	0.866
Body mass index (BMI)	0.450	0.195	0.004	0.015	0.814
Sodium	1.594	0.342	0.000	0.016	0.493
Chloride	−1.798	−0.373	0.000	0.017	0.462
Frequency of smoking consumption	−1.705	−0.137	0.030	0.013	0.929
Magnesium	8.862	0.122	0.069	0.025	0.836

R of the model: 0.644.

In the multivariate analysis for women, we observed many associated variables (Table 9) that formed a robust model (R = 0.768), with the following positive associated variables with DBP: uric acid, LDH, hemoglobin, age, daily free hours, sleep satisfaction and BMI; and the following negatively correlated variables with DBP: phosphorus, with romantic partner, daily physical activity hours, personal growth, triglycerides, WHR, chloride, with children and frequency of smoking consumption.

Table 9. Multivariate regression analysis for diastolic blood pressure in women.

Variable	B	Beta Coefficient	Significance	Change in R^2	Tolerance
Constant	137.064	-	0.001	-	-
Uric acid	2.304	0.303	0.001	0.070	0.768
Lactate dehydrogenase (LDH)	0.066	0.276	0.001	0.083	0.887
Phosphorus	−3.916	−0.256	0.007	0.048	0.658
With partner	−3.910	−0.258	0.005	0.042	0.689
Daily physical activity hours	−2.783	−0.337	0.000	0.043	0.780
Hemoglobin	1.839	0.286	0.001	0.041	0.808

Table 9. Cont.

Variable	B	Beta Coefficient	Significance	Change in R^2	Tolerance
Personal growth	−1.796	−0.228	0.010	0.036	0.749
Age	0.452	0.622	0.000	0.032	0.257
Daily free hours	0.806	0.235	0.007	0.045	0.787
Sleep satisfaction	0.874	0.166	0.053	0.026	0.776
Triglycerides	−0.051	−0.293	0.003	0.025	0.590
Body mass index (BMI)	0.560	0.274	0.008	0.019	0.545
Waist-to-hip ratio (WHR)	−27.736	−0.175	0.078	0.022	0.575
Chloride	−0.840	−0.194	0.017	0.022	0.875
With children	−4.526	−0.263	0.051	0.021	0.313
Frequency of smoking consumption	−1.589	−0.138	0.092	0.016	0.854

R of the model: 0.768.

In the multivariate analysis for DBP in men, the positively correlated variables with DBP were with children, total proteins, magnesium, self-motivation and AST, while the negatively correlated variable with DBP was quality of food intake. The R of the model was 0.591 (Table 10).

Table 10. Multivariate regression analysis for diastolic blood pressure in men.

Variable	B	Beta Coefficient	Significance	Change in R^2	Tolerance
Constant	−1.733	-	0.937	-	-
With children	10.350	0.363	0.001	0.135	0.848
Total proteins	6.194	0.242	0.021	0.064	0.846
Quality of food intake	−1.011	−0.244	0.013	0.042	0.965
Magnesium	14.325	0.202	0.057	0.046	0.818
Self-motivation	1.538	0.187	0.055	0.033	0.977
Aspartate aminotransferase (AST)	0.045	0.181	0.072	0.030	0.907

R of the model: 0.591.

4. Discussion

4.1. Sex Differences in Blood Pressure

In the present study, we observed that most personal (including BMI) variables were similar between the sexes, which makes both groups comparable in BP parameters. We showed that both SBP and DBP were significantly higher in men and were correlated by different factors in both sexes. The higher values of SBP and DBP in men coincide with previous reports showing higher levels of pre-hypertension (for SBP) in men when compared with women in the adult population of China (71.1% vs. 44.6%) [27] and the university population of Spain (56.5% vs. 13.0%) [1]. These results coincide with ours, where higher levels of hypertension (11.2% vs. 2.2%) and mainly pre-hypertension of SBP (47.5% vs. 4.4%) were found in men when compared with women. These results are more similar to that found by Ortiz-Galeano et al. in Spain [1]. This is explained by the higher similitude between our study and their study, being both populations mainly comprised of young people, where sex differences are more pronounced. The differences in BP observed between the sexes have been explained by the biological effects of sex chromosomes, including sex hormones and reproductive events [4]. However, there is evidence that cardiovascular complications start at lower BP levels in females than in males [4], questioning the current practice of using the same BP threshold for the identification of hypertension in both sexes [28,29]. In addition, in the elderly, hypertensive women double the number of men [30]; this can be partly explained by hormonal and hemodynamic changes that occur after menopause, including a higher sympathetic activity and vasoconstrictor responsiveness [31].

4.2. Personal and Biochemical Factors in SBP

In the bivariate correlations performed in the whole sample, we observed that male sex was the variable most associated with SBP (Table 4), which coincides with the sex differences of SBP previously mentioned. In addition, we observed that many biochemical and some psychological variables were positively and negatively correlated with SBP and DBP.

In the case of SBP, in the multivariate regression analysis for the global sample, we observed that male sex, BMI and age were the most positively correlated variables with SBP, followed by schooling, which was negatively correlated with SBP. BMI and age are well-known variables related to high SBP, which, in the case of BMI, is explained by the role that adiposity plays in the physiopathology of hypertension [5]. This variable, along with age, was positively correlated with SBP in the whole sample, as well as in the women's sample (Tables 5 and 6), which suggests that their association, although present in both sexes, is higher in women than in men. In the case of the negative correlation of schooling with SBP, a possible explanation is that people with higher schooling remain sited or physically inactive more often, which negatively impacts SBP (when adjusted for BMI and the rest of the searched variables). This variable was also seen in men's and women's subsamples (Tables 6 and 7) and coincides with the positive correlation of the variable daily physical activity hours with SBP in the men's sample. These findings coincide with a previous report performed in normotensive men, where significant correlations between SBP, physical activity and left ventricle mass were found [32]. Different to that found in hypertensive men in whom physical activity is associated with reduced BP [33], the coincidence between these findings and our results is explained by the fact that most men included in this study were normotensive or pre-hypertensive, and only 8.8% were hypertensive. These findings indicate the importance of personal and behavioral variables in BP variations of a relatively healthy population. We also observed that the personal variable "sleep satisfaction" was marginally and positively correlated with SBP in the whole sample (Table 5), which suggests that restful sleep is needed in order to maintain a healthy BP and avoid hypotension. In addition, it has been shown that poor sleep patterns are related to a higher probability of presenting hypertension [34]. Therefore, it seems that sleep quality has an important role in BP regulation.

We also observed that the biochemical variables albumin and total proteins were positively correlated with SBP in the multiple regression analyses of global and men's samples (Tables 5 and 7), which is probably due to the oncotic pressure that albumin exerts [35]. Additionally, these results coincide with the bivariate correlations between total proteins and albumin with SBP in the whole sample (Table 4). On the other hand, the serum electrolytes were also correlated with SBP in the multivariate regression analyses, where phosphorus and potassium were negatively correlated with it in the global and men's samples (Tables 5 and 7). These findings coincide with previous reports, showing that phosphorus and potassium supplementation are related to lower levels of SPB [3,6]. In the men's sample, we also observed that iron was negatively correlated with SBP, while calcium was marginally positively correlated with SBP (Table 7). The negative correlation between iron and SBP in men coincides with a report showing that intake of non-heme iron is inversely related to BP [36]. It is interesting that this correlation was observed only in men and opposed the bivariate correlation between SBP and iron in the global sample, which suggests that men are mainly affected by the influence of iron in SBP, although additional studies should corroborate it. In addition, the marginal positive correlation between calcium and SBP in men, which, although coincides with the bivariate correlations in the global sample, contrasts with this last study that found that calcium intake was also inversely correlated with BP [36] and with a report showing a low negative correlation between calcium in serum with SBP and DBP in patients with type 2 diabetes [37]. However, a previous report performed in Pakistan showed that people with essential hypertension had higher concentrations of many electrolytes, including calcium when compared with normotensives [38]. Therefore, more studies searching the relationship between calcium concentration and BP are needed.

We also observed that the global and women's samples showed that monocytes were positively correlated with SBP, while eosinophils were negatively correlated with it (Tables 5 and 6). These findings coincide with a previous report showing a positive association of monocytes and neutrophils with higher levels of SBP and eosinophils with lower levels of SBP [39]. This is an interesting finding that needs to be further explored and which suggests a role of inflammatory mechanisms in SBP levels. Finally, a positive correlation between creatinine and SBP in the whole sample was observed (Table 5), which coincides with the positive significant bivariate correlations between creatinine and SBP and DBP in the global sample (Table 4) and suggests that renal function plays an important role on SBP.

4.3. Psychological Factors in SBP

With respect to the psychological variables studied, we found that there were no psychological factors associated with SBP in the global sample; however, in the sex-specific analysis, the psychological variable "emotion perception" was negatively associated with SBP in both sexes in the multivariate analyses (Tables 6 and 7); in addition, in the men's sample, there was a positive correlation between the psychological variable "autonomy" with SBP in the multivariate analysis (Table 7). The negative correlation with "emotion perception" coincides with a previous report showing a higher ability of emotion recognition in normotensive subjects when compared with pre-hypertensive and hypertensive subjects [9] and with a study that showed that anxiety disorders and depression were associated with resistant hypertension [10], considering that emotion perception was inversely related to symptoms of anxiety and depression, with moderate negative correlations. However, it is of interest that we did not find a significant correlation between anxiety and depression variables with SBP or DBP in the multivariate analyses. This suggests that these negative psychological variables can affect SBP only when they are present as clinical disorders and not when they are measured with symptomatic scales, as in this case. In addition, these variables have been associated with the presence of hypertension and not with BP variations in a relatively healthy population.

The positive correlation between the psychological variable "autonomy" with SBP in the men's sample could be related to the fact that this variable is related to being less influenced by other's opinions in one own's life, as well as with a higher ability to defend one own's rights. Therefore, men with higher levels of this ability can be prone to having higher levels of SBP because they have a "stronger" character and willpower; however, further studies evaluating the influence of this variable on SBP in each sex are needed.

4.4. Personal and Biochemical Factors in DBP

The results of DBP showed that some similar and many different personal and biochemical variables were significantly associated with it. As observed in SBP, BMI and age were positively correlated with DBP in the global and women's samples (Tables 8 and 9), suggesting that these two variables (age and BMI) influence women more than men.

The positive correlations of hemoglobin, sodium and magnesium and the negative correlations of chloride with DBP are of interest. In the case of hemoglobin, the results coincide with a report showing that higher hemoglobin levels are related to an increase in SBP and DBP in both sexes [40]. Data coincide with the bivariate analyses in this study, where moderate significant correlations were found between hemoglobin and SBP and DBP in the global sample (Table 4), and also coincide with positive correlations between SBP and DBP with erythrocytes and hematocrit. This correlation has been explained by the effects of hemoglobin in the increase in blood viscosity, which, in turn, is related to increased peripheral resistance and BP; in addition, higher hemoglobin levels have been related to less secretion of B-type natriuretic peptide, which is related to natriuresis and aldosterone inhibition, leading to reduced BP. Therefore, by an opposite mechanism, an increase in hemoglobin levels would increase BP [40]. It is interesting that hemoglobin appeared in the multivariate analyses of DBP but not of SBP, for which the bivariate correlation with hemoglobin is higher (Table 4). It is possible that with larger sample sizes, hemoglobin could also be correlated with SBP, as in the previous report [40]. With respect to the negative correlation between chloride and DBP in the global sample, we observed that these results coincide with a previous report showing that serum chloride levels were inversely correlated with SBP and DBP [41]. The positive correlation with sodium coincides with a report showing that high sodium intake is related to an increase in BP [13] and with a report that demonstrated higher levels of sodium in hypertensive people [12]; in addition, the marginally positive correlation between magnesium and DBP coincides with the low but significant positive correlation between magnesium levels and DBP in the global sample of the bivariate analysis (Table 4), although differing from a study showing that magnesium intake was inversely related with BP [36], and with another study showing that magnesium supplementation is related to BP reduction in patients with mild hypertension [42]; however, a study performed in persons with essential hypertension showed higher levels of magnesium in this population when compared with normotensive persons [38]. These discrepancies can be explained by the type of population studied in each report, suggesting that serum magnesium could be positively correlated with DBP in a relatively healthy population. However, only larger studies will clarify this relationship. Finally, in the multivariate analysis for DBP in the whole sample, we found that BUN was negatively correlated with it in a significant way. The study of this relationship was not found in previous reports; therefore, future research will clarify the role of BUN in DBP.

When we observed the variables associated with DBP in each sex, uric acid was the most associated variable with DBP in women (Table 9), which coincides with a previous report showing that serum uric acid levels were only associated with BP in women [43]. In addition, as previously reported [12,43], we observed a positive correlation between fasting glucose with SBP and DBP in the global samples (Tables 5 and 8) and with SBP in the women's sample (Table 6), indicating that the association between glucose and BP is higher in women than in men, as previously suggested [43].

The positive correlation between LDH and DPB in the multivariate analysis of women, as well as the positive correlation between AST and DBP in the men's sample, suggest that liver function and its specific enzymes play a role in DBP; however, more studies are needed in order to determine their influence, considering that no related reports were found. Similarly, the negative correlation between triglycerides and DBP and the marginal negative correlation between WHR with DBP in the women's sample require further research that discards or corroborates these findings.

4.5. Behavioral and Psychological Factors in DBP

Interestingly, the frequency of smoking consumption was negatively correlated with DBP after adjusting for confounders, and this coincides with a cross-sectional study performed in men that showed that current smokers have lower DBP when compared with nonsmokers [44]. With respect to other sociodemographic and behavioral variables, we observed that different variables were associated with each sex; for example, in women, the variables of having a romantic partner, having children and daily physical activity hours were negatively correlated with DBP, while daily free hours was positively correlated with it (Table 9). The variable having children was positively correlated with DBP in men, in whom the quality of food intake was negatively correlated with DPB (Table 10). These results suggest that personal variables influence DBP more than SBP and should be considered in studies researching variables associated with DBP.

Although no psychological variables were associated with DBP in the multivariate analysis of the global sample, the subscale "personal growth" of the scale "psychological well-being" was negatively correlated with DBP in women, and the subscale "self-motivation" of the TEIQUE scale of emotional intelligence was marginally and positively correlated with DBP in men. The variable personal growth is related to questions like "I have the feeling that over time, I have developed a lot as a person", and its relationship with lower DPB in women can be related to a more calmed mood and higher mental health. In addition, the variable self-motivation is related to questions like: "On the whole, I'm a highly motivated person", which could contribute positively to levels of BP and, in this case, DBP. Nevertheless, further studies will clarify this relationship.

The main limitation of the study is the sample size, which, if larger, would have permitted us to perform analyses separated by normotensives, pre-hypertensives and hypertensives in each sex and would have diminished the possible bias by including many independent variables in the multivariate analyses; in addition, the non-random sampling method did not permit us to perform a generalization to all in the Mexican population, and neither to the population of all ages, considering that most participants were young people. The usage of electronic questionnaires can also diminish the accurate understanding of the questions, which could have affected the answers of the participants. Another limitation is the cross-sectional nature of the study, which cannot permit us to determine causal relations between the variables studied and BP. However, the main strength is the inclusion of many independent variables, including personal, biochemical, anthropometric, behavioral and psychological variables, which led us to detect the influence of each one of these factors in a more accurate way.

In conclusion, we observed that men showed higher levels of SBP and DBP than women, with more differences for SBP. In addition, we reported that many personal and psychological variables were associated with these variables, with some differences between the sexes. Among the personal variables, BMI and age were significantly and positively correlated with SBP and DBP, with more correlation in the women's sample. Among the biochemical factors and SBP, we found that albumin and monocytes were positively correlated with it, while potassium, phosphorus and eosinophils were negatively correlated with it. Additionally, schooling was a constant variable negatively correlated with SBP in all samples (global, men and women). Among the psychological variables, we observed that emotional perception was negatively correlated with SBP in men's and women's samples, while autonomy was positively correlated with SBP in the men's sample; however, the association was less when compared with personal and biochemical variables. With regard to DBP, we observed that the biochemical variables, hemoglobin, sodium, uric acid and glucose, were positively correlated with DBP in the global sample, while chloride and BUN were negatively correlated with it. In addition, many personal and behavioral variables, including BMI, age and smoking consumption frequency, also correlated with DBP in the global sample. In addition, many other personal variables were differently correlated with DBP in each sex. All these results indicate that BP is a variable that presents multiple correlations with different factors, including the sex, and these correlations in each sex are different; therefore, studies aimed at identifying or studying BP should consider the effect of sex. Further longitudinal studies with larger sample sizes will corroborate or discard these results.

Supplementary Materials: The following supporting information can be downloaded at: https://www.mdpi.com/article/10.3390/jcm13020378/s1.

Author Contributions: Conceptualization, B.E.R.-G., A.M.S.-C. and A.J.L.B.-T.; Methodology, A.J.L.B.-T.; Validation, A.M.S.-C.; Formal analysis, A.J.L.B.-T.; Investigation, B.E.R.-G., A.M.S.-C., S.G.G.-M. and A.J.L.B.-T.; Data curation, S.G.G.-M.; Writing—original draft, B.E.R.-G., A.M.S.-C. and A.J.L.B.-T.; Writing—review & editing, B.E.R.-G. All authors have read and agreed to the published version of the manuscript.

Funding: This research was funded by PRO-SNI program of the University of Guadalajara, grant number PRO-SNI 2019-2022.

Institutional Review Board Statement: The study was conducted in accordance with the Declaration of Helsinki, and approved by the Institutional Review Board of the ethics committee of the Health Sciences University Center of the University of Guadalajara (protocol code 19-21, date of approval, 14 October 2019).

Informed Consent Statement: Informed consent was obtained from all subjects involved in the study.

Data Availability Statement: The raw data presented in this study are available on request to the corresponding author. The data are not publicly available due to the database has a specific codification that needs to be explained by the researcher responsible of the study. In addition, all sensible data of the participants in the database must be eliminated from it in order to be send to another researcher.

Conflicts of Interest: The authors declare no conflict of interest.

References

1. Galeano, I.O.; Franquelo-Morales, P.; Notario-Pacheco, B.; Rodríguez, J.A.N.; Cañete, M.U.; Martínez-Vizcaíno, V. Prehipertensión arterial en adultos jóvenes. *Rev. Clin. Esp.* **2012**, *212*, 287–291. [CrossRef] [PubMed]
2. Trudel-Fitzgerald, C.; Gilsanz, P.; Mittleman, M.A.; Kubzansky, L.D. Dysregulated Blood Pressure: Can Regulating Emotions Help? *Curr. Hypertens. Rep.* **2015**, *17*, 92. [CrossRef] [PubMed]
3. Filippini, T.; Naska, A.; Kasdagli, M.; Torres, D.; Lopes, C.; Carvalho, C.; Moreira, P.; Malavolti, M.; Orsini, N.; Whelton, P.K.; et al. Potassium intake and bood pressure: A Dose-Response Meta-Analysis of Randomized Controlled Trials. *J. Am. Heart Assoc.* **2020**, *9*, e015719. [CrossRef] [PubMed]
4. Yanes, L.L.; Romero, D.G.; Iliescu, R.; Zhang, H.; Davis, D.; Reckelhoff, J.F. Postmenopausal hypertension: Role of the renin-angiotensin system. *Hypertension* **2010**, *56*, 359–363. [CrossRef] [PubMed]
5. Casilimas, G.A.G.; Martin, D.; Martínez, M.A.; Merchán, C.R.; Mayorga, C.; Barragán, A.F. Fisiopatología de la hipertensión arterial secundaria a obesidad. *Arch. Cardiol. México* **2017**, *87*, 336–344. [CrossRef] [PubMed]
6. McClure, S.T.; Rebholz, C.M.; Mitchell, D.C.; Selvin, E.; Appel, L.J. The association of dietary phosphorus with blood pressure: Results from a secondary analysis of the PREMIER trial. *J. Hum. Hypertens.* **2019**, *34*, 132–142. [CrossRef] [PubMed]
7. Scalco, A.Z.; Scalco, M.Z.; Azul, J.B.S.; Neto, F.B. Hypertension and depression. *Clinics* **2005**, *60*, 241–250. [CrossRef]
8. Brugnera, A.; Compare, A.; Omboni, S.; Greco, A.; Carrara, S.; Tasca, G.; Poletti, B.; Parati, G. Psychological covariates of blood pressure among patients with hypertension and metabolic syndrome. *Health Psychol.* **2022**, *41*, 946–954. [CrossRef]
9. Shukla, M.; Pandey, R.; Jain, D.; Lau, J.Y.F. Poor emotional responsiveness in clinical hypertension: Reduced accuracy in the labelling and matching of emotional faces amongst individuals with hypertension and prehypertension. *Psychol. Health* **2017**, *33*, 765–782. [CrossRef]
10. Handan, D.; Hakan, D.; Puşuroğlu, M.; Seyda Yılmaz, A. Anxiety disorders and depression are associated with resistant hypertension. *Adv. Clin. Exp. Med.* **2022**. [CrossRef]
11. Auer, A.; von Känel, R.; Lang, L.L.; Thomas, L.; Zuccarella-Hackl, C.; Degroote, C.; Gideon, A.; Wiest, R.; Wirtz, P.H. Do Hypertensive Men Spy with an Angry Little Eye? Anger Recognition in Men with Essential Hypertension—Cross-sectional and Prospective Findings. *Ann. Behav. Mes.* **2022**, *56*, 875–889. [CrossRef] [PubMed]
12. Baker, L.A.A.; Aldin, S.Z.J. Association of some biochemical parameters and blood pressure among males with hypertension in the camps of Nineveh province-Iraq. *J. Popul. Ther. Clin. Pharmacol.* **2022**, *29*, e167–e176. [CrossRef] [PubMed]
13. Baldo, M.P.; Brant, L.C.C.; Cunha, R.S.; Del Carmen Bisi Molina, M.; Griep, R.H.; Barreto, S.M.; Lotufo, P.A.; Bensenor, I.M.; Mill, J.G. The association between salt intake and arterial stiffness is influenced by a sex-specific mediating effect through blood pressure in normotensive adults: The ELSA-Brasil study. *J. Clin. Hypertens.* **2019**, *21*, 1771–1779. [CrossRef] [PubMed]
14. Díaz-Pértegas, S.; Pita-Fernández, S. Determinación del tamaño muestral para calcular la significación del coeficiente de correlación lineal. *Cad. Aten. Primaria* **2022**, *9*, 209–211.
15. Bobes-García, J.; González, G.; Portilla, P.; Sáiz-Martínez, D.A.; Bascarán-Fdez, M.; Iglesias-Álvarez, G.; Fdez-Domínguez, J.M. Propiedades psicométricas del cuestionario de Oviedo de Sueño. *Psicothema* **2000**, *12*, 107–112.
16. Bernal-Orozco, M.; Badillo-Camacho, N.; Macedo-Ojeda, G.; González-Gómez, M.; Orozco-Gutiérrez, J.; Prado-Arriaga, R.; Márquez-Sandoval, F.; Altamirano-Martínez, M.; Vizmanos, B. Design and Reproducibility of a Mini-Survey to Evaluate the Quality of Food Intake (Mini-ECCA) in a Mexican Population. *Nutrients* **2018**, *10*, 524. [CrossRef] [PubMed]

17. Márquez-Sandoval, Y.F.; Salazar-Ruiz, E.N.; Macedo-Ojeda, G.; Altamirano-Martínez, M.B.; Bernal-Orozco, M.F.; Salas-Salvadó, J.; Vizmanos, B. Design and validation of a questionnaire to assess dietary behavior in Mexican students in the area of health. *Nutr. Hosp.* **2014**, *30*, 153–164. [CrossRef]
18. Radloff, L. The CES-D Scale: A self-report depression scale for research in the general population. *Appl. Psychol. Meas.* **1977**, *1*, 385–401. [CrossRef]
19. Bojorquez-Chapela, L.; Salgado de Snyder, N. Características psicométricas de la escala Center for Epidemiological Studies-Depression (CES-D), versiones de 20 y 10 reactivos en mujeres de una zona rural mexicana. *Salud Ment.* **2009**, *32*, 297–307.
20. Garcia-Campayo, J.; Zamorano, E.; Ruiz, M.A.; Pardo, A.; Perez-Paramo, M.; Lopez-Gomez, V.; Freire, O.; Rejas, J. Cultural adaptation into Spanish of the generalized anxiety disorder-7 (GAD-7) scale as a screening tool. *Health Qual. Life Outcomes* **2010**, *8*, 8. [CrossRef]
21. Cortina-Guzmán, L.G.; Berenzon-Gom, S. Traducción al español y propiedades picométricas del instrumento "positivity self test". *Psicol. Iberoam.* **2013**, *21*, 53–64. [CrossRef]
22. Diaz, D.; Rodriguez-Carvajal, R.; Blanco, A.; Moreno-Jimenez, B.; Gallardo, I.; Valle, C.; Van Dierendonck, D. Adaptación española de las escalas de bienestar psicológico de Ryff. *Psicothema* **2006**, *18*, 572–577. [PubMed]
23. Ferrando, P.J.; Chico, E.; Tous, J.M. Propiedades psicométricas del test de Optimismo Life Orientation Test. *Psicothema* **2002**, *14*, 673–680.
24. Chirumbolo, A.; Picconi, L.; Morelli, M.; Petrides, K.V. The Assessment of Trait Emotional intelligence: Psychometric Characteristics of the TEIQue-Full Form in a Large Italian Adult Sample. *Front. Psychol.* **2019**, *9*, 2786. [CrossRef]
25. Chobanian, A.V.; Bakris, G.L.; Black, H.R.; Cushman, W.C.; Green, L.A.; Izzo, J.L., Jr. The seventh report of the Joint National Committee on prevention, detection, evaluation, and treatment of high blood pressure: The JNC 7 report. *J. Am. Med. Assoc.* **2003**, *289*, 2560–2572. [CrossRef]
26. Lear, S.A.; James, P.T.; Ko, G.T.; Kumanyika, S.K. Appropriateness of waist circumference and waist-to-hip ratio cutoffs for different ethnic groups. *Eur. J. Clin. Nutr.* **2010**, *64*, 42–61. [CrossRef]
27. Dong, G.; Wang, D.H.; Liu, M.; Liu, Y.; Zhao, Y.; Yang, M.; Meng, X.; Tian, S.; Meng, X.; Zhang, H. Sex difference of the prevalence and risk factors associated with prehypertension among urban Chinese adults from 33 communities of China. *J. Hypertens.* **2012**, *30*, 485–491. [CrossRef]
28. Kringeland, E.; Tell, G.S.; Midtbo, H.; Igland, J.; Haugsgjerd, T.R.; Gerdts, E. Stage 1 hypertension, sex, and acute coronary syndromes during midlife: The Hordaland health study. *Eur. J. Prev. Cardiol.* **2022**, *29*, 147–154. [CrossRef]
29. Ji, H.; Niiranen, T.J.; Rader, F.; Henglin, M.; Kim, A.; Ebinger, J.E.; Claggett, B.; Merz, C.N.B.; Cheng, S. Sex differences in blood pressure associations with cardiovascular outcomes. *Circulation* **2021**, *143*, 761–763. [CrossRef]
30. Nwankwo, T.; Yoon, S.S.; Burt, V.; Gu, Q. *Hypertension among Adults in the United States: National Health and Nutrition Examination Survey, 2011–2012*; NCHS Data Brief; National Center for Health Statistics: Hyattsville, MD, USA, 2013; pp. 1–8.
31. Joyner, M.J.; Wallin, B.G.; Charkoudian, N. Sex differences and blood pressure regulation in humans. *Exp. Physiol.* **2015**, *101*, 349–355. [CrossRef]
32. Molina, L.; Elosúa, R.; Marrugat, J.; Pons, S. Relation of maximum blood pressure during exercise and regular physical activity in normotensive men with left ventricular mass and hypertrophy. *Am. J. Cardiol.* **1999**, *84*, 890–893. [CrossRef] [PubMed]
33. Anonymous. The sixth report of the Joint National Committee on prevention, detection, evaluation, and treatment of high blood pressure. *Arch. Intern. Med.* **1997**, *157*, 2413–2446. [CrossRef]
34. Li, C.; Shang, S. Relationship between Sleep and Hypertension: Findings from the NHANES (2007–2014). *Int. J. Environ. Res. Public Health* **2021**, *18*, 7867. [CrossRef] [PubMed]
35. Shan, M.M.; Mandiga, P. *Psyshiology, Plasma, Osmolality and Oncotic Pressure*; StatPearsPublising: Treasure Island, FL, USA, 2022; pp. 154–196.
36. Chan, Q.; Stamler, J.; Griep, L.M.O.; Daviglus, M.L.; Van Horn, L.; Elliott, P. An update on nutrients and blood pressure. *J. Atheroscler. Thromb.* **2016**, *23*, 276–289. [CrossRef] [PubMed]
37. Behradmanesh, S.; Nasri, H. Association of serum calcium with level of blood pressure in type 2 diabetic patients. *J. Nephropathol.* **2013**, *2*, 254–257. [CrossRef] [PubMed]
38. Farsana, Y.; Samad, N. REPORT-Association between serum electrolytes and erythrocytes Na+, K+ in hypertensive and normotensive male compared to female. *Pak. J. Pharmacol. Sci.* **2020**, *33*, 32122850.
39. Siedlinski, M.; Józefczuk, E.; Xu, X.; Teumer, A.; Evangelou, E.; Schnabel, R.B.; Welsh, P.; Maffia, P.; Erdmann, J.; Tomaszewski, M.; et al. White blood cells and blood pressure. *Circulation* **2020**, *141*, 1307–1317. [CrossRef]
40. Lee, S.; Rim, J.H.; Kim, J. Association of hemoglobin levels with blood pressure and hypertension in a large population-based study: The Korea National Health and Nutrition Examination Surveys 2008–2011. *Clin. Chim. Acta* **2015**, *438*, 12–18. [CrossRef] [PubMed]
41. De Bacquer, D.; De Backer, G.; De Buyzere, M.; Kornitzer, M. Is low serum chloride level a risk factor for cardiovascular mortality? *J. Cardiovasc. Risk* **1998**, *5*, 177–184. [CrossRef]
42. Hatzistavri, L.; Sarafidis, P.A.; Georgianos, P.I.; Tziolas, I.M.; Aroditis, C.P.; Zebekakis, P.; Pikilidou, M.; Lasaridis, A.N. Oral magnesium supplementation reduces ambulatory blood pressure in patients with mild hypertension. *Am. J. Hypertens.* **2009**, *22*, 1070–1075. [CrossRef]

43. Bawazier, L.A.; Sja'bani, M.; Irijanto, F.; Zulaela, Z.; Widiatmoko, A.; Kholiq, A.; Tomino, Y. Association of serum uric acid, morning home blood pressure and cardiovascular risk factors in a population with previous prehypertension: A cross-sectional study. *BMJ Open* **2020**, *10*, e038046. [CrossRef] [PubMed]
44. Li, G.; Wang, H.; Wang, K.; Wang, W.; Dong, F.; Qian, Y.; Gong, H.; Hui, C.; Xu, G.; Li, Y.; et al. The association between smoking and blood pressure in men: A cross-sectional study. *BMC Public Health* **2017**, *17*, 797. [CrossRef] [PubMed]

Disclaimer/Publisher's Note: The statements, opinions and data contained in all publications are solely those of the individual author(s) and contributor(s) and not of MDPI and/or the editor(s). MDPI and/or the editor(s) disclaim responsibility for any injury to people or property resulting from any ideas, methods, instructions or products referred to in the content.

Article

Evolution of Cardiovascular Risk Factors in Post-COVID Patients

Irina Mihaela Abdulan [1,2,†], Veronica Feller [2], Andra Oancea [1,2,*], Alexandra Mаștaleru [1,2,*], Anisia Iuliana Alexa [3], Robert Negru [1], Carmen Marinela Cumpăt [1,2,†] and Maria Magdalena Leon [1,2]

1. Department of Medical Specialties I, "Grigore T. Popa" University of Medicine and Pharmacy, 700115 Iasi, Romania; irina.abdulan@umfiasi.ro (I.M.A.); robert.negru@umfiasi.ro (R.N.); marinela.cumpat@umfiasi.ro (C.M.C.); maria.leon@umfiasi.ro (M.M.L.)
2. Clinical Rehabilitation Hospital, 700661 Iasi, Romania; veronica.feller@gmx.de
3. Department of Surgery II, Discipline of Ophthalmology, "Grigore T. Popa" University of Medicine and Pharmacy, 700115 Iasi, Romania; anisia-iuliana.alexa@umfiasi.ro
* Correspondence: andra.radulescu@yahoo.com (A.O.); alexandra.mastaleru@umfiasi.ro (A.M.)
† These authors contributed equally to this work.

Abstract: (1) Background: SARS-CoV-2 infection has been a subject of extensive discussion in the medical field, particularly in relation to the risk factors and effective treatment strategies for reducing the negative health outcomes associated with the virus. However, researchers indicate that individuals in the recovery phase after COVID-19 experience a range of symptoms that significantly impact their overall well-being and quality of life. At present, there is insufficient evidence to substantiate the claim that patients in the post-acute phase of COVID-19 are at an elevated risk of developing new-onset hypertension or even metabolic syndrome. The current study aimed to assess the risk of cardiovascular diseases after COVID-19 and the optimal treatment of these conditions. (2) Methods: This research was conducted at the Cardiovascular Rehabilitation Clinic of the Iasi Clinical Rehabilitation Hospital (Romania) between the 1st of September and 31st of December 2022. From a total of 551 patients hospitalized in that period, 70 patients with multiple comorbidities were selected. This study included patients over 18 years old who were diagnosed with COVID-19 within the past 30 days. (3) Results: The included patients were mostly women (62.9%) from the urban area (61.4%). Comparing the post-COVID-19 period to the pre-COVID-19 one, it was observed that the risk of hypertension increased from 69.57% to 90% among the subjects ($p = 0.005$). Risk factors for the new onset of hypertension were identified as age, female gender, and an elevated body mass index. Moreover, the number of patients with dyslipidemia doubled, and a higher body mass index was noted. (4) Conclusions: Our findings suggest that patients affected by COVID-19 are at an increased risk of developing hypertension and related disorders.

Keywords: COVID-19; hypertension; obesity; dyslipidemia; long COVID-19

1. Introduction

The COVID-19 pandemic continues to be a significant global health issue, even after more than three years since the first cases were reported. While most patients recover from mild to moderate respiratory illness without needing specialized treatment, it is essential to note that older individuals and those with underlying conditions like cardiovascular diseases, diabetes, chronic respiratory diseases, or neoplasia are at a higher risk of experiencing complications [1].

Patients with underlying cardiovascular disease are particularly vulnerable to the effects of COVID-19. Pre-existing cardiovascular conditions in COVID-19 patients are associated with a higher risk of mortality. Additionally, COVID-19 itself can lead to various cardiovascular complications, such as myocardial injury, arrhythmias, acute coronary syndrome (ACS), and venous thromboembolism (VTE) [2].

Several systematic reviews have explored the connections between cardiovascular disease (CVD) and outcomes in COVID-19 patients. Among these reviews, the largest study conducted by Luo et al. revealed that individuals with CVD had 2.65 times higher odds of mortality when infected with COVID-19 [3].

Not only patients with cardiovascular disease are affected by this infection. Studies show that COVID-19 may lead to the development of hypertension and related diseases [4–7]. Elevated blood pressure [7,8] and hypertension as post-acute sequelae of COVID-19 have been reported in several studies [9,10]. This suggests that COVID-19 could have long-term implications for cardiovascular health. However, further research is needed to fully understand the causal relationship between COVID-19 and the evolution of hypertension and related conditions [7].

The repercussions of infection with COVID-19 can be observed not only immediately, but also at a distance from the infection, months after the acute episode, leading to various symptoms. The most common ones include palpitations and chest pain. Less frequently, individuals may experience late arterial and venous thromboembolism, heart failure, strokes, or transient ischemic attacks, and myopericarditis [11].

The purpose of this study was to evaluate the impact of SARS-CoV-2 infection on cardiovascular diseases as well as on specific treatments.

2. Materials and Methods

2.1. Study Design and Participants

This research was conducted at the Cardiovascular Rehabilitation Clinic of the Iasi Clinical Rehabilitation Hospital (Romania), where patients with SARS-CoV-2 infection were admitted during the pandemic. Later, they were promptly taken over by our clinic in order to initiate cardio-pulmonary rehabilitation programs. From a total of 551 patients hospitalized between the 1st September and 31st December 2022, 70 patients with multiple comorbidities were selected.

The inclusion criteria were an age of over 18 and the presence of COVID infection in the last 30 days. We excluded from the research the patients who did not have a confirmed infection in their medical history, or who went through the disease more than 30 days before recruitment. We also eliminated those who had a previous admission more than three months ago, due to the fact that any acute episode could destabilize the patient's general condition and influence the results of the analyses; those with liver failure, chronic kidney disease with a creatinine clearance less than 15 mL/min/1.73 m^2, or cardiac pacemakers; or those who did not want to participate. The flow chart of the study group selection can be observed in Figure 1.

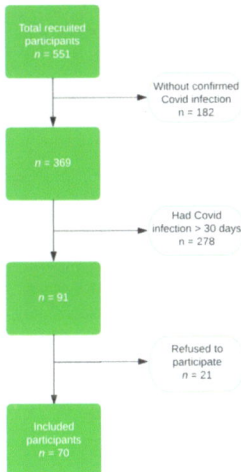

Figure 1. Flow chart of the study group selection.

2.2. Patient Evaluation

We collected data regarding the gender, age, demographic data, BMI, comorbidities (cardiovascular, pulmonary, and metabolic conditions), and current medication (the interest was on cardiovascular antihypertensive medication and on types of drugs). The patients' previous medical history was taken from the medical records of their prior hospitalization.

2.3. Ethical Approval

In order to be enrolled in the research, all of the patients had to complete a written informed consent form. Our study received approval from the Ethics Committee of the Iasi Clinical Rehabilitation Hospital (certificate of approval dated 5 May 2022).

2.4. Statistical Data

Data analysis was performed using SPSS 20.0 (Statistical Package for the Social Sciences, Chicago, IL, USA). The normality of the distribution was assessed for continuous variables by using the Shapiro–Wilk test. The continuous variables that had a normal distribution were presented as a mean ± standard deviation (SD), or as a number of cases (n) with a percent frequency (%) for categorical variables. The independent samples t-test was used when two continuous normally distributed samples were compared, while the one-way ANOVA test was applied when comparing more than two samples. When comparing categorical variables, the Fisher's exact test or chi-square test was used in cases where the expected values of any of the contingency table cells were below 5. A two-sided p-value < 0.05 was considered significant for all statistical analyses.

3. Results

The studied group included 70 patients, mostly women (62.9%), with an average age of 60.84 ± 12.32. The mean body mass index was 29.39 ± 5.05, and 20% of the patients were smokers (Table 1).

Table 1. General characteristics according to the form of the disease in the study group.

General Characteristics	Total (n = 70)	Mild (n = 19)	Medium (n = 39)	Severe (n = 12)	p-Value
Age, years (mean ± SD)	60.84 ± 12.32	62.52 ± 12.29	59.69 ± 10.95	61.91 ± 16.72	0.681
Gender, n (%)					
Male	26 (37.1)	8 (42.1)	14 (35.9)	4 (33.3)	0.866
Female	44 (62.9)	11 (57.9)	25 (64.1)	8 (66.7)	
BMI, kg/m^2 (mean ± SD)	29.39 ± 5.05	29.35 ± 3.79	29.35 ± 5.68	29.59 ± 4.99	0.989
Smoking	14 (20%)	4 (21.1)	8 (20.5)	2 (16.7)	0.791
Place of origin					
Rural	27 (38.6)	6 (31.6)	18 (46.2)	3 (25.0)	0.912
Urban	43 (61.4)	13 (68.4)	21 (53.8)	9 (75.0)	

BMI—body mass index.

All cardiovascular comorbidities were considered. The most significant differences were observed in the cases of chronic kidney disease, dyslipidemia, and obesity status. Additionally, there was a statistically significant increase in the number of patients diagnosed with hypertension or chronic venous insufficiency after COVID-19 infection (Table 2).

Table 2. Comorbidities in the studied group, before and after infection.

Comorbidities	Pre-COVID (n = 70)	Post-COVID (n = 70)	p-Value
Hypertension, n (%)	48 (68.57)	63 (90)	0.005
Chronic ischemic heart disease, n (%)	10 (14.28)	17 (24.3)	0.198
Tricuspid regurgitation, n (%)	3 (4.28)	9 (12.85)	0.128
Mitral regurgitation, n (%)	7 (10)	18 (25.71)	0.037
Chronic cardiac failure, n (%)	10 (14.28)	15 (21.42)	0.378
By-pass, n (%)	5 (7.14)	5 (7.14)	1.000
Atrial fibrillation, n (%)	6 (8.57)	5 (7.1)	1.000
Transient ischemic attack, n (%)	7 (10)	7 (10)	1.000
Arteriosclerosis obliterans, n (%)	2 (2.85)	8 (11.42)	0.166
Chronic venous insufficiency, n (%)	9 (12.85)	21 (30)	0.022
Dyslipidemia, n (%)	16 (22.85)	33 (47.14)	0.004
Obesity, n (%)	13 (18.57)	46 (65.71)	<0.001
Diabetes mellitus, n (%)	13 (18.57)	13 (18.57)	1.000
Asthma, n (%)	2 (2.85)	2 (2.85)	1.000
Chronic obstructive pulmonary disease, n (%)	4 (5.51)	4 (5.51)	1.000
Chronic kidney disease, n (%)	4 (5.71)	69 (98.57)	<0.001

The data obtained led us to detail the results according to the form of infection (Table 3).

Table 3. Comorbidities in the studied group, depending on the form of the disease.

	Mild			Medium			Severe		
	Pre-COVID	Post-COVID	p-Value	Pre-COVID	Post-COVID	p-Value	Pre-COVID	Post-COVID	p-Value
HBP, n (%)									
1	3 (15.8)	4 (21.1)	0.138	3 (7.7)	8 (20.5)	0.033	2 (16.7)	3 (25)	0.590
2	6 (31.6)	5 (26.3)		13 (33.3)	14 (35.9)		2 (16.7)	3 (25)	
3	5 (26.3)	9 (47.4)		9 (23.1)	12 (30.8)		5 (41.7)	5 (41.7)	
CHD, n (%)	2 (10.5)	6 (31.6)	0.232	8 (20.5)	10 (25.6)	0.789	0 (0)	1 (8.3)	1.000
TR, n (%)									
Mild	1 (5.3)	1 (5.3)	1.000	0 (0)	4 (10.3)	0.021	1 (8.3)	2 (16.7)	1.000
Moderate	0 (0)	0 (0)		0 (0)	1 (2.6)		1 (8.3)	1 (8.3)	
MR, n (%)									
Mild	2 (10.5)	4 (21.1)	0.660	4 (10.3)	10 (25.6)	0.138	1 (8.3)	2 (16.7)	0.246
Moderate	0 (0)	0 (0)		0 (0)	0 (0)		0 (0)	2 (16.7)	
CHF, n (%)									
NYHA I	0 (0)	0 (0)		0 (0)	0 (0)		1 (8.3)	1 (8.3)	
NYHA II	1 (5.3)	3 (15.8)	0.660	3 (7.7)	5 (12.8)	0.347	2 (16.7)	1 (8.3)	1.000
NYHA III	1 (5.3)	1 (5.3)		0 (0)	2 (5.1)		1 (8.3)	1 (8.3)	
NYHA IV	0 (0)	0 (0)		1 (2.6)	0 (0)		0 (0)	0 (0)	
By-pass, n (%)									
1	0 (0)	0 (0)		2 (5.1)	1 (2.6)		0 (0)	0 (0)	-
3	1 (5.3)	1 (5.3)	1.000	2 (5.1)	2 (5.2)	1.000	0 (0)	0 (0)	
4	0 (0)	0 (0)		0 (0)	1 (2.6)		0 (0)	0 (0)	
AF, n (%)	1 (5.3)	0 (0)	-	3 (7.7)	4 (10.3)	1.000	2 (16.7)	1 (8.3)	1.000
TIA, n (%)	1 (5.3)	1 (5.3)	1.000	3 (7.7)	3 (7.7)	1.000	3 (25)	3 (25)	1.000

Table 3. Cont.

	Pre-COVID	Mild Post-COVID	p-Value	Pre-COVID	Medium Post-COVID	p-Value	Pre-COVID	Severe Post-COVID	p-Value
AO, n (%)									
I	0 (0)	0 (0)	-	0 (0)	3 (7.7)	0.313	0 (0)	0 (0)	0.478
II	0 (0)	0 (0)		1 (2.6)	2 (5.1)		0 (0)	2 (16.7)	
IV	0 (0)	0 (0)		1 (2.6)	1 (2.6)		0 (0)	0 (0)	
CVI, n (%)									
CEAP 1	0 (0)	0 (0)		0 (0)	1 (1)		1 (8.3)	0 (0)	
CEAP 2	2 (10.5)	3 (15.8)		1 (2.6)	3 (7.7)		0 (0)	1 (8.3)	
CEAP 3	1 (5.3)	2 (10.5)	0.447	0 (0)	4 (10.3)	0.160	0 (0)	3 (25)	-
CEAP 4	0 (0)	1 (5.3)		3 (7.7)	3 (7.7)		0 (0)	0 (0)	
CEAP 6	0 (0)	0 (0)		1 (2.6)	0 (0)		0 (0)	0 (0)	
HC, n (%)	5 (26.3)	10 (52.6)	0.184	7 (17.9)	17 (43.6)	0.026	4 (33.3)	6 (50)	0.680
BMI, n (%)									
Overweight	2 (10.5)	6 (31.6)		1 (2.6)	7 (17.9)		0 (0)	3 (25)	
I	2 (10.5)	7 (36.8)	0.012	4 (10.3)	11 (28.2)	<0.001	0 (0)	3 (25)	0.012
II	0 (0)	1 (5.3)		1 (2.6)	4 (10.3)		0 (0)	1 (8.3)	
III	1 (5.3)	0 (0)		1 (2.6)	2 (5.1)		1 (8.3)	1 (8.3)	
DM, n (%)	2 (10.5)	2 (10.5)	1.000	7 (17.9)	8 (20.5)	1.000	4 (33.3)	4 (33.3)	1.000
Asthma, n (%)	1 (5.3)	1 (5.3)	1.000	1 (2.6)	1 (2.6)	1.000	12 (100)	12 (100)	1.000
COPD, n (%)	1 (5.3)	2 (10.5)	1.000	2 (5.1)	2 (5.1)	1.000	1 (8.3)	1 (8.3)	1.000
CKD, n (%)									
1	0 (0)	2 (10.5)		0 (0)	1 (2.6)		0 (0)	2 (17.7)	
2	0 (0)	11 (57.9)	<0.001	0 (0)	27 (69.2)	<0.001	0 (0)	6 (50)	<0.001
3	0 (0)	6 (31.6)		2 (5.1)	10 (25.6)		1 (8.3)	3 (25)	
4	1 (5.3)	0 (0)		0 (0)	0 (0)		0 (0)	1 (8.3)	

HBP—high blood pressure; CHD—coronary heart disease; TR—tricuspid regurgitation; MR—mitral regurgitation; CF—cardiac failure; AF—atrial fibrillation; TIA—transient ischemic attack; AO—arteriosclerosis obliterans; CVI—chronic venous insufficiency; HC—hypercholesterolemia; BMI—body mass index; DM—diabetes mellitus; COPD—chronic obstructive pulmonary disease; and CKD—chronic kidney disease.

In the case of the patients with a mild form, a statistically significant decrease in renal function was observed, as well as an increase in body mass index. The number of patients with dyslipidemia doubled, but the data were not statistically significant.

The patients with a medium form of infection showed the most differences: an increase in the degree of arterial hypertension, the presence of mild tricuspid insufficiency, and an increase in body mass index. As in the case of the previous group, the most significant differences were observed in the case of renal function.

Severe infection was statistically associated with an increased body mass index and decreased kidney function.

We observed statically significant differences between age and the degree of hypertension. Moreover, even if it was without statistical significance, we noted that BMI increased in those with second- and third-degree hypertension (Table 4).

Table 4. Risk factors associated with hypertension.

	Without	First-Degree	Second-Degree	Third-Degree	
Age	53.42 ± 5.79	50.00 ± 10.70	64.72 ± 11.69	65.80 ± 10.35	<0.001
BMI	25.80 ± 2.74	27.97 ± 4.34	30.05 ± 5.26	30.63 ± 5.29	0.080

Using the Games–Howell post hoc test, we evaluated the differences between age and hypertension. Statistically significant differences were observed between those without hypertension and those with second-degree hypertension ($p = 0.013$), and, respectively, those with third-degree hypertension ($p = 0.003$). Regarding the BMI, using the same test, we observed statistically significant differences between those without hypertension and the patients diagnosed with third-degree hypertension ($p = 0.018$).

Analyzing the patients' medication before and after the infectious episode (Table 5), statistically significant differences were obtained only in the administration of ACE inhibitors in people who went through the medium form of the disease. Even so, several aspects are worth mentioning:

- Patients with a mild form required more drugs to control cardiovascular symptoms.
- Those with a medium form were the category where beta-blockers and calcium channel blockers were most supplemented.
- In the case of those with a severe form, a slight increase was observed in those who required beta-blocker medication and a decrease in the use of sartans.

Table 5. Cardiovascular medication before and after the infection.

Medication	Mild Pre-COVID	Mild Post-COVID	p-Value	Medium Pre-COVID	Medium Post-COVID	p-Value	Severe Pre-COVID	Severe Post-COVID	p-Value
ACE inhibitors, n (%)	3 (15.8)	5 (26.3)	0.693	6 (15.4)	1 (2.6)	0.048	2 (16.7)	2 (16.7)	1.000
Sartans, n (%)	2 (10.5)	3 (15.8)	1.000	5 (12.8)	8 (20.5)	0.545	6 (50)	3 (25)	0.400
Beta-blockers, n (%)	7 (36.8)	8 (42.1)	1.000	16 (41)	24 (61.5)	0.112	6 (50)	8 (66.7)	0.680
Calcium channel blockers, n (%)	7 (36.8)	9 (47.4)	0.743	6 (15.4)	13 (33.3)	0.112	5 (41.7)	6 (50)	1.000
Diuretic, n (%)	5 (26.3)	4 (21.1)	0.157	10 (25.7)	6 (15.4)	0.516	5 (41.7)	5 (41.7)	1.000
Central blockers, n (%)	1 (5.3)	1 (5.3)	1.000	1 (2.6)	2 (5.1)	1.000	1 (8.3)	1 (8.3)	1.000

4. Discussion

Ever since the identification of the COVID-19 outbreak, research efforts have been focused on evaluating optimal therapeutic interventions to attenuate COVID-19-related mortality. Similarly, studies have aimed to identify predictive factors that independently correlate with mortality in patients diagnosed with COVID-19 infection [12]. Nevertheless, information regarding the post-acute and enduring sequelae after the acute phase of COVID-19 remains limited [13]. Considering this, the present study was designed to assess both the influence of COVID-19 on cardiovascular diseases and the efficacy of specific treatments to mitigate morbidity and mortality.

Within the COVID-19 pandemic era, researchers have focused more on hypertension and its associated pathologies [7]. For instance, in their comprehensive review, Shibata et al. investigated the relationship between COVID-19 and hypertension, elucidating that complications of this infection can be recognized as vascular disorders [14]. Furthermore, the spectrum of hypertensive disorders, encompassing cardiovascular disease and chronic kidney disease, have been identified as significant risk factors, predisposing individuals to more severe COVID-19-associated outcomes [4,5]. Over time, multiple researchers have evaluated the potential risk of hypertension after COVID-19. Notably, Zuin et al., through their meta-analysis, highlighted that the patients recovering after COVID-19 exhibited an increased risk of developing new-onset hypertension, as opposed to individuals who were not diagnosed with this infection [15]. However, compared to prior studies based on the general population, wherein the incidence ranges between 15.3 and 47.3 [16,17], this meta-analysis demonstrated a lower rate of new-onset hypertension [15]. Another study that aimed to investigate the frequency of new or worsened existing hypertension, conducted on a cohort of 200 patients, indicated that hypertension is a relatively common occurrence, with an incidence rate of approximately 16%. Additionally, the same study revealed that the patients affected by this disease had a significant risk of developing new-onset hypertension or experiencing a worsening of their existing hypertension condition. In fact, the research estimated that approximately one in every seven people affected by COVID-19 is at risk of such complications [18].

In accordance with previous studies, our analysis demonstrated an increased rate of hypertension after COVID ($p < 0.001$). Moreover, the risk was influenced by female gender ($p = 0.050$), older age, and a higher BMI.

Currently, there is still no consensus on the underlying mechanisms contributing to the emergence of new-onset hypertension following COVID-19. The existing literature data consider dysregulation within the renin–angiotensin–aldosterone system, viral persistence, pre-existing autoimmune conditions, the delayed resolution of inflammation, or residual organ damage as key mechanisms [15,19].

In our research, we made additional observations regarding the medication requirements of the patients. Specifically, we found that the patients with medium and severe forms of COVID-19 required an increased use of beta-blocker medication. This finding can be attributed to the mechanisms of action of these drugs and their role in the pathology of COVID-19 infection. For instance, researchers report that beta-blockers have an anti-inflammatory effect by inhibiting the release of pro-inflammatory cytokines, which helps to diminish the progression of cytokine storms in patients with severe forms of the disease. Furthermore, beta-blockers have been found to inhibit the release of catecholamines caused by the infection, thereby diminishing the development of sympathetic storms. Both cytokine storms and sympathetic storms can lead to complications in patients with severe forms of COVID-19, such as acute lung injury, acute respiratory distress syndrome, and multiple organ failure. Thus, the use of this medication, by interrupting this interaction, has the potential to reduce mortality caused by this pathology [20]. According to Heriansyah T et al., beta-blockers have been identified as beneficial due to their ability to modulate the function of juxtaglomerular cells in the kidneys, thereby blocking the entry gate of the virus. This regulation leads to a decrease in the activity of the renin–angiotensin–aldosterone system pathway and a subsequent reduction in ACE2 levels [21].

In the patients diagnosed with a moderate form of COVID-19, an increased utilization of calcium channel blockers (CCBs) was observed. The role of this medication in reducing morbidity and mortality in patients diagnosed with COVID-19 was demonstrated in a series of studies. A study conducted on 77 hospitalized COVID-19 patients showed that antihypertensive treatment with amlodipine or nifedipine was associated with reduced intubation or mechanical ventilation risk. Moreover, the patients receiving treatment with CCBs had a lower mortality risk than the control group [22]. A meta-analysis further supported these findings, which demonstrated that using CCBs is associated with a reduced mortality rate in hypertensive patients diagnosed with COVID-19 [23]. These outcomes can be attributed to the mechanism of action of CCBs. Studies demonstrated that CCBs can inhibit viral entry without affecting ACE2 expression or activity [24]. This effect is achieved by blocking the calcium ions required for fusion in cell membranes mediated by the spike protein [23]. Additionally, CCBs have a pharmacological effect on the relaxation of the pulmonary smooth muscle, thereby producing pulmonary vasodilatation. As a result, this medication helps alleviate hypoxic conditions in patients with COVID-19 [22].

According to statistical data, the use of ACE inhibitors (ACEis) or sartans is one of the most used therapeutic approaches for patients with hypertension. However, at the onset of the COVID-19 pandemic, there were controversies surrounding the use of these medication classes in hypertensive patients with COVID-19 [25]. Due to the interaction of ACEis or ARBs with the bradykinin pathway, concerns were raised regarding the potential increased mortality risk in hypertensive COVID-19 patients. Nevertheless, a meta-analysis conducted by Gnanenthiran et al., including 14 randomized control trials, suggested that initiating or continuing treatment with ACEis or ARBs is safe in COVID-19 hypertensive patients. Furthermore, the study revealed a lower risk of myocardial infarction among patients treated with inhibitors of the renin–angiotensin system [26]. Similarly, another meta-analysis involving 2823 patients with COVID-19 aimed to compare the effects of continuing or interrupting treatment with ACEIs/ARBs. The study observed a reduction of 41.1% in all-cause hospital mortality in patients who continued the treatment with this class of medication. The same study indicated that ACEis or ARRBs have multiple roles in inhibiting inflammation induced by the renin–angiotensin–aldosterone system axis, contributing to their beneficial effects on increasing survival rates in COVID-19 patients [27].

According to the World Health Organization, obesity has become a global health problem, with the number of affected individuals tripling between 1975 and 2016. In 2016, approximately 40% of the worldwide population was classified as overweight or obese [28]. The COVID-19 pandemic has presented a significant challenge, as individuals who are overweight or obese are at a higher risk of developing severe COVID-19 [29]. In the US, obesity alone accounts for 20% of COVID-19 hospitalizations, while the combination of obesity with type 2 diabetes and hypertension contributes to 60% of all COVID-19 hospitalizations [30]. In our study, we observed an increase in BMI after COVID-19 infection across all forms of the disease. This rise in obesity can be attributed to significant changes in daily routines, such as reduced physical activity and negative alterations in eating habits [29]. A systematic review involving 5,681,813 participants identified a few more risk factors for an increased BMI, including sedentarism, depression, anxiety, unhealthy lifestyle behaviors, excessive stress, sex, and being from an ethnic minority [31].

In line with the prevailing trend of obesity, our study demonstrated a twofold increase in the number of patients with dyslipidemia. The results align with the existing literature regarding the risk of these patients. For instance, Evan Xu et al. conducted a study to evaluate the risk of dyslipidemia in patients following COVID-19 infection. The researchers included three cohorts: 51,919 patients diagnosed with COVID-19 who survived the initial 30 days of infection, 2647 patients with no history of infection, and a historical contemporary control group consisting of 22,539,941 patients. None of the patients in these cohorts had a prior diagnosis of dyslipidemia. The study demonstrated that the patients diagnosed with COVID-19 had increased risks and burdens of incident dyslipidemia [32]. The potential mechanism underlying this association may involve the immune and inflammatory responses triggered by the infection, which could impact hepatic lipoprotein metabolism. Furthermore, changes in the oral and gut microbiomes, as well as proteomic and metabolomic profiles in patients with COVID-19, may contribute to these effects [33–37]. Given that COVID-19 patients experienced an increase in BMI due to changes in diet, exercise, anxiety, and depression, there may be a correlation between these two conditions [32]. However, further studies are needed to determine whether obesity may mediate the incidence of dyslipidemia, or the opposite.

Numerous studies have indicated that COVID-19 patients are at an increased risk of experiencing a decline in kidney function following the acute phase of the infection [38]. Our study yielded similar findings, highlighting the importance of further research to elucidate the underlying mechanism driving this effect and to identify potential therapeutic interventions aimed to slow the progression of CKD.

The high prevalence of patients diagnosed with COVID-19 who require intense care measures has emphasized the need for better preventive measures to reduce the risk of complications associated with this virus, especially among patients with underlying comorbidities. Therefore, a series of vaccines became globally available, but there was a lot of debate regarding their safety and effectiveness. In Romania, patients were encouraged to receive COVID-19 vaccination, although the decision was voluntary, affording patients the autonomy to make choices regarding vaccination and their preferred vaccine. The decision was influenced by several factors, including the limited information currently available on the vaccine's effectiveness and its potential impacts in the short-, medium-, and long-term. Due to confidentiality and privacy policies, our study did not include information on whether the patients were vaccinated against COVID-19 or not. The patients' responses to this question were often vague, and they were evasive in providing details about their vaccination status, the type of vaccine they received, or how many doses they had. In a meta-analysis conducted by Xu et al., which analyzed 22 randomized control trials, it was demonstrated that vaccination is effective both in preventing COVID-19 infection and in reducing the risk of COVID-19 morbidity and mortality in elderly people. Moreover, the study revealed that those who received both vaccine doses had a lower risk of developing the disease. Although there were some adverse reactions to vaccination, the incidence was low, highlighting the benefits of vaccines in preventing the development of severe illness and reducing the mortality risk associated with COVID-19 [39].

In accordance with WHO data, 66.1% of the worldwide population has been administered the last dose of the primary vaccination series, while roughly 32% have received at least one booster or supplementary dose [40]. Thus, with the increasing number of individuals receiving COVID-19 vaccinations, a range of complications associated with the vaccine have been documented. Among these complications, cardiovascular issues have been identified as a significant concern. Notably, there has been growing attention to the potential of COVID-19 vaccination to induce an increased risk of developing hypertension [41].

To explore the prevalence and mechanisms of COVID-19 vaccination-induced blood pressure elevation, Angeli et al. conducted a meta-analysis that analyzed six studies, resulting in a sample size of 357,387 subjects. The authors identified 13,444 events of abnormal or elevated blood pressure among the vaccinated individuals. Furthermore, the researchers revealed a wide range of hypertensive risks associated with COVID-19 vaccination, with estimates ranging from 0.93% to 23.72%. The pooled point estimate was calculated to be 3.91%. Additionally, the study revealed that 0.6% of the vaccinated population experienced stage III hypertension, hypertensive urgencies, and hypertension emergencies [42].

The relationship between COVID-19 vaccines and the increased risk of developing hypertension remains uncertain and necessitates further investigation to understand the underlying mechanisms [41]. Some authors suggested that the potential link may involve the dysfunction of the counter-regulatory renin–angiotensin system axis. Moreover, studies have indicated that the increase in blood pressure after COVID-19 vaccination, mediated by the interaction between the spike protein and the angiotensin-converting enzyme 2, may be more frequent in younger subjects [43]. However, it is important to note that not all studies support this explanation, due to variability in age ranges [44–46]. Another hypothesis suggests that excipients present in the vaccine (e.g., polyethylene glycol) could play a role, although their concentration is considered insignificant [41,47]. The lockdown period during the COVID-19 pandemic should also be considered to contribute to the risk of developing hypertension. In this period, there was an increase in risk factors for hypertension, such as a sedentary lifestyle, unhealthy diet, anxiety, depression, and increased body mass index.

5. Limitations of the Study

The strong point of this study is the fact that we evaluated the patients' short-term outcomes after the infections, many of them being lost from the record in other centers where cardio-respiratory recovery is not performed.

The present research was performed on a small group of patients. We still do not have data related to the impact of the infection on cardiovascular diseases, mainly on arterial hypertension, so we can comment only on the changes that occurred one month after the acute episode.

6. Conclusions

Over the last few years, infection with COVID-19 has become a widely debated topic in the medical literature due to its consequences across various systems.

The effects of the infection observed in this study were an increase in the degree of hypertension and the need to change treatment by choosing medication to control the heart rate (beta-blockers and calcium blockers). One month after the infection, a higher BMI, deterioration of renal function, and alteration of the lipid profile were observed.

Our conclusions lead to the idea of the infection amplifying cardiovascular risk factors, in addition to the direct effect that the infection has on blood pressure.

The implication of this increased risk on the global burden of cardiovascular diseases, as well as its impact on the healthcare system and costs, will require further investigation and the need for the longer-term follow-up of patients with comorbidities and added risk factors.

Author Contributions: Conceptualization, V.F. and M.M.L.; methodology, I.M.A. and C.M.C.; software, A.M.; validation, I.M.A., A.O. and A.M.; investigation, R.N.; resources, A.I.A.; writing—original draft preparation, V.F., I.M.A. and A.O.; writing—review and editing, A.M.; visualization, M.M.L.; supervision, M.M.L. All authors have read and agreed to the published version of the manuscript. All authors have contributed equally to this work.

Funding: This research received no external funding.

Institutional Review Board Statement: This study was conducted in accordance with the Declaration of Helsinki and approved by the Ethics Committee of the Iasi Clinical Rehabilitation Hospital (certificate of approval dated 5 May 2022).

Informed Consent Statement: Informed consent was obtained from all subjects involved in the study.

Data Availability Statement: The data presented in this study are available upon request from the corresponding author.

Conflicts of Interest: The authors declare no conflict of interest.

References

1. World Health Organization. Coronavirus Disease (COVID-19). Available online: https://www.who.int/health-topics/coronavirus#tab=tab_1 (accessed on 11 July 2023).
2. Nishiga, M.; Wang, D.W.; Han, Y.; Lewis, D.B.; Wu, J.C. COVID-19 and cardiovascular disease: From basic mechanisms to clinical perspectives. *Nat. Rev. Cardiol.* **2020**, *17*, 543–558. [CrossRef]
3. Luo, L.; Fu, M.; Li, Y.; Hu, S.; Luo, J.; Chen, Z.; Yu, J.; Li, W.; Dong, R.; Yang, Y.; et al. The potential association between common comorbidities and severity and mortality of coronavirus disease 2019: A pooled analysis. *Clin. Cardiol.* **2020**, *43*, 1478–1493. [CrossRef] [PubMed]
4. Su, Y.; Yuan, D.; Chen, D.; Ng, R.; Wang, K.; Choi, J.; Li, S.; Hong, S.; Zhang, R.; Xie, J.; et al. Multiple early factors anticipate post-acute COVID-19 sequelae. *Cell* **2022**, *185*, 881–895.e20. [CrossRef] [PubMed]
5. Shibata, S.; Kobayashi, K.; Tanaka, M.; Asayama, K.; Yamamoto, E.; Nakagami, H.; Hoshide, S.; Kishi, T.; Matsumoto, C.; Mogi, M.; et al. COVID-19 pandemic and hypertension: An updated report from the Japanese Society of Hypertension project team on COVID-19. *Hypertens. Res.* **2023**, *46*, 589–600. [CrossRef] [PubMed]
6. Cohen, K.; Ren, S.; Heath, K.; Dasmariñas, M.C.; Jubilo, K.G.; Guo, Y.; Lipsitch, M.; Daugherty, S.E. Risk of persistent and new clinical sequelae among adults aged 65 years and older during the post-acute phase of SARS-CoV-2 infection: Retrospective cohort study. *BMJ* **2022**, *376*, e068414. [CrossRef]
7. Matsumoto, C.; Shibata, S.; Kishi, T.; Morimoto, S.; Mogi, M.; Yamamoto, K.; Kobayashi, K.; Tanaka, M.; Asayama, K.; Yamamoto, E.; et al. Long COVID and hypertension-related disorders: A report from the Japanese Society of Hypertension Project Team on COVID-19. *Hypertens. Res.* **2023**, *46*, 601–619. [CrossRef] [PubMed]
8. Saeed, S.; Tadic, M.; Larsen, T.H.; Grassi, G.; Mancia, G. Coronavirus disease 2019 and cardiovascular complications: Focused clinical review. *J. Hypertens.* **2021**, *39*, 1282–1292. [CrossRef]
9. Al-Aly, Z.; Xie, Y.; Bowe, B. High-dimensional characterization of post-acute sequelae of COVID-19. *Nature* **2021**, *594*, 259–264. [CrossRef]
10. Daugherty, S.E.; Guo, Y.; Heath, K.; Dasmariñas, M.C.; Jubilo, K.G.; Samranvedhya, J.; Lipsitch, M.; Cohen, K. Risk of clinical sequelae after the acute phase of SARS-CoV-2 infection: Retrospective cohort study. *BMJ* **2021**, *373*, n1098. [CrossRef]
11. Raman, B.; Bluemke, D.A.; Lüscher, T.F.; Neubauer, S. Long COVID: Post-acute sequelae of COVID-19 with a cardiovascular focus. *Eur. Heart J.* **2022**, *43*, 1157–1172. [CrossRef]
12. Medetalibeyoglu, A.; Emet, S.; Kose, M.; Akpinar, T.S.; Senkal, N.; Catma, Y.; Kaytaz, A.M.; Genc, S.; Omer, B.; Tukek, T. Serum Endocan Levels on Admission Are Associated With Worse Clinical Outcomes in COVID-19 Patients: A Pilot Study. *Angiology* **2021**, *72*, 187–193. [CrossRef]
13. Akpek, M. Does COVID-19 Cause Hypertension? *Angiology* **2022**, *73*, 682–687. [CrossRef]
14. Shibata, S.; Arima, H.; Asayama, K.; Hoshide, S.; Ichihara, A.; Ishimitsu, T.; Kario, K.; Kishi, T.; Mogi, M.; Nishiyama, A.; et al. Hypertension and related diseases in the era of COVID-19: A report from the Japanese Society of Hypertension Task Force on COVID-19. *Hypertens. Res.* **2020**, *43*, 1028–1046. [CrossRef]
15. Zuin, M.; Rigatelli, G.; Bilato, C.; Pasquetto, G.; Mazza, A. Risk of Incident New-Onset Arterial Hypertension After COVID-19 Recovery: A Systematic Review and Meta-analysis. *High Blood Press. Cardiovasc. Prev.* **2023**, *30*, 227–233. [CrossRef] [PubMed]
16. Colangelo, L.A.; Yano, Y.; Jacobs, D.R., Jr.; Lloyd-Jones, D.M. Association of Resting Heart Rate With Blood Pressure and Incident Hypertension over 30 Years in Black and White Adults: The CARDIA Study. *Hypertension* **2020**, *76*, 692–698. [CrossRef] [PubMed]

17. Aladin, A.I.; Al Rifai, M.; Rasool, S.H.; Keteyian, S.J.; Brawner, C.A.; Michos, E.D.; Blaha, M.J.; Al-Mallah, M.H.; McEvoy, J.W. The Association of Resting Heart Rate and Incident Hypertension: The Henry Ford Hospital Exercise Testing (FIT) Project. *Am. J. Hypertens.* **2016**, *29*, 251–257. [CrossRef]
18. Delalić, Ð.; Jug, J.; Prkačin, I. Arterial hypertension following COVID-19: A retrospective study of patients in a central european tertiary care center. *Acta Clin. Croat.* **2022**, *61*, 23–27. [CrossRef] [PubMed]
19. Mehandru, S.; Merad, M. Pathological sequelae of long-haul COVID. *Nat. Immunol.* **2022**, *23*, 194–202. [CrossRef]
20. Al-Kuraishy, H.M.; Al-Gareeb, A.I.; Mostafa-Hedeab, G.; Kasozi, K.I.; Zirintunda, G.; Aslam, A.; Allahyani, M.; Welburn, S.C.; Batiha, G.E. Effects of β-Blockers on the Sympathetic and Cytokines Storms in COVID-19. *Front. Immunol.* **2021**, *12*, 749291. [CrossRef]
21. Heriansyah, T.; Nur Chomsy, I.; Febrianda, L.; Farahiya Hadi, T.; Andri Wihastuti, T. The Potential Benefit of Beta-Blockers for the Management of COVID-19 Protocol Therapy-Induced QT Prolongation: A Literature Review. *Sci. Pharm.* **2020**, *88*, 55. [CrossRef]
22. Solaimanzadeh, I. Nifedipine and Amlodipine Are Associated With Improved Mortality and Decreased Risk for Intubation and Mechanical Ventilation in Elderly Patients Hospitalized for COVID-19. *Cureus* **2020**, *12*, e8069. [CrossRef]
23. Alsagaff, M.Y.; Mulia, E.P.B.; Maghfirah, I.; Luke, K.; Nugraha, D.; Rachmi, D.A.; Septianda, I.; A'yun, M.Q. Association of calcium channel blocker use with clinical outcome of COVID-19: A meta-analysis. *Diabetes Metab. Syndr.* **2021**, *15*, 102210. [CrossRef] [PubMed]
24. Fang, L.; Karakiulakis, G.; Roth, M. Are patients with hypertension and diabetes mellitus at increased risk for COVID-19 infection? *Lancet Respir. Med.* **2020**, *8*, e21. [CrossRef] [PubMed]
25. Kumar, S.; Nikravesh, M.; Chukwuemeka, U.; Randazzo, M.; Flores, P.; Choday, P.; Raja, A.; Aseri, M.; Shivang, S.; Chaudhuri, S.; et al. Safety of ACEi and ARB in COVID-19 management: A retrospective analysis. *Clin. Cardiol.* **2022**, *45*, 759–766. [CrossRef]
26. Gnanenthiran, S.R.; Borghi, C.; Burger, D.; Caramelli, B.; Charchar, F.; Chirinos, J.A.; Cohen, J.B.; Cremer, A.; Di Tanna, G.L.; Duvignaud, A.; et al. Renin-Angiotensin System Inhibitors in Patients With COVID-19: A Meta-Analysis of Randomized Controlled Trials Led by the International Society of Hypertension. *J. Am. Heart Assoc.* **2022**, *11*, e026143. [CrossRef]
27. Liu, Q.; Fu, W.; Zhu, C.J.; Ding, Z.H.; Dong, B.B.; Sun, B.Q.; Chen, R.C. Effect of continuing the use of renin–angiotensin system inhibitors on mortality in patients hospitalized for coronavirus disease 2019: A systematic review, meta-analysis, and meta-regression analysis. *BMC Infect Dis.* **2023**, *23*, 53. [CrossRef]
28. World Health Organization (WHO). Obesity and Overweight. 2017. Available online: https://www.who.int/news-room/fact-sheets/detail/obesity-and-overweight (accessed on 10 August 2023).
29. Steenblock, C.; Hassanein, M.; Khan, E.G.; Yaman, M.; Kamel, M.; Barbir, M.; Lorke, D.E.; Everett, D.; Bejtullah, S.; Lohmann, T.; et al. Obesity and COVID-19: What are the Consequences? *Horm. Metab. Res.* **2022**, *54*, 496–502. [CrossRef]
30. O'Hearn, M.; Liu, J.; Cudhea, F.; Micha, R.; Mozaffarian, D. Coronavirus Disease 2019 Hospitalizations Attributable to Cardiometabolic Conditions in the United States: A Comparative Risk Assessment Analysis. *J. Am. Heart Assoc.* **2021**, *10*, e019259. [CrossRef] [PubMed]
31. Nour, T.Y.; Altintaş, K.H. Effect of the COVID-19 pandemic on obesity and its risk factors: A systematic review. *BMC Public Health* **2023**, *23*, 1018. [CrossRef]
32. Xu, E.; Xie, Y.; Al-Aly, Z. Risks and burdens of incident dyslipidaemia in long COVID: A cohort study. *Lancet Diabetes Endocrinol.* **2023**, *11*, 120–128. [CrossRef]
33. Zhang, S.; Luo, P.; Xu, J.; Yang, L.; Ma, P.; Tan, X.; Chen, Q.; Zhou, M.; Song, S.; Xia, H.; et al. Plasma Metabolomic Profiles in Recovered COVID-19 Patients without Previous Underlying Diseases 3 Months after Discharge. *J. Inflamm. Res.* **2021**, *14*, 4485–4501. [CrossRef]
34. Sorokin, A.V.; Karathanasis, S.K.; Yang, Z.H.; Freeman, L.; Kotani, K.; Remaley, A.T. COVID-19-Associated dyslipidemia: Implications for mechanism of impaired resolution and novel therapeutic approaches. *FASEB J.* **2020**, *34*, 9843–9853. [CrossRef] [PubMed]
35. Roccaforte, V.; Daves, M.; Lippi, G.; Spreafico, M.; Bonato, C. Altered lipid profile in patients with COVID-19 infection. *J. Lab. Precis. Med.* **2020**, *6*, 2. [CrossRef]
36. Ren, Z.; Wang, H.; Cui, G.; Lu, H.; Wang, L.; Luo, H.; Chen, X.; Ren, H.; Sun, R.; Liu, W.; et al. Alterations in the human oral and gut microbiomes and lipidomics in COVID-19. *Gut* **2021**, *70*, 1253–1265. [CrossRef]
37. Chen, Y.; Yao, H.; Zhang, N.; Wu, J.; Gao, S.; Guo, J.; Lu, X.; Cheng, L.; Luo, R.; Liang, X.; et al. Proteomic Analysis Identifies Prolonged Disturbances in Pathways Related to Cholesterol Metabolism and Myocardium Function in the COVID-19 Recovery Stage. *J. Proteome Res.* **2021**, *20*, 3463–3474. [CrossRef]
38. Schiffl, H.; Lang, S.M. Long-term interplay between COVID-19 and chronic kidney disease. *Int. Urol. Nephrol.* **2023**, *55*, 1977–1984. [CrossRef]
39. Xu, K.; Wang, Z.; Qin, M.; Gao, Y.; Luo, N.; Xie, W.; Zou, Y.; Wang, J.; Ma, X. A systematic review and meta-analysis of the effectiveness and safety of COVID-19 vaccination in older adults. *Front. Immunol.* **2023**, *14*, 1113156. [CrossRef] [PubMed]
40. Available online: https://covid19.who.int/table (accessed on 29 September 2023).
41. Buso, G.; Agabiti-Rosei, C.; Muiesan, M.L. The relationship between COVID-19 vaccines and increased blood pressure: A word of caution. *Eur. J. Intern. Med.* **2023**, *111*, 27–29. [CrossRef]
42. Angeli, F.; Reboldi, G.; Trapasso, M.; Santilli, G.; Zappa, M.; Verdecchia, P. Blood Pressure Increase following COVID-19 Vaccination: A Systematic Overview and Meta-Analysis. *J. Cardiovasc. Dev. Dis.* **2022**, *9*, 150. [CrossRef] [PubMed]

43. Angeli, F.; Zappa, M.; Reboldi, G.; Gentile, G.; Trapasso, M.; Spanevello, A.; Verdecchia, P. The spike effect of acute respiratory syndrome coronavirus 2 and coronavirus disease 2019 vaccines on blood pressure. *Eur. J. Intern. Med.* **2023**, *109*, 12–21. [CrossRef]
44. Zappa, M.; Verdecchia, P.; Spanevello, A.; Visca, D.; Angeli, F. Blood pressure increase after Pfizer/BioNTech SARS-CoV-2 vaccine. *Eur. J. Intern. Med.* **2021**, *90*, 111–113. [CrossRef] [PubMed]
45. Tran, V.N.; Nguyen, H.A.; Le, T.T.A.; Truong, T.T.; Nguyen, P.T.; Nguyen, T.T.H. Factors influencing adverse events following immunization with AZD1222 in Vietnamese adults during first half of 2021. *Vaccine* **2021**, *39*, 6485–6491. [CrossRef] [PubMed]
46. Jeet Kaur, R.; Dutta, S.; Charan, J.; Bhardwaj, P.; Tandon, A.; Yadav, D.; Islam, S.; Haque, M. Cardiovascular Adverse Events Reported from COVID-19 Vaccines: A Study Based on WHO Database. *Int. J. Gen. Med.* **2021**, *14*, 3909–3927. [CrossRef]
47. Bouhanick, B.; Montastruc, F.; Tessier, S.; Brusq, C.; Bongard, V.; Senard, J.M.; Montastruc, J.L.; Herin, F. Hypertension and COVID-19 vaccines: Are there any differences between the different vaccines? A safety signal. *Eur. J. Clin. Pharmacol.* **2021**, *77*, 1937–1938. [CrossRef] [PubMed]

Disclaimer/Publisher's Note: The statements, opinions and data contained in all publications are solely those of the individual author(s) and contributor(s) and not of MDPI and/or the editor(s). MDPI and/or the editor(s) disclaim responsibility for any injury to people or property resulting from any ideas, methods, instructions or products referred to in the content.

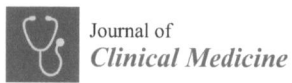

Article

Changes in Metabolic Health and Sedentary Behavior in Obese Children and Adolescents

Maciej Kochman [1,*], Marta Brzuszek [2] and Mirosław Jabłoński [3]

1. Physiotherapy Department, Institute of Health Sciences, College of Medical Sciences, University of Rzeszów, Marszałkowska 24, 35-215 Rzeszów, Poland
2. Institute of Health Sciences, College of Medical Sciences, University of Rzeszów, Kopisto 2a, 35-959 Rzeszów, Poland
3. Chair of Rehabilitation and Physiotherapy, Faculty of Health Sciences, Medical University of Lublin, Jaczewskiego 8 Street, 20-090 Lublin, Poland
* Correspondence: mkochman@ur.edu.pl

Abstract: Obesity is becoming more common among children and adolescents. As in adults, obesity in the pediatric population is associated with an increased risk of metabolic disorders and diseases. In the related literature, little attention has been devoted to evaluating how metabolic health and sedentary behavior change in the obese pediatric population. Therefore, this study aimed to assess changes in metabolic health and sedentary behavior in obese children aged 7–12 and adolescents aged 13–17. For this single-center hospital-based prospective observational study, we included 202 Polish children and adolescents aged 7–17 years. We performed blood pressure measurements and collected blood samples to assess metabolic health markers. Based on the performed measurements, we also calculated additional indexes and ratios: BMI, WHtR, ABSI, VAI, and HOMA-IR. The analysis of the results showed clear and significant differences between the study groups. The older boys and girls were identified with higher values of anthropometric ratios, blood pressure, time spent sitting, and lower HDL cholesterol values ($p < 0.05$). The analysis also revealed a strong-to-moderate correlation between age and anthropometric ratios, blood pressure, HDL cholesterol, and sitting time ($p < 0.05$). Obese children and adolescents included in this study represent poor metabolic health and are at great risk of developing other metabolic diseases such as type 2 diabetes, hypertension, or metabolic syndrome. This risk increases with age; therefore, a number of preventive and therapeutic actions should be taken in overweight and obese children and adolescents to avoid further metabolic complications.

Keywords: obesity; metabolic disorders; cardiometabolic risk factors; children; adolescents

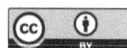

1. Introduction

Obesity is a chronic metabolic disease with complex interactions between genetic, environmental, and biological factors. It has been recognized as one of the diseases of affluence and is a real threat to human health worldwide [1]. The excess of adipose tissue that accumulates in the body is caused by a disturbance in the proportion between food supply and energy expenditure, resulting from the mutual and complicated interaction of environmental and genetic factors [2]. The appearance of obesity is significantly correlated with the risk of many other diseases, such as metabolic syndrome, type 2 diabetes, metabolic dysfunction-associated fatty liver disease (MAFLD), nonalcoholic steatohepatitis (NASH), selected cancers, or cardiovascular disease [3,4]. According to World Health Organization (WHO) reports, obesity is becoming more common among children and adolescents [5]. In the pediatric population, as in adults, obesity is associated with an increased risk of metabolic disorders and diseases [5,6], such as increased blood pressure and cholesterol levels [7], impaired glucose tolerance, insulin resistance, and type 2 diabetes [8], fatty liver [8,9], accelerated puberty in girls [10], or psychological and social problems [11–13].

In both epidemiological studies and the clinical environment, various anthropometric ratios assessing general and abdominal obesity have been proposed. The classic and most commonly used method for assessing body mass is the body mass index (BMI). Despite its simple measurement and ease of assessment, BMI is not the best and most appropriate way to assess obesity because it does not take into account individual body composition or body fat distribution [14]. For this purpose, different measurements are used, such as waist circumference and waist-to-height ratio (WHtR) [15,16], a body shape index (ABSI), and visceral adiposity index (VAI) [17,18]. There are also special methods to accurately assess the amount of body fat, such as body electrical bioimpedance; however, specific devices are needed for this purpose [19]. From a clinical point of view, it is important to diagnose abdominal obesity, because this type of obesity is strongly correlated with the occurrence of other diseases, such as hypertension, dyslipidemia, coronary artery disease [20], or type 2 diabetes [21].

The development of metabolic disorders is also contributed to by a sedentary lifestyle. Sedentary behavior leads to a reduction in the level of physical activity and, when combined with inadequate nutrition, becomes an important predictor of obesity in children. Decreasing time spent in a sitting position and undertaking regular physical activity have many beneficial effects, such as decreasing the risk of cardiovascular disease through reducing cholesterol and lipid levels [22].

As described above, impaired metabolic health increases serious complications and mortality; therefore, monitoring of metabolic health parameters should be crucial in public health policy, especially in the pediatric population. In the related literature, there are many reports concerning associations between obesity and metabolic disorders in the pediatric population; however, little attention has been devoted to evaluating how metabolic health changes in the obese pediatric population, especially in Poland. Therefore, this study aimed to assess changes in metabolic health in obese children aged 7–12 and adolescents aged 13–17. By conducting this research, we wanted to answer the following questions: (1) What are the differences between the study groups in the lipid profile, fasting glucose level, blood pressure, anthropometric measures, and sedentary behavior? (2) Which metabolic health markers are correlated with age?

2. Materials and Methods

2.1. Study Design and Ethics Approval

The protocol of this single-center hospital-based prospective observational study was approved by the Ethics Committee of the Medical University of Lublin (ref. No. KE-0254/13/2018) and the examinations were carried out in compliance with the Declaration of Helsinki. Before the start of the study, each participant and their parent or legal guardian were informed of the examination procedures. After that, each participant and their parent or legal guardian gave their written informed consent to participate in the study.

2.2. Participants

For this observational study, we recruited 283 obese children and adolescents aged 7–17 years living in the Subcarpathian region, Poland, who were referred to the 2nd Department of Pediatrics and Pediatric Endocrinology at the Clinical Hospital No. 2 in Rzeszow, Poland, from January 2018 to April 2019 due to diagnostic obesity. We excluded 81 people from the study due to their not meeting inclusion criteria (49 persons); refusal to participate or fear of examination (32 persons); therefore, for this study we included 202 participants. The following were the inclusion criteria: (1) obtained informed consent; (2) central obesity criteria according to IDF guidelines: waist circumference above the 90th percentile; (3) no genetic or hormonal disease leading to obesity (e.g., Prader Willi syndrome, Bardet–Biedl syndrome, Cushing syndrome, hypothyroidism); (4) no other neurological and orthopedic diseases or learning disabilities. We excluded participants who (1) did not consent to the study or were afraid of study procedures at any stage of the study, (2) with waist circumference below the s90th percentile, (3) with any genetic or hormonal disease affecting obesity, or (4) with other neurological or orthopedic diseases and learning disabilities. The study group was divided into two subgroups: the younger group aged 7–12 and the older group aged 13–17. The younger group consisted of 100 participants (32 girls and 68 boys) and the older group consisted of 102 participants (44 girls and 58 boys). The detailed characteristics of the groups are shown in Table 1.

Table 1. Characteristics of the study group.

Variable		Group Aged 7–12 (n = 100)		Group Aged 13–17 (n = 102)		Total (n = 202)	
		Mean	SD	Mean	SD	Mean	SD
Age	Girls	10	1.67	14.82	1.42	12.79	2.83
	Boys	10.57	1.15	14.53	1.35	12.4	2.34
	Total	10.39	1.36	14.66	1.38	12.55	2.54
Body mass [kg]	Girls	61.09	14.76	84.7	12.97	74.76	18.01
	Boys	69.36	18.7	93.41	20.11	80.43	22.73
	Total	66.72	17.89	89.65	17.85	78.3	21.21
Height [m]	Girls	1.5	0.12	1.64	0.07	1.58	0.12
	Boys	1.54	0.11	1.72	0.1	1.63	0.14
	Total	1.53	0.12	1.68	0.1	1.61	0.13

2.3. Anthropometric and Metabolic Health Measures

Anthropometric measurements were performed by a qualified physiotherapist. Body weight and height were measured using a calibrated Seca scale with a height gauge. The participants were weighed in the clothes they were currently wearing during their stay at the clinic. They were weighed without shoes and outer clothing and the results were recorded to the nearest 0.1 kg. Height was measured with an accuracy of 0.1 cm [23]. Waist circumference was measured twice using a measuring tape. During the measurement, participants were asked to remain in a standing position. The waist circumference was measured in the middle of the distance between the last free rib and the upper edge of the iliac crest with an accuracy of 0.1 cm. The arithmetic mean of two measurements was included in the statistical analysis [24].

Blood samples were collected via phlebotomy from fasting patients (at least 8 h of fasting) in the morning (between 7 and 9 am) of the second day of stay at the clinic by qualified nurses using an S-Monovette blood collection system. Blood analysis was performed after centrifugation of the blood samples. The level of total cholesterol, HDL cholesterol, LDL cholesterol, and triglycerides was analyzed by Trinder reaction-based assays (Atellica CH Analyzer). The level of fasting glucose was analyzed by enzymatic hexokinase and glucose-6-phosphate dehydrogenase methods (Atellica CH Analyzer), and insulin was analyzed by chemiluminometric sandwich immunoassay (Atellica IM Analyzer). Blood analysis was performed in a clinical hospital laboratory meeting the accreditation and quality requirements for a clinical hospital.

Blood pressure was measured in the seated position by qualified nurses using a non-invasive Mindray BeneView T5 cardiomonitor according to standard blood pressure measurement procedures. This device has age-specific cuff widths dedicated for newborns, children and adults. Participants were asked to rest for 5 min before their blood pressure was measured. Three blood pressure measurements were taken and the arithmetic mean of all measurements was included in the statistical analysis [25].

Based on the performed measurements, we also calculated additional indexes and ratios: Body mass index (BMI) was calculated as BMI = weight (kg)/height (m)^2; Waist to height ratio (WHtR) was calculated as WHtR = WC (m)/height (m); Body shape index (ABSI) was calculated as ABSI = WC (m)/(BMI$^{2/3}$ × height (m)$^{1/2}$); Visceral adiposity index (VAI) was calculated separately for boys and girls according to the following formulas:

VAI (boys) = (WC/(1.88 × BMI + 39.68)) × (TG/1.03) × (1.31/HDL) and VAI (girls) = (WC/(1.89 × BMI + 36.58)) × (TG/0.81) × (1.52/HDL); HOMA-IR was calculated as follows: HOMA-IR = (fasting insulin (mU/mL) × fasting glucose (mg/dL))/405 [26–28].

Finally, we conducted a short survey on the time spent daily in a sitting position during the common school day. Questions included information about school time and homework, time devoted to computer games, watching television, as well as spontaneous and organized activities during the past week in hours and minutes.

2.4. Statistical Analysis

Statistical analysis was performed using Statistica 13.3 software. The Shapiro–Wilk test revealed that the investigated variables were not normally distributed; therefore, nonparametric tests were used for further statistical analysis. Statistical significance was assumed if $p < 0.05$. The Mann–Whitney U test was used to compare quantitative data corresponding to blood tests, anthropometric measures, and sitting time. The relationships between age, sitting time, and metabolic health markers were evaluated using the Spearman's rank correlation coefficient. Statistical significance was assumed if $p < 0.05$.

A sample size calculator was used to determine the minimum sample size for the population studied. A fraction size of 0.5 was applied with a maximum error of 5%, and as a result a sample size of 173 people was obtained. Finally, 202 individuals were enrolled in the study group.

3. Results

The evaluation of anthropometric measurements and ratios showed significant differences in BMI, WHtR, ABSI, and VAI between gender-specific age groups. Girls aged 7–12 were identified with lower mean and median values of BMI (26.91 ± 3.44 and 25.81 vs. 31.63 ± 4.5 and 30.8) and greater mean and median values of ABSI (0.077 ± 0.003 and 0.077 vs. 0.074 ± 0.003 and 0.074) compared to girls aged 13–17. In boys aged 7–12, lower mean and median values of BMI, WHtR, VAI, and greater values of ABSI were also found in those aged 7–12 (28.6 ± 4.5 and 27.11 vs. 31.21 ± 4.6 and 30.57; 0.59 ± 0.05 and 0.6 vs. 0.57 ± 0.056 and 0.56; 3.63 ± 3.16 and 2.5 vs. 4.06 ± 2.3 and 3.15; 0.079 ± 0.004 and 0.079 vs. 0.076 ± 0.005 and 0.075, respectively). Similar results were obtained comparing age groups regardless of gender.

According to metabolic health markers, significant differences were identified between study groups in systolic and diastolic blood pressure, total cholesterol, HDL—cholesterol, LDL—cholesterol, and HOMA-IR. In girls aged 7–12, the mean and median values of systolic (114.56 ± 14.08 and 113 vs. 126.63 ± 13.93 and 128) and diastolic blood pressure (70.11 ± 7.42 and 71 vs. 76.27 ± 7.17 and 76.67) were lower and the values of total cholesterol (184.62 ± 22.56 and 184 vs. 168.93 ± 27.54 and 171) and LDL—cholesterol (117.21 ± 18.75 and 117 vs. 103.5 ± 24.91 and 105.5) were higher compared to the girls aged 13–17. Boys aged 7–12 were found with lower mean and median values of HOMA-IR (2.48 ± 1.47 and 1.9 vs. 2.76 ± 1.08 and 2.84) and systolic blood pressure (121 ± 10.74 and 120.33 vs. 130.11 ± 13.53 and 129.33) and greater values of HDL (46.4 ± 9.31 and 48 vs. 43.53 ± 7.87 and 43) and LDL—cholesterol (112.94 ± 29.96 and 112.5 vs. 102.81 ± 36.08 and 100) compared to boys aged 13–17. The analysis of age groups regardless of gender showed similar differences.

A comparison of sitting time revealed that both girls and boys aged 13–17 spent significantly more time in a sitting position than the younger group (615.95 ± 133.91 and 600 vs. 531.94 ± 154.51 and 540; 592.07 ± 124.64 and 600 vs. 532.16 ± 127.97 and 540, respectively). Detailed results are shown in Table 2.

We also evaluated the relationship between age and anthropometric measurements and ratios, as well as metabolic health markers. We observed strong-to-weak correlations between analyzed parameters. This relationship is presented separately for the gender-specific age groups and the entire population studied.

Table 2. Comparison of anthropometric measurements, metabolic health markers, and sitting time between groups.

Variable	Gender	Group Aged 7–12 (N = 100)		Group Aged 13–17 (N = 102)		Z	p
		Mean (SD)	Median	Mean (SD)	Median		
BMI	Girls	26.91 (3.44)	25.81	31.63 (4.5)	30.8	−4.68	<0.0001
	Boys	28.6 (4.5)	27.11	31.21 (4.6)	30.57	−3.81	<0.0001
	Total	28.06 (4.25)	27	31.39 (4.54)	30.78	−5.81	<0.0001
WHtR	Girls	0.57 (0.05)	0.55	0.58 (0.06)	0.57	−0.43	0.668
	Boys	0.59 (0.05)	0.6	0.57 (0.056)	0.56	2.73	0.006
	Total	0.59 (0.05)	0.58	0.57 (0.06)	0.56	1.93	0.05
ABSI	Girls	0.077 (0.003)	0.077	0.074 (0.003)	0.074	5.05	<0.0001
	Boys	0.079 (0.004)	0.079	0.076 (0.005)	0.075	4.52	<0.0001
	Total	0.079 (0.003)	0.077	0.075 (0.004)	0.074	6.73	<0.0001
VAI	Girls	4.54 (2.45)	3.94	4.78 (3.16)	3.98	−0.05	0.96
	Boys	3.63 (3.16)	2.5	4.06 (2.3)	3.15	−2.29	0.02
	Total	3.89 (2.99)	3.28	4.36 (2.7)	3.28	−2.14	0.03
HOMA-IR	Girls	3.48 (2.44)	2.74	3.33 (2.42)	2.48	0.55	0.58
	Boys	2.48 (1.47)	1.9	2.76 (1.08)	2.84	−1.89	0.06
	Total	2.8 (1.88)	2.11	3.01 (1.81)	2.69	−1.37	0.172
SBP	Girls	114.56 (14.08)	113	126.63 (13.93)	128	−3.31	0.001
	Boys	121 (10.74)	120.33	130.11 (13.53)	129.33	−3.65	0.0002
	Total	118.97 (12.2)	118.67	128.57 (13.74)	128.33	−4.71	<0.0001
DBP	Girls	70.11 (7.42)	71	76.27 (7.17)	76.67	−3.31	0.0009
	Boys	75.58 (5.95)	75	77.79 (9.95)	78	−1.3	0.192
	Total	73.85 (6.9)	74.67	77.12 (8.82)	77	−2.62	0.009
CL [mg/dL]	Girls	184.62 (22.56)	184	168.93 (27.54)	171	2.06	0.04
	Boys	182.12 (36.89)	181.5	173.72 (39.9)	168	1.72	0.086
	Total	182.87 (33.16)	183	171.71 (3516)	171	2.62	0.009
HDL-C [mg/dL]	Girls	46.28 (9.22)	47	43.83 (8.46)	42	1.2	0.228
	Boys	46.4 (9.31)	48	43.53 (7.87)	43	1.96	0.05
	Total	46.36 (9.24)	47	43.66 (8.08)	42	2.47	0.013
LDL-C [mg/dL]	Girls	117.21 (18.75)	117	103.5 (24.91)	105.5	2.67	0.008
	Boys	112.94 (29.96)	112.5	102.81 (36.08)	100	2.34	0.019
	Total	114.22 (27.07)	116	103.1 (31.73)	100.5	3.28	0.001
TG [mg/dL]	Girls	105.59 (43.75)	102	108 (60.58)	90.5	0.37	0.708
	Boys	120.99 (72.66)	102.5	130.69 (57)	114	−1.84	0.066
	Total	116.38 (65.53)	102	121.16 (59.31)	107.5	−1.01	0.31

Table 2. Cont.

Variable	Gender	Group Aged 7–12 (N = 100)		Group Aged 13–17 (N = 102)		Z	p
		Mean (SD)	Median	Mean (SD)	Median		
FG [mg/dL]	Girls	83.56 (6.03)	84.5	82.21 (10.73)	81	0.8	0.424
	Boys	84.01 (9.76)	83	85.86 (11.9)	85	−0.77	0.439
	Total	83.87 (8.71)	83	84.29 (11.5)	83	−0.1	0.921
ST [min]	Girls	531.94 (154.51)	540	615.95 (133.91)	600	−1.99	0.046
	Boys	532.16 (127.97)	540	592.07 (124.64)	600	−2.48	0.013
	Total	532.09 (136.11)	540	602.1 (128.49)	600	−3.32	0.001

N—number of participants; Z–z-score; BMI—body mass index; WC–waist circumference; WHtR—waist to height ratio; ABSI–a body shape index; VAI—visceral adiposity index; HOMA-IR—homeostatic model assessment of insulin resistance; SBP—systolic blood pressure; DBP—diastolic blood pressure; CL—total cholesterol; HDL-C—HDL cholesterol; LDL-C—LDL cholesterol; TG—triglycerides; FG—fasting glucose; ST—sitting time.

For the girls aged 7–12, a highly significant, positive, and strong-to-moderate correlation was identified between age and VAI (R = 0.61, $p < 0.001$), HOMA-IR (R = 0.56; $p = 0.001$), triglycerides (R = 0.59, $p < 0.001$), sitting time (R = 0.4, $p = 0.025$) and fasting glucose (R = 0.38, $p = 0.031$). A significant and moderate but negative correlation was identified between age and WHtR (R = −0.46, $p = 0.011$) and HDL cholesterol (R = −0.46, $p = 0.011$). In boys aged 7–12, the only correlation was found between age and HOMA-IR (R = 0.33, $p = 0.006$). For the entire group aged 7–12, a highly significant, weak, and positive correlation was observed between age and BMI (R = 0.23, $p = 0.022$), HOMA-IR (R = 0.38, $p = 0.0001$), systolic blood pressure (R = 0.29, $p < 0.004$), and sitting time (R = 0.3, $p = 0.003$). In addition, a significant, weak but negative correlation was found between age and HDL cholesterol (R = −0.28, $p = 0.005$).

For the girls aged 13–17, a significant, positive, and moderate correlation was identified between age and BMI (R = 0.35; $p = 0.021$) and a moderate but negative correlation between age and HOMA-IR (R = 0.45, $p = 0.003$) and fasting glucose (R = −0.57, $p < 0.0001$). For the boys aged 13–17, a highly significant, positive, and moderate correlation was observed between age and BMI (R = 0.39, $p = 0.003$), VAI (R = 0.42, $p = 0.001$), systolic blood pressure (R = 0.41, $p = 0.002$), triglycerides (R = 0.33, $p = 0.012$) and sitting time (R = 0.43, $p = 0.0009$). A moderate but negative correlation was found between age and ABSI (R = −0.26, $p = 0.045$), and HDL cholesterol (R = −0.38, $p = 0.003$). For the entire group aged 13–17, a highly significant, moderate, and positive correlation was identified between age and BMI (R = 0.38, $p < 0.0001$), VAI (R = 0.23, $p = 0.02$), systolic blood pressure (R = 0.26, $p = 0.01$), and sitting time (R = 0.25, $p = 0.014$). A significant, moderate but negative correlation was found between age and HDL cholesterol (R = −0.21, $p = 0.037$), fasting glucose (R = −0.2, $p = 0.0497$), and ABSI (R = −0.29, $p = 0.003$).

For the entire group of girls, a highly significant, moderate, and positive correlation was identified between age and BMI (R = 0.58, $p < 0.0001$), systolic (R = 0.37, $p = 0.001$) and diastolic blood pressure (R = 0.29, $p = 0.011$), and sitting time (R = 0.27, $p = 0.021$). A significant, strong-to-moderate, but negative correlation was found between ABSI (R = −0.61, $p < 0.0001$) and LDL cholesterol (R = −0.27, $p = 0.022$). For the entire group of boys, a highly significant, positive, and moderate correlation was found in BMI (R = 0.44, $p < 0.0001$), VAI (R = 0.26, $p = 0.004$), HOMA-IR (R = 0.29, $p = 0.001$), systolic blood pressure (R = 0.42, $p < 0.0001$) and sitting time (R = 0.36, $p < 0.0001$). A negative and moderate correlation was found between age and ABSI (R = −0.42, $p < 0.0001$) and HDL cholesterol (R = −0.3, $p = 0.0006$). As in the group of boys, similar relationships were found when we analyzed the entire studied population regardless of gender. These results are shown in Table 3.

Table 3. Correlation of age vs. anthropometric measurements, ratios, metabolic health markers, and sitting time.

		Aged 7–12 (N = 100)		Aged 13–17 (N = 102)		Total (N = 202)	
		R	p	R	p	R	p
BMI	Girls	0.21	0.251	0.35	0.021	0.58	<0.0001
	Boys	0.23	0.057	0.39	0.003	0.44	<0.0001
	Total	0.23	0.022	0.38	<0.0001	0.49	<0.0001
WHtR	Girls	−0.46	0.011	0.21	0.18	0.06	0.611
	Boys	0.16	0.203	0.01	0.951	−0.17	0.0612
	Total	−0.01	0.948	0.1	0.314	−0.09	0.206
ABSI	Girls	0.01	0.988	−0.29	0.062	−0.61	<0.0001
	Boys	−0.09	0.469	−0.26	0.045	−0.42	<0.0001
	Total	−0.01	0.91	−0.29	0.003	−0.49	<0.0001
VAI	Girls	0.61	0.0007	−0.06	0.706	0.07	0.581
	Boys	0.04	0.772	0.42	0.001	0.26	0.004
	Total	0.16	0.122	0.23	0.02	0.22	0.002
HOMA-IR	Girls	0.56	0.001	−0.45	0.003	−0.1	0.409
	Boys	0.33	0.006	0.16	0.259	0.29	0.001
	Total	0.38	0.0001	−0.15	0.151	0.16	0.027
SBP	Girls	0.27	0.137	0.1	0.54	0.37	0.001
	Boys	0.24	0.053	0.41	0.002	0.42	<0.0001
	Total	0.29	0.004	0.26	0.01	0.4	<0.0001
DBP	Girls	0.01	0.983	−0.1	0.536	0.29	0.011
	Boys	0.02	0.844	−0.05	0.722	0.08	0.41
	Total	0.1	0.33	−0.1	0.322	0.15	0.035
CL	Girls	0.08	0.675	−0.03	0.873	−0.21	0.078
	Boys	−0.03	0.825	0.223	0.093	−0.1	0.247
	Total	0.01	0.946	0.11	0.264	−0.14	0.055
HDL-C	Girls	−0.46	0.011	−0.01	0.956	−0.2	0.092
	Boys	−0.21	0.086	−0.38	0.003	−0.3	0.0006
	Total	−0.28	0.005	−0.21	0.037	−0.28	<0.0001
LDL-C	Girls	−0.09	0.646	0.05	0.74	−0.27	0.022
	Boys	−0.01	0.988	0.26	0.051	−0.14	0.131
	Total	−0.02	0.859	0.16	0.104	−0.17	0.015
TG	Girls	0.59	0.0007	−0.06	0.703	0.03	0.785
	Boys	−0.04	0.759	0.33	0.012	0.19	0.03
	Total	0.19	0.06	0.11	0.293	0.13	0.06
FG	Girls	0.38	0.031	−0.57	<0.0001	−0.23	0.051
	Boys	0.01	0.956	0.14	0.286	0.09	0.307
	Total	0.13	0.204	−0.2	0.0497	−0.01	0.845

Table 3. *Cont.*

		Aged 7–12 (N = 100)		Aged 13–17 (N = 102)		Total (N = 202)	
		R	p	R	p	R	p
ST	Girls	0.4	0.025	−0.01	0.971	0.27	0.021
	Boys	0.23	0.059	0.43	0.0009	0.36	<0.0001
	Total	0.3	0.003	0.25	0.014	0.34	<0.0001

N—number of participants; R—Spearman correlation coefficient; BMI—body mass index; WC—waist circumference; WHtR—waist to height ratio; ABSI—a body shape index; VAI—visceral adiposity index; HOMA-IR—homeostatic model assessment of insulin resistance; SBP—systolic blood pressure; DBP—diastolic blood pressure; CL—total cholesterol; HDL-C—HDL cholesterol; LDL-C—LDL cholesterol; TG—triglycerides; FG—fasting glucose; ST—sitting time.

4. Discussion

In this study, we evaluated how metabolic health changes between obese children aged 7–12 and adolescents aged 13–17 years. We observed significant differences between gender-specific age groups in analyzed anthropometric and metabolic health parameters. The values of BMI and blood pressure were higher in both older boys and girls, while the values of ABSI and LDL cholesterol were higher in younger boys and girls. Girls aged 7–12 were identified with greater values of total cholesterol while only boys with HDL cholesterol were identified. The comparison of metabolic parameters between the age groups regardless of gender revealed similar results, as the older group was identified with greater values of BMI, blood pressure, WHtR, and VAI, while the values of ABSI, HDL, and LDL cholesterol and total cholesterol were higher in the younger group. We did not observe differences in levels of triglycerides and fasting glucose between groups. As is commonly known, the human body changes with age, especially during puberty. In this period, there are dynamic changes in the external appearance of boys and girls, and the whole body and its proportions change due to growth and weight gain [29]. However, higher values of anthropometric parameters and lower values of HDL cholesterol in the older group are a cause for concern, as in the literature there is strong evidence of associations of these factors with diabetic complications [30], cardiovascular [31], and cardiometabolic risks [32]. Moreover, HDL cholesterol plays a critical protective and antiatherogenic role [33]. We also observed higher values of total cholesterol and LDL cholesterol in the younger group. These parameters are also a cause for concern, as they correlate with hypertension [34] and atherosclerotic cardiovascular disease [35].

The above results are also consistent with the correlations we performed between age and anthropometric ratios, as well as metabolic health markers. Our results showed strong-to-weak positive correlations between age and BMI, HOMA-IR, VAI, and systolic blood pressure. The negative strong-to-weak correlations were noticed between age and HDL cholesterol level and ABSI. These results indicate that the metabolic health of the study group may deteriorate in the future unless preventive actions are taken to stop or reverse this process [36,37]. In some studies, authors observed a relationship between the stage of puberty and the development of metabolic disorders. According to Boyne et al., an earlier onset of puberty is associated with increased cardiometabolic risk only in girls. Their study showed that earlier menarche and greater breast development in girls were related to higher fasting glucose and the pubarchal stage was associated with systolic blood pressure [38].

Sedentary behavior, as well as insufficient physical activity, passive leisure activities, high-calorie diets, and unhealthy eating habits, may lead to metabolic disorders and various health problems [39–41]. In this study, the comparison of sitting time revealed that both girls and boys aged 13–17 spent significantly more time in a sitting position than the younger boys and girls. We also observed a positive and moderate correlation between age and sitting time in almost every analyzed group. This has been also observed in a longitudinal study by Janssen et al. of English children and adolescents [42]. According to Martinez-

Gomez et al., the time spent in sedentary activities can play a critical role in the development of cardiovascular risk during adolescence. The results of their study suggest the need to take into account a reduction in sedentary behavior as an additional preventive strategy for the premature development of cardiovascular risk in infancy and adolescence, as well as the promotion of physical activity and improvements in eating habits [43]. The study results of Govindan et al. indicate that increased time spent watching television was significantly related to obesity for both boys and girls aged 10–12 and this relationship was influenced by corresponding decreased physical activity. The authors suggest that interventions reducing sedentary behaviors may be an important component of reducing childhood obesity [44]. This has also been confirmed in other studies [45,46]. The cohort study carried out by Aljahdali et al. showed that sedentary time was related to cardiometabolic risk factors in Mexican children and adolescents. The authors indicated that replacing sedentary time with higher intensities improves cardiometabolic markers [45]. The study conducted by Velde et al. revealed that sedentary time was positively associated with BMI z-score and waist circumference in Dutch primary school children aged 7–12 years [46].

The results of this research are alarming and should be taken into account by governments and national health systems to promote preventive, educational, and therapeutic actions and health programs, especially in overweight and obese children and adolescents, and their parents. This study may also have clinical applications for primary care physicians and other clinical specialists during routine health check-ups in children and adolescents. Finally, as the study participants were primary and high school students, this study may have an educational impact on schoolteachers and principals to better understand the health-related problems of students.

We must admit that this study has some limitations. The primary limitation of our study is that the study groups were unequal. In both age groups, there were fewer girls and that could disturb the comparison between groups. Because this was a hospital-based study, we were also unable to include a control group to prove whether changes in metabolic health were related to the obesity or age-related growth of children. Finally, it could be beneficial to include physical activity and nutritional assessments to further investigate the metabolic health status of study participants.

5. Conclusions

In our study, we observed critical changes between gender-specific age groups in anthropometric and metabolic health parameters. The comparison of metabolic parameters between the age groups regardless of gender revealed that the older group was identified with greater values of BMI, blood pressure, WHtR, and VAI, while the values of ABSI, HDL and LDL cholesterol, and total cholesterol were higher in the younger group. The comparison of gender-specific age groups indicated that the values of BMI and blood pressure were higher in both older boys and girls, while the values of ABSI and LDL cholesterol were higher in younger boys and girls. Girls aged 7–12 were identified with greater values of total cholesterol while boys were identified with HDL cholesterol. We also demonstrated strong-to-weak positive correlations between age and BMI, HOMA-IR, VAI, and systolic blood pressure, but also negative strong-to-weak correlations between age and HDL cholesterol level and ABSI. We also observed that sedentary behavior worsens with age in both boys and girls. The correlation between age and sitting time was positive and moderate in almost every analyzed group. Obese children and adolescents are at great risk of developing further metabolic diseases such as type 2 diabetes, hypertension, or metabolic syndrome. The risk increases with age; therefore, a number of preventive and therapeutic actions should be taken in overweight and obese children and adolescents to avoid further metabolic complications. They should also be encouraged to follow a healthy lifestyle, including a healthy and low-calorie diet, and engage in various forms of physical activity to reduce sitting time and ultimately improve their metabolic health status. Because obesity is now considered a worldwide epidemic increasing comorbidities' prevalence and metabolic disorders, it is important to monitor the metabolic health parameters, especially in the pediatric population. Further studies including control groups, physical activity and nutritional assessments are needed in this area.

Author Contributions: Conceptualization, M.K. and M.J.; methodology, M.K. and M.J.; software, M.K. and M.B; validation, M.K. and M.B.; formal analysis, M.K.; investigation, M.K. and M.B.; resources, M.B.; data curation, M.K. and M.B.; writing—original draft preparation, M.K.; writing—review and editing, M.J. and M.K.; visualization, M.K.; supervision, M.J.; project administration, M.K. and M.B.; funding acquisition, M.J. All authors have read and agreed to the published version of the manuscript.

Funding: This research received no external funding.

Institutional Review Board Statement: The study was conducted in accordance with the Declaration of Helsinki, and approved by the Ethics Committee of the Medical University of Lublin (ref. no. KE-0254/13/2018).

Informed Consent Statement: Informed consent was obtained from all subjects involved in the study.

Data Availability Statement: The datasets used during the current study are available from the corresponding author on reasonable request.

Acknowledgments: The authors would like to thank all the participants who committed their time to this study.

Conflicts of Interest: The authors declare no conflict of interest.

References

1. Kumar, S.; Kaufman, T. Childhood Obesity. *Panminerva Med.* **2018**, *60*, 200–212. [CrossRef] [PubMed]
2. Lin, X.; Li, H. Obesity: Epidemiology, Pathophysiology, and Therapeutics. *Front. Endocrinol.* **2021**, *12*, 706978. [CrossRef]
3. Kawai, T.; Autieri, M.V.; Scalia, R. Adipose Tissue Inflammation and Metabolic Dysfunction in Obesity. *Am. J. Physiol.-Cell Physiol.* **2021**, *320*, C375–C391. [CrossRef] [PubMed]
4. Gutiérrez-Cuevas, J.; Santos, A.; Armendariz-Borunda, J. Pathophysiological Molecular Mechanisms of Obesity: A Link between MAFLD and NASH with Cardiovascular Diseases. *Int. J. Mol. Sci.* **2021**, *22*, 11629. [CrossRef] [PubMed]
5. World Health Organization. *Report of the Commission Ending Childhood Obesity*; WHO: Geneva, Switzerland, 2016.
6. Lee, E.Y.; Yoon, K.-H. Epidemic Obesity in Children and Adolescents: Risk Factors and Prevention. *Front. Med.* **2018**, *12*, 658–666. [CrossRef]
7. Umer, A.; Kelley, G.A.; Cottrell, L.E.; Giacobbi, P.; Innes, K.E.; Lilly, C.L. Childhood Obesity and Adult Cardiovascular Disease Risk Factors: A Systematic Review with Meta-Analysis. *BMC Public Health* **2017**, *17*, 683. [CrossRef]
8. Valaiyapathi, B.; Gower, B.; Ashraf, A.P. Pathophysiology of Type 2 Diabetes in Children and Adolescents. *Curr. Diabetes Rev.* **2020**, *16*, 220–229. [CrossRef]
9. Mann, J.; Valenti, L.; Scorletti, E.; Byrne, C.; Nobili, V. Nonalcoholic Fatty Liver Disease in Children. *Semin. Liver Dis.* **2018**, *38*, 001–013. [CrossRef]
10. Reinehr, T.; Roth, C.L. Is There a Causal Relationship between Obesity and Puberty? *Lancet Child Adolesc. Health* **2019**, *3*, 44–54. [CrossRef]
11. Rankin, J.; Matthews, L.; Cobley, S.; Han, A.; Sanders, R.; Wiltshire, H.D.; Baker, J.S. Psychological Consequences of Childhood Obesity: Psychiatric Comorbidity and Prevention. *Adolesc. Health Med. Ther.* **2016**, *7*, 125–146. [CrossRef]
12. Sahoo, K.; Sahoo, B.; Choudhury, A.; Sofi, N.; Kumar, R.; Bhadoria, A. Childhood Obesity: Causes and Consequences. *J. Fam. Med. Prim. Care* **2015**, *4*, 187. [CrossRef]
13. Smith, J.D.; Fu, E.; Kobayashi, M.A. Prevention and Management of Childhood Obesity and Its Psychological and Health Comorbidities. *Annu. Rev. Clin. Psychol.* **2020**, *16*, 351–378. [CrossRef]
14. Rothman, K.J. BMI-Related Errors in the Measurement of Obesity. *Int. J. Obes.* **2008**, *32*, S56–S59. [CrossRef]
15. Lu, Y.; Liu, S.; Qiao, Y.; Li, G.; Wu, Y.; Ke, C. Waist-to-Height Ratio, Waist Circumference, Body Mass Index, Waist Divided by Height0.5 and the Risk of Cardiometabolic Multimorbidity: A National Longitudinal Cohort Study. *Nutr. Metab. Cardiovasc. Dis.* **2021**, *31*, 2644–2651. [CrossRef]
16. Ashwell, M.; Gunn, P.; Gibson, S. Waist-to-Height Ratio Is a Better Screening Tool than Waist Circumference and BMI for Adult Cardiometabolic Risk Factors: Systematic Review and Meta-Analysis. *Obes. Rev.* **2012**, *13*, 275–286. [CrossRef] [PubMed]
17. Krakauer, N.; Krakauer, J. Untangling Waist Circumference and Hip Circumference from Body Mass Index with a Body Shape Index, Hip Index, and Anthropometric Risk Indicator. *Metab. Syndr. Relat. Disord.* **2018**, *16*, 160–165. [CrossRef]
18. Hourani, H.; Alkhatib, B. Anthropometric Indices of Obesity as Predictors of High Blood Pressure among School Children. *Clin. Exp. Hypertens.* **2021**, *44*, 11–19. [CrossRef]

19. Kochman, M.; Kasperek, W.; Guzik, A.; Drużbicki, M. Body Composition and Physical Fitness: Does This Relationship Change in 4 Years in Young Adults? *Int. J. Environ. Res. Public Health* **2022**, *19*, 1579. [CrossRef]
20. Gutiérrez-Cuevas, J.; Sandoval-Rodriguez, A.; Meza-Rios, A.; Monroy-Ramírez, H.C.; Galicia-Moreno, M.; García-Bañuelos, J.; Santos, A.; Armendariz-Borunda, J. Molecular Mechanisms of Obesity-Linked Cardiac Dysfunction: An Up-Date on Current Knowledge. *Cells* **2021**, *10*, 629. [CrossRef] [PubMed]
21. Chen, R.; Ji, L.; Chen, Y.; Meng, L. Weight-to-Height Ratio and Body Roundness Index Are Superior Indicators to Assess Cardio-Metabolic Risks in Chinese Children and Adolescents: Compared with Body Mass Index and a Body Shape Index. *Transl. Pediatr.* **2022**, *11*, 318–329. [CrossRef]
22. Pope, Z.C.; Huang, C.; Stodden, D.; McDonough, D.J.; Gao, Z. Effect of Children's Weight Status on Physical Activity and Sedentary Behavior during Physical Education, Recess, and After School. *J. Clin. Med.* **2020**, *9*, 2651. [CrossRef] [PubMed]
23. Zhang, F.-L.; Ren, J.-X.; Zhang, P.; Jin, H.; Qu, Y.; Yu, Y.; Guo, Z.-N.; Yang, Y. Strong Association of Waist Circumference (WC), Body Mass Index (BMI), Waist-to-Height Ratio (WHtR), and Waist-to-Hip Ratio (WHR) with Diabetes: A Population-Based Cross-Sectional Study in Jilin Province, China. *J. Diabetes Res.* **2021**, *2021*, 8812431. [CrossRef]
24. Dyrstad, S.M.; Edvardsen, E.; Hansen, B.H.; Anderssen, S.A. Waist Circumference Thresholds and Cardiorespiratory Fitness. *J. Sport Health Sci.* **2019**, *8*, 17–22. [CrossRef] [PubMed]
25. Velázquez-López, L.; Santiago-Díaz, G.; Nava-Hernández, J.; Muñoz-Torres, A.V.; Medina-Bravo, P.; Torres-Tamayo, M. Mediterranean-Style Diet Reduces Metabolic Syndrome Components in Obese Children and Adolescents with Obesity. *BMC Pediatr.* **2014**, *14*, 175. [CrossRef]
26. Vizzuso, S.; Del Torto, A.; Dilillo, D.; Calcaterra, V.; Di Profio, E.; Leone, A.; Gilardini, L.; Bertoli, S.; Battezzati, A.; Zuccotti, G.V.; et al. Visceral Adiposity Index (VAI) in Children and Adolescents with Obesity: No Association with Daily Energy Intake but Promising Tool to Identify Metabolic Syndrome (MetS). *Nutrients* **2021**, *13*, 413. [CrossRef] [PubMed]
27. Lee, H.J.; Lim, Y.-H.; Hong, Y.-C.; Shin, C.H.; Lee, Y.A. Body Mass Index Changes and Insulin Resistance at Age 4: A Prospective Cohort Study. *Front. Endocrinol.* **2022**, *13*, 872591. [CrossRef]
28. Barazzoni, R.; Gortan Cappellari, G.; Semolic, A.; Ius, M.; Zanetti, M.; Gabrielli, A.; Vinci, P.; Guarnieri, G.; Simon, G. Central Adiposity Markers, Plasma Lipid Profile and Cardiometabolic Risk Prediction in Overweight-Obese Individuals. *Clin. Nutr.* **2019**, *38*, 1171–1179. [CrossRef]
29. Best, O.; Ban, S. Adolescence: Physical Changes and Neurological Development. *Br. J. Nurs.* **2021**, *30*, 272–275. [CrossRef] [PubMed]
30. Wan, H.; Wang, Y.; Xiang, Q.; Fang, S.; Chen, Y.; Chen, C.; Zhang, W.; Zhang, H.; Xia, F.; Wang, N.; et al. Associations between Abdominal Obesity Indices and Diabetic Complications: Chinese Visceral Adiposity Index and Neck Circumference. *Cardiovasc. Diabetol.* **2020**, *19*, 118. [CrossRef]
31. Ben-Aicha, S.; Badimon, L.; Vilahur, G. Advances in HDL: Much More than Lipid Transporters. *Int. J. Mol. Sci.* **2020**, *21*, 732. [CrossRef]
32. Amato, M.C.; Giordano, C.; Galia, M.; Criscimanna, A.; Vitabile, S.; Midiri, M.; Galluzzo, A.; for the AlkaMeSy Study Group. Visceral Adiposity Index: A reliable indicator of visceral fat function associated with cardiometabolic risk. *Diabetes Care* **2010**, *33*, 920–922. [CrossRef]
33. Bonacina, F.; Pirillo, A.; Catapano, A.L.; Norata, G.D. HDL in Immune-Inflammatory Responses: Implications beyond Cardiovascular Diseases. *Cells* **2021**, *10*, 1061. [CrossRef]
34. Calderón-García, J.F.; Roncero-Martín, R.; Rico-Martín, S.; De Nicolás-Jiménez, J.M.; López-Espuela, F.; Santano-Mogena, E.; Alfageme-García, P.; Sánchez Muñoz-Torrero, J.F. Effectiveness of Body Roundness Index (BRI) and a Body Shape Index (ABSI) in Predicting Hypertension: A Systematic Review and Meta-Analysis of Observational Studies. *Int. J. Environ. Res. Public Health* **2021**, *18*, 11607. [CrossRef]
35. Ferhatbegović, L.; Mršić, D.; Kušljugić, S.; Pojskić, B. LDL-C: The Only Causal Risk Factor for ASCVD. Why Is It Still Overlooked and Underestimated? *Curr. Atheroscler. Rep.* **2022**, *24*, 635–642. [CrossRef] [PubMed]
36. López-Galisteo, J.P.; Gavela-Pérez, T.; Mejorado-Molano, F.J.; Pérez-Segura, P.; Aragón-Gómez, I.; Garcés, C.; Soriano-Guillén, L. Prevalence and Risk Factors Associated with Different Comorbidities in Obese Children and Adolescents. *Endocrinol. Diabetes Nutr. (Engl. Ed.)* **2022**, *69*, 566–575. [CrossRef]
37. Bendor, C.D.; Bardugo, A.; Pinhas-Hamiel, O.; Afek, A.; Twig, G. Cardiovascular Morbidity, Diabetes and Cancer Risk among Children and Adolescents with Severe Obesity. *Cardiovasc. Diabetol.* **2020**, *19*, 79. [CrossRef]
38. Boyne, M.; Thame, M.; Osmond, C.; Fraser, R.; Gabay, L.; Taylor-Bryan, C.; Forrester, T. The Effect of Earlier Puberty on Cardiometabolic Risk Factors in Afro-Caribbean Children. *J. Pediatr. Endocrinol. Metab.* **2014**, *27*, 453–460. [CrossRef] [PubMed]
39. de Oliveira, R.G.; Guedes, D.P. Physical Activity, Sedentary Behavior, Cardiorespiratory Fitness and Metabolic Syndrome in Adolescents: Systematic Review and Meta-Analysis of Observational Evidence. *PLoS ONE* **2016**, *11*, e0168503. [CrossRef]
40. de Rezende, L.F.M.; Rodrigues Lopes, M.; Rey-López, J.P.; Matsudo, V.K.R.; do Carmo Luiz, O. Sedentary Behavior and Health Outcomes: An Overview of Systematic Reviews. *PLoS ONE* **2014**, *9*, e105620. [CrossRef] [PubMed]
41. Bell, A.C.; Richards, J.; Zakrzewski-Fruer, J.K.; Smith, L.R.; Bailey, D.P. Sedentary Behaviour—A Target for the Prevention and Management of Cardiovascular Disease. *Int. J. Environ. Res. Public Health* **2022**, *20*, 532. [CrossRef]

42. Janssen, X.; Mann, K.D.; Basterfield, L.; Parkinson, K.N.; Pearce, M.S.; Reilly, J.K.; Adamson, A.J.; Reilly, J.J. Development of Sedentary Behavior across Childhood and Adolescence: Longitudinal Analysis of the Gateshead Millennium Study. *Int. J. Behav. Nutr. Phys. Act.* **2016**, *13*, 88. [CrossRef]
43. Martínez-Gómez, D.; Eisenmann, J.C.; Gómez-Martínez, S.; Veses, A.; Marcos, A.; Veiga, O.L. Sedentary Behavior, Adiposity, and Cardiovascular Risk Factors in Adolescents. The AFINOS Study. *Rev. Esp. Cardiol. (Engl. Ed.)* **2010**, *63*, 277–285. [CrossRef]
44. Govindan, M.; Gurm, R.; Mohan, S.; Kline-Rogers, E.; Corriveau, N.; Goldberg, C.; DuRussel-Weston, J.; Eagle, K.A. Gender Differences in Physiologic Markers and Health Behaviors Associated With Childhood Obesity. *Pediatrics* **2013**, *132*, 468–474. [CrossRef] [PubMed]
45. Aljahdali, A.A.; Baylin, A.; Ruiz-Narvaez, E.A.; Kim, H.M.; Cantoral, A.; Tellez-Rojo, M.M.; Banker, M.; Peterson, K.E. Sedentary Patterns and Cardiometabolic Risk Factors in Mexican Children and Adolescents: Analysis of Longitudinal Data. *Int. J. Behav. Nutr. Phys. Act.* **2022**, *19*, 143. [CrossRef] [PubMed]
46. ten Velde, G.; Plasqui, G.; Willeboordse, M.; Winkens, B.; Vreugdenhil, A. Associations between Physical Activity, Sedentary Time and Cardiovascular Risk Factors among Dutch Children. *PLoS ONE* **2021**, *16*, e0256448. [CrossRef]

Disclaimer/Publisher's Note: The statements, opinions and data contained in all publications are solely those of the individual author(s) and contributor(s) and not of MDPI and/or the editor(s). MDPI and/or the editor(s) disclaim responsibility for any injury to people or property resulting from any ideas, methods, instructions or products referred to in the content.

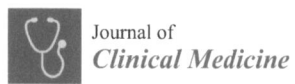

Systematic Review

Examining the Link between Air Quality (PM, SO$_2$, NO$_2$, PAHs) and Childhood Obesity: A Systematic Review

Barbara Siewert [1], Agata Kozajda [1], Marta Jaskulak [2,*] and Katarzyna Zorena [2]

[1] Environment and Health Scientific Circle, Medical University of Gdańsk, 80-210 Gdańsk, Poland; barbara.siewert@gumed.edu.pl (B.S.); a.kozajda@gumed.edu.pl (A.K.)
[2] Department of Immunobiology and Environment Microbiology, Medical University of Gdańsk, 80-210 Gdańsk, Poland; katarzyna.zorena@gumed.edu.pl
* Correspondence: marta.jaskulak@gumed.edu.pl

Abstract: Background/Objectives: Childhood obesity has emerged as a global health concern with profound implications for long-term health outcomes. In recent years, there has been increasing interest in the potential role of environmental factors in the development of childhood obesity. This comprehensive review aims to elucidate the intricate relationship between various components of air pollution and childhood obesity. **Methods:** We systematically analyze the existing literature from the past 5 years to explore the mechanistic pathways linking air pollution, including particulate matter (PM), nitrogen oxides (NO$_x$), sulfur dioxide (SO$_2$), and polycyclic aromatic hydrocarbons (PAHs), to childhood obesity. This systematic review examines 33 epidemiological studies on the link between air pollution and childhood obesity, published from 1 January 2018, to 31 January 2024. **Results:** Studies from counties with low overall air pollution noticed only low to no impact of the exposure to childhood obesity, unlike studies from countries with higher levels of pollution, suggesting that the mitigation of air pollutants can reduce the chance of it being a negative factor for the development of obesity. This relationship was noticed for PM$_{2.5}$, PM$_1$, PM$_{10}$, NO$_x$, and SO$_2$ but not for PAHs, which showed a negative effect on children's health across 10 out of 11 studies. **Conclusions:** This review underscores the need for interdisciplinary approaches to address both environmental and socio-economic determinants of childhood obesity. Efforts aimed at reducing air pollution levels and promoting healthy lifestyle behaviors are essential for safeguarding the health and well-being of children worldwide.

Keywords: particulate matter (PM); PM$_{10}$; PM$_{2.5}$; PM$_1$; NO$_x$; SO$_x$; PAHs; children; adolescents; obesity

Citation: Siewert, B.; Kozajda, A.; Jaskulak, M.; Zorena, K. Examining the Link between Air Quality (PM, SO$_2$, NO$_2$, PAHs) and Childhood Obesity: A Systematic Review. *J. Clin. Med.* **2024**, *13*, 5605. https://doi.org/10.3390/jcm13185605

Academic Editors: Justyna Wyszyńska and Piotr Matłosz

Received: 1 August 2024
Revised: 11 September 2024
Accepted: 13 September 2024
Published: 21 September 2024

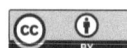

Copyright: © 2024 by the authors. Licensee MDPI, Basel, Switzerland. This article is an open access article distributed under the terms and conditions of the Creative Commons Attribution (CC BY) license (https://creativecommons.org/licenses/by/4.0/).

1. Introduction

In the 21st century, overweight and obesity in both adults and children are becoming a global epidemic. The World Health Organization (WHO) officially recognized obesity as "a chronic condition that requires treatment, promotes the development of other diseases and is associated with increased mortality" [1]. Obese individuals experience both short-term and long-term consequences. Even children, despite their young age, are at risk for dyslipidemia, hypertension, diabetes mellitus, non-alcoholic fatty liver disease, obstructive sleep apnea, psychosocial disturbances, an impaired quality of life, and a shorter life expectancy [2]. In the world population, obesity occurs in approximately 20% of children, adolescents, and adults. The prevalence of obesity in most developed societies has increased over the last 20 years. The latest results showed that childhood obesity is a major health problem, and the prevalence of overweight and obesity in school-age children in 2010 was 21–22% [3]. In the developmental age population, the data are as follows: approximately 155 million school-age children are overweight and obese; 30–45 million are children and adolescents aged 5 to 17, and 22 million are children under 5 years of age. There has been a significant increase in the incidence of obesity among preschool children [3]. However, among school-age children, excessive body weight was found to be more common in boys than in girls [4].

However, it is believed that, nowadays, genetic factors are responsible for the occurrence of obesity in only 25 to 45% [4,5], while changes in people's lifestyle as well as global trends have a huge impact on the development of overweight and obesity. While there are two significant causes of childhood obesity, it would be an understatement to attribute the phenomenon solely to a sedentary lifestyle and an inappropriate diet. Overall, the greatest impact on the development of obesity has non-genetic factors—primarily environmental ones [6–12]. Urbanization, industrialization, and globalization contribute to the multifactorial character of civilization diseases. Urbanization heightens substantial health risks including air pollution and chemical, biological, and physical hazards that bring about illnesses. Simultaneously, it triggers changes in occupational activities and reinforces disproportions of socioeconomic status and social structures that can promote illnesses and inequalities in healthcare access [13].

According to statistics, the highest percentage of obese people occurs among those with a lower socio-economic status [1]. Among such people, the awareness of the problem of obesity, its causes, and its consequences is often lower. Rather intuitively, overweight and obesity were reported to occur in economically developed countries due to a greater supply of food and reduced physical activity [13]. However, the disparities between countries resulting from recent urbanization or urban sprawl dictate the obesity growth rates. They have flattened or started decreasing in the majority of High-Income Countries, whereas in Low- and Middle-Income Countries, drastic increases have been seen in recent years [13].

According to the WHO, environmental risks cause 12% of the global burden of disease, with air pollution ranking first [14–16]. It exists as a burning problem leading to numerous health problems in low- and middle-income countries, where 92% of air pollution-related deaths occur. Air pollution may be regarded as an obesogenic factor and constitutes a common threat worldwide [16]. Most important air pollutants include particulate matter (PM_1, $PM_{2.5}$, PM_{10}, etc.), carbon monoxide (CO), nitrogen oxides (NO_x), sulfides, and Polycyclic Aromatic Hydrocarbons (PAHs) [17].

There is growing evidence showing that air pollution may be associated with obesity development [2]. Several mechanisms for this have been postulated, including changes in the basal metabolism, inducing systemic inflammation, oxidative stress, and hormone disruption [1,2,18], increases in brain inflammation, including microglial activation and anxiety, leading to increased caloric intake [3], and influences on child behavior, such as physical activity levels and eating habits [2]. In humans, outdoor and indoor air pollution is the root of morbidity, influencing respiratory diseases as well as inducing inflammation, cardiovascular diseases, obesity, diabetes, cancer, Alzheimer's Disease, and premature mortality [19]. Moreover, once obesity, hypertension, or diabetes is developed in an individual, they become more susceptible to air pollution exposure, showing more drastic increases in markers of inflammation (Table 1) [20].

Table 1. Significance of PM, SO_2, NO_2, and PAHs reflected by their cover environmental and industrial sources, routes of exposure, and adverse health effects [19–24].

Air Pollutant	Source	Routes of Exposure	Health Effects
PM_1	emissions from factories, vehicle exhaust, tire particles from vehicle use, wildfires or indoor wood-burning	ingestion and inhalation	heart attacks, lung cancer, dementia, emphysema, edema

Table 1. *Cont.*

Air Pollutant	Source	Routes of Exposure	Health Effects
$PM_{2.5}$	motor combustion, power plant combustion, industrial processes, stoves, fireplaces, and home wood burning, smoke from fireworks and wildfires, smoking, dust, soot, dirt, windblown salt	ingestion, inhalation, dermal contact	heart and lung disease, bronchitis emphysema, nonfatal heart attacks, irregular heartbeat, asthma and more intense flareups, decreased lung function, early death
PM_{10}	smoke, dust and dirt from unsealed road, construction, landfill, and agriculture mold, smoke from wildfire and waste burning, power generation, motor vehicle exhaust	inhalation	lung tissue damage, asthma, heart failure, cancer, adverse birth outcomes, chronic obstructive pulmonary disease (COPD), premature death
NO_x	combustion of fossil fuels, road transport	inhalation	premature death, cardiopulmonary effects, decreased lung function growth in children, respiratory symptoms, allergic responses.
SO_2	fossil fuels combustion, smelting of mineral ores	Inhalation	Bronchitis, cardiovascular disease
PAHs	coal gasification plants, smokehouses, municipal incinerators	ingestion, inhalation, and dermal contact	cataracts, kidney and liver damage, and jaundice, skin inflammation

Since children have relatively weaker lung defenses and immunity, they are even more susceptible to the negative effects of air pollution than adult individuals [24,25], notwithstanding the fact that they may be exposed to higher levels of air pollutants due to their increased outdoor time and higher levels of physical activity out there [26]. In such polluted environments, the beneficial effects of outdoor physical activity are diminished and have no impact on cardiopulmonary fitness or any health benefits whatsoever [27,28]. Moreover, they lack control over their diet, surroundings, and living conditions and may have little understanding of the consequences of developing obesity [4].

In this way, they reflect faulted social, economic, education, and urban planning and agricultural policies; thus, this childhood obesity should be taken seriously into account and managed more efficiently to provide early prevention [28].

Despite some developments in preventative measures encompassing technological solutions and spreading environmental awareness in many countries across the world, air pollution poses a tremendous threat to mankind [15]. Our previous research showed that high exposure to gaseous pollutants and particulate matter in ambient air may be one of the factors contributing to the risk of developing diabetes mellitus type 1 (T1DM) in children [29,30]. Currently, our systematic review provides a valuable summary of the newest knowledge about the association between air pollution and childhood obesity. The primary aim of this review article is to comprehensively investigate and analyze the association between various components of air pollution, including particulate matter (PM), sulfur dioxide (SO_2), nitrogen dioxide (NO_2), and polycyclic aromatic hydrocarbons (PAHs), and childhood obesity. Understanding this relationship is of paramount importance due to the rising prevalence of childhood obesity worldwide.

2. Methods

The systematic review takes into consideration a wide variety of studies that explore the connection between air pollution and childhood obesity. The focus was on the articles published between 1 January 2018 and 31 January 2024 (a 5-year overview of findings).

Criteria for Defining Childhood Obesity: In the included studies, childhood obesity was defined using various criteria. Most studies utilized Body Mass Index (BMI) percentiles specific to age and sex, as recommended by the Centers for Disease Control and Prevention (CDC) and the World Health Organization (WHO). Specifically, children with a BMI at or above the 95th percentile for their age and sex were classified as obese [31,32].

Search Strategy: the literature search was conducted using the PubMed, Scopus, and WebOfScience databases. The search strategy employed specific keywords related to air pollutants and childhood obesity, including both full terms and abbreviations. The search terms included "PM" or "particulate matter" (1, 2.5, and 10 μm), "NO_x" or "nitrogen oxides", "SOx" or "sulfate oxides", and "PAH" or "polycyclic aromatic hydrocarbons" combined with "children obesity", "child obesity", or "adolescent(s) obesity".

Inclusion Criteria:

- Language: Only studies published in English were considered.
- Publication Date: Studies published between 1 January 2018, and 31 January 2024.
- Population: Participants under 18 years of age.

Study Design: Original research studies including clinical, longitudinal, and cross-sectional studies that provided real-life observational data were prioritized. High-quality review articles, such as systematic reviews and meta-analyses, were only included in the introduction to offer a broader context or explain the possible mechanisms of action, provided they met the same inclusion criteria.

Focus: The studies had to explicitly investigate the relationship between air pollution and childhood obesity.

Exclusion Criteria: Studies in which obesity was considered a secondary outcome without clear or correlated measurement parameters related to air pollution; non-peer-reviewed articles, editorials, and opinion pieces; and studies relying solely on computer models or animal experiments.

Study Selection and Data Extraction: The study selection process was carried out by two independent reviewers. Discrepancies were resolved through discussion or, when necessary, consultation with a third reviewer. The PRISMA flow diagram (Figure 1) illustrates the study selection process. Data extraction was performed using a standardized form, capturing study characteristics, population details, exposure metrics, outcome measures, and key findings. Quality assessment of the included studies was conducted using established criteria, ensuring the reliability of the evidence.

Data Synthesis: The studies were then categorized by the type of air pollutant and analyzed both chronologically and by the strength of their reported effects. The data were synthesized to identify patterns and draw conclusions regarding the relationship between various air pollutants and childhood obesity.

Quality Assessment: Each study included in the review underwent a quality assessment to evaluate the risk of bias. This assessment was based on predefined criteria tailored to the study designs included, such as the sample size, methodology robustness, and accuracy of exposure and outcome measurements. To assess the quality of the included studies, we employed the Newcastle–Ottawa Scale (NOS) for non-randomized studies, which evaluates studies based on three broad criteria: the selection of study groups, the comparability of groups, and the ascertainment of either the exposure or outcome of interest [33]. The NOS assigns a maximum of nine stars, with higher scores indicating higher quality. Studies scoring seven or more stars were considered of high quality, while those with fewer stars were evaluated for potential bias. These results are discussed in the context of the overall findings in the tables and the Section 4.

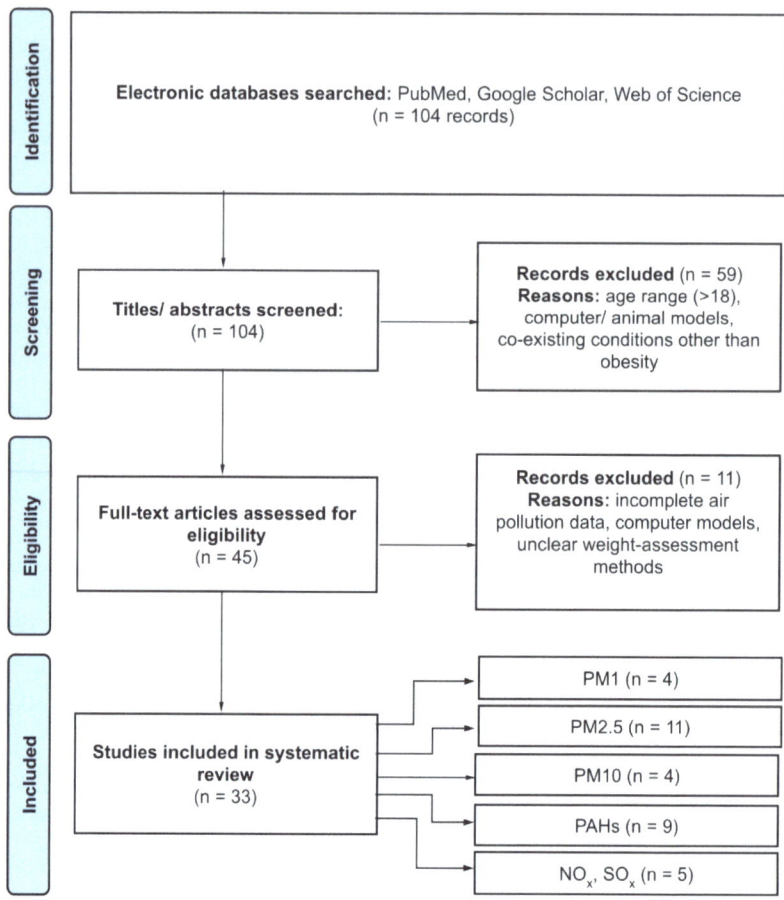

Figure 1. PRISMA flowchart [34].

3. Associations between the Exposure to Air Pollution and Childhood Obesity

3.1. $PM_{2.5}$

The distinct properties of $PM_{2.5}$ make it particularly harmful when compared to larger particles such as PM_{10}. Due to its small size, $PM_{2.5}$ can penetrate deep into the lungs and enter the bloodstream, allowing it to travel to various organs [35]. This characteristic enables $PM_{2.5}$ to have a more widespread and profound impact on the body, contributing to systemic inflammation, oxidative stress, and endocrine disruption. These mechanisms are increasingly being linked to metabolic changes and the development of obesity, particularly in children, who are more vulnerable to environmental pollutants. Figure 2 shows potential sites of absorbance of air contaminants into the system [36].

The significant attention $PM_{2.5}$ has received from researchers is driven by its global prevalence in the environment and its demonstrated adverse health effects [17]. Numerous epidemiological studies have linked $PM_{2.5}$ exposure to a range of health outcomes, including respiratory and cardiovascular diseases, as well as metabolic disorders like obesity [2,20]. The emerging evidence connecting $PM_{2.5}$ to childhood obesity has sparked particular concern due to the long-term health implications for affected children, such as an increased risk of developing chronic diseases later in life [25].

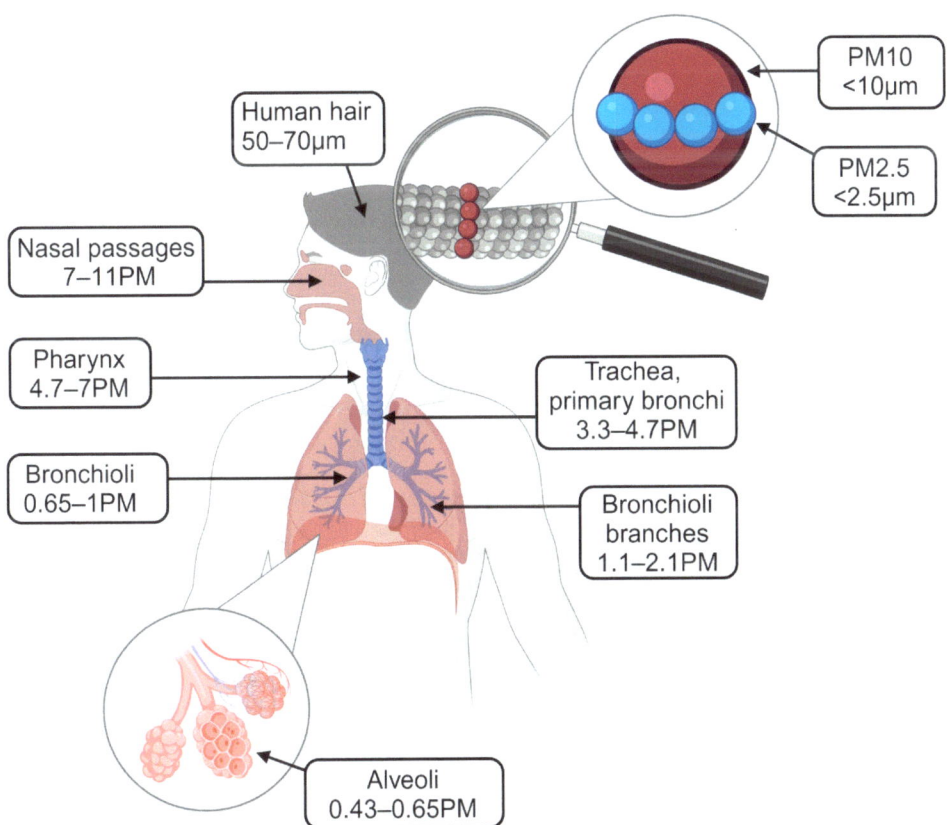

Figure 2. Comparison of PMs' perimeters and areas where PMs penetrate the respiratory system [36]. PM_{10} is known to penetrate the nasopharynx and start inflammatory reactions in the upper levels of the respiratory tract. $PM_{2.5}$ appears to have a particularly adverse effect due to its size and ability to travel deep within the respiratory system. PM_1 is thought to penetrate the lowest portions of the respiratory system (such as the bronchioli and alveoli), although many details of its nature and mechanisms are still to be explored. [Created with BioRender.com accessed on 6 April 2024. This figure is licensed under BioRender's Academic License Terms and is intended for use in this publication only. Agreement number: MQ278AXY29].

The main epidemiological studies that explored the potential association of $PM_{2.5}$ exposure and childhood obesity in the past 5 years are presented in Table 2 [37–46].

A cohort study conducted by Tong et al. [47] has demonstrated a dose–response relationship between the $PM_{2.5}$ level and obesity in children aged 6 to 8 years, with a particularly strong link to central obesity. Similarly, exposure to $PM_{2.5}$ among school-age children was associated with an increased BMI Z-score, waist circumference and waist-to-height ratio, and higher prevalence of not only central but also general obesity. The results were more pronounced in boys than in girls, except for general obesity. Interestingly, reductions in $PM_{2.5}$ levels after the launch of environmental protection measures showed that the risk of overweight/obesity decreased by 8% with a 1 µg/m³ increment in $PM_{2.5}$, but the likelihood of obesity was smaller in females than in males (Liang et al., 2022) [48]. Two studies in Mexico discovered links between exposure to $PM_{2.5}$ of similar levels and obesity as well as glucose dysregulation [34,47]. The average concentration of 22.4 µg/m³ $PM_{2.5}$ has led to changes in the levels of HbA1c. Each 10 µg/m³ increase in $PM_{2.5}$ was likely to double the probability of developing obesity in adolescents. A large-scale study of Peruvian children aged 0.5 to 5 years has suggested that intrauterine and extrauterine exposures of an increment of 10 µg/m^3 significantly increase the odds of overweightness or obesity using the WHO reference value for the sex and height scheme [48]. However, Fioravanti et al. (2008) found no relationship between exposure to PM$_{2.5}$ of a time-averaged concentration of 19.5 µg/m^3 assessed by geocoding and overweightness or obesity in a group of 500 children at 4-year and 8-year follow-ups measuring the waist circumference, waist-to-hip ratio, and total and HDL cholesterol [49].

In contrast, a study focusing on the Boston area, with a much lower postnatal exposure to PM$_{2.5}$ (the concentration being only 8.5 µg/m^3, on average) has modified the weight trajectory in the first 5 years of life: there was stronger association between weight and age in males [35]. Moreover, as a result of an investigation of 3460 participants, a positive association between the exposure and weight was observed in the first 3 years of life, becoming negative afterwards. Interestingly, low-birth-weight infants were found to be more vulnerable to normal-weight babies [50]. In another study, similar conclusions have been drawn concerning preterm babies [51]. A positive correlation between prenatal airborne pollution exposure and weight for length and body mass indices was found among 1-year-old children. In light of Zhang's Chinese cross-national study, average levels of PM$_{2.5}$ pollution ranging from 46.9 to 81.0 µg/m^3 show no evidence for an association between airborne pollution and hypertension-elevated HDL-C or TG levels; nevertheless, they impacted the odds of developing metabolic syndrome as well as abdominal obesity, which were even higher than those in the former study [38].

Table 2. Associations between PM$_{2.5}$ exposure and childhood obesity.

Author, Year	Location	Age [Years]	Cohort Size	Biomarkers	Main Findings
Fioravanti, 2018 [49]	Italy	0 follow up at 4 and 8	500	waist circumference, waist-to-hip ratio, total and HDL cholesterol	No evidence of an association was found between exposure to air pollutants and overweight/obesity in children.
Moody, 2019 [52]	Mexico	0–7	365	HbA1c levels	Prenatal and perinatal exposures to PM$_{2.5}$ are associated with changes in HbA1c, which are indicative of glucose dysregulation, in early childhood.
Tamayo-Ortiz, 2021 [35]	Mexico	-	2219	weight and height were measured, following the cut-off points in the WHO guidelines, and for children and adolescents, age-specific guidelines from the Mexican Social Security Institute that follow age-specific WHO guidelines were used.	An almost twofold increase in the odds of obesity for each 10 µg/m^3 of PM$_{2.5}$. The association was strongest for adolescents.
Zhang, 2021 [53]	China	10–18	9897	glucose oxidase, TG, FBG, HDL-C, abdominal obesity	No positive associations between air pollutants and hypertension, HDL-C, or TG; MetS subjects were more likely to be boys, to have a higher BMI, and to have a family history of type 2 diabetes, hypertension, obesity, or cerebrovascular disease when compared to participants without MetS. The odds ratio of MetS is associated with a 10 µg/m^3 increase in the two-year average of 1.31 for abdominal obesity.

Table 2. Cont.

Author, Year	Location	Age [Years]	Cohort Size	Biomarkers	Main Findings
Zhou, 2021 [51]	China	0–1	10,547	weight and length, weight for length (WFL), and body mass index (BMI), with overweight and obesity (OWOB) defined based on WHO Standards	Positive associations of prenatal PM_1 and $PM_{2.5}$ exposure with the WFL and BMI Z-score for one-year-old children, which could be partly explained by preterm birth. 10 $\mu g/m^3$ increase in prenatal exposure to $PM_{2.5}$. It was significantly associated with an increase in the WFL Z-score for one-year-old children. Similar associations were found for the BMI Z-score.
Zhang, 2021 [38]	China	7–18	44,718	BMI Z-score, waist circumference, waist-to-height ratio	Exposure to $PM_{2.5}$ was associated with an increased BMI Z-score, waist circumference, and WHtR and a higher prevalence of both general and central obesity. Stronger associations were observed for particles, especially PM_1 and $PM_{2.5}$, than for gaseous pollutants, e.g., NO_2. The results were more pronounced in boys than in girls, except for general obesity.
Wu, 2022 [39]	China (SNEC)	6–18	47,990	child age- and sex-specific z-scores for body mass index (BMI Z-score) and weight status were generated using the WHO growth reference	Exposure was associated with a greater childhood BMI Z-score and a higher likelihood of obesity. Similar associations were observed for PM_1, $PM_{2.5}$, and PM_{10} and were greater in boys and children living close to roadways.
Paz-Aparicio, 2022 [37]	Peru	0.5–5	65,232	values for height and weight for each sex assessed using the WHO guideline	A significant association between O/O and extrauterine and intrauterine $PM_{2.5}$ exposure for an increment of 10 $\mu g/m^3$.
Vanoli, 2022 [50]	USA	0–5	3460	weight	$PM_{2.5}$ significantly modified the association between age and weight in males, with a positive association in children younger than 3 years and a negative association afterwards. Low-birthweight babies are more susceptible than normal-weight infants
Liang, 2022 [48]	China	7	2105	BMI: the standards from the growth charts of the China Centers for Disease Control (CDC) were then used to calculate the BMI z score (BMIz); overweight and obesity were diagnosed based on sex-specific BMI-for-age growth charts from the China CDC.	The results showed that the risk of overweight/obesity decreased with a 1 $\mu g/m^3$ decrease in $PM_{2.5}$ after adjusting for covariates. The reduction in the risk of obesity was larger in females than in males
Tong, 2022 [47]	China	6–8	4284	BMI	Higher levels of accumulating exposure to $PM_{2.5}$ were associated with an increased childhood obesity index, and the effect was the most significant for WHtR compared to BMI and BMIz. This effect was more pronounced in boys than in girls, except for WHtR, and it was the most significant under the $PM_{2.5}$ exposure period from pregnancy to 6 years old. Dose–response relationship between $PM_{2.5}$ exposure and childhood obesity, especially central obesity

3.2. PM_1

The main studies that explored the potential relationship between the exposure to PM_1 and childhood obesity within the past 5 years are presented in Table 3 [37,50–52]. An exposure to PM_1 of an average concentration of 50.8 µg/m^3 induced short-term effects among participants aged 9–18: the associations between PM_1 and systolic blood pressure and diastolic blood pressure were more pronounced in females, younger individuals, participants already overweight or obese, and those with insufficient physical activity (Wu et al., 2020) [39]. Accordingly, in a Wu et al. study from 2022, increments of 10 mg/m^3 resulted in an increase in the systolic pressure of 2.56 mmHg and, in turn, increased the probability of hypertension by 61% [40]. Zhang et al. found out that PM_1 is a leading agent among air pollutants (at a concentration of 46.9 µg/m^3) in causing an increased BMI Z-score, waist circumference and weight-to-height ratio, along with a higher prevalence of both general and central obesity [53]. Zhang et al. found no evidence of a correlation between developing metabolic syndrome and PM_1 levels; however, a 10 µg/m^3 increase in PM_1 was linked with elevated FBG measures among the 10–18 age group of 9897 participants (Zhang et al., 2021) [38]. A 10 µg/m^3 increase in prenatal exposure to PM_1 was significantly associated with a 0.105 increase in the WFL Z-score for one-year-old children. In another Chinese study, the positive associations of prenatal PM_1 exposure with WFL and the BMI Z-score for one-year-old children, although moderated by preterm birth, were not negligible (Zhou et al., 2021) [53] (Table 3).

Table 3. Associations between PM_1 exposure and childhood obesity.

Author, Year	Location	Age [Years]	Cohort Size	Biomarkers	Main Findings
Zhang, 2021 [53]	China	10–18	9897	Glucose oxidase, TG, FBG, HDL-C, Abdominal obesity	Odds ratio of MetS was associated with a 10 µg/m^3 increase in the two-year average—1.20 higher for abdominal obesity; a 10 µg/m^3 increase in PM_1 and NO_2 was associated with a prevalence of FBG
Zhou, 2021 [51]	China	0–1	10,547	Weight and length, weight for length (WFL), and body mass index (BMI), followed by the definition of overweight and obesity (OWOB)	Positive associations of prenatal PM_1 and $PM_{2.5}$ exposure with WFL and BMI Z-scores for one-year-old children, which could be partly explained by preterm birth. A 10 µg/m^3 increase in prenatal exposure to PM_1 was significantly associated with a 0.105 increase in the WFL Z-score for one-year-old children. Similar associations were found for the BMI Z-score.
Zhang, 2021 [38]	China	7–18	44,718	BMI, waist circumference, WHtR, BMI Z-score	Exposure to PM_1, associated with an increased BMI Z-score, waist circumference, and WHtR and a higher prevalence of both general and central obesity. Stronger associations were observed for particles, especially PM_1, than for gaseous pollutants, e.g., NO_2. Generally, particles with a smaller diameter had greater effect estimates than larger particles.
Wu, 2022 [39]	China	6–18	47,990	Child age- and sex-specific z-scores for body mass index (BMI Z-score) and weight status	Exposure was associated with a greater childhood BMI Z-score and a higher likelihood of obesity. Similar associations were observed for PM_1, $PM_{2.5}$, and PM_{10} and were greater in boys and children living close to roadways

3.3. PM_{10}

The main studies that explored the potential relationship between the exposure to PM_{10} and childhood obesity within the past 5 years are presented in Table 4 [43,44,51,54].

Table 4. Associations between PM_{10} exposure and childhood obesity.

Author, Year	Country	Age [Years]	Cohort Size	Biomarkers	Main Findings
Fioravanti, 2018 [49]	Italy	infants, 4- and 8-year checkup	719	BMI Z-scores, waist circumference, waist-to-hip ratio, and total and HDL cholesterol measured at 8 years.	No association between exposure to vehicular traffic and exposure to pollutants on obesity-related parameters such as BMI, blood lipids, and abdominal adiposity during childhood.
de Bont, 2019 [41]	Spain	7–10	2660	Child weight and height and age- and sex-specific z-scores for body mass index (zBMI)	An IQR increase in PM_{10}-home (5.6 µg/m^3) was associated with a 10% increase in the odds of being overweight or obese.
de Bont, 2021 [46]	Spain	2–5	416,955	Height and weight measures.	A total of 142,590 (34.2%) children developed overweight or obesity. Increased exposure to PM_{10} was associated with a 2–3% increased risk of developing overweight and obesity. For all air pollutants, associations were stronger among children living in the most deprived areas compared to the least deprived areas.
Zhang, 2021 [53]	China	7–18	44,718	Body mass index (BMI), waist circumference, WHtR, and the prevalence of general and central obesity	Exposure to PM_{10} was associated with an increased BMI Z-score, waist circumference, and WHtR and a higher prevalence of both general and central obesity. Particles with a smaller diameter had greater effect estimates than larger particles. The associations were more pronounced in boys than in girls, except for general obesity.

de Bont and his co-workers, in 2019, examined over 2500 children aged 7–10 years in Barcelona, Spain [41]. More than three-quarters of the participants were exposed to PM_{10} levels higher than the WHO official recommendation, being <20 µg/m^3. According to the acquired z-BMI scores, a 5.6 µg/m^3 increase in PM_{10} at-home levels was associated with a 10% increase in the odds of being overweight. A study conducted by the same author in 2021 confirmed the previous findings. Having examined over 400,000 children aged 2 to 5, it was thought that the increased exposure to PM_{10} is connected with a 2–3% risk of obesity development (which seems to be much more detailed of a finding than the previous study). A similar percentage of participants experienced the PM_{10} pollution level exceeding WHO guidelines. Interestingly, the correlation between air pollutants and obesity was visibly stronger for children from more deprived areas compared to those of the middle class. A study performed by Zhang et al. in 2021 on almost 45,000 Chinese children under 18 shows similar results [38]. Not only the BMI-score but also the waist-to-height ratio is considered to be influenced by PM_{10}. The increase in the BMI z-score was 0.11 per 10 µg/m^3 increment in annual average concentrations of PM_{10}. The association seemed to be more visible in the boys' groups than in girls, except for general obesity (even distribution of results). However, particles of a smaller diameter such as $PM_{2.5}$ and PM_1 were found to have a greater effect than PM_{10}, possibly due to their ability to penetrate deeper parts of the pulmonary system. Huang et al. (2022) provides results largely consistent with previous findings [42]. The study additionally considered the skinfold thickness and body fat percentage in order to classify participants as overweight or obese. It is suggested that PM_{10} with 10 µg/m³ increment has the potential to elevate the risk of obesity globally (Lin et al., 2022) [43]. Although other authors indicate that the significant changes occur when the concentration exceeds 20 µg/m³, Zheng et al. (2024) presents the outlook that the significant rise in the risk of obesity takes place at the point of 50 µg/m³, considerably higher than what was established by previous authors [44]. It is indicated that PM_{10} exposure increases the probability of being overweight or obese, especially in Asia, which can be caused by a cultural-based difference in the definition of obesity.

Parasin et al. (2021) found an increase in the risk of developing obesity in children caused by PMs exposure, and the effects of PM_{10} after the follow-up period of 4 years were found to be statistically insignificant [45]. The author points to the wide variety of mechanisms involved in $PM_{2.5}$ and PM_1 exposures compared to PM_{10}. Similarly, no association between exposure to pollutants and obesity was found in an Italian birth cohort [49]. The study used various obesity-related parameters like BMI, waist circumference, waist-to-hip ratio, and total and HDL cholesterol, and none were proven to consistently change with PM_{10} exposure. The conclusion is that the knowledge of the obesogenic qualities of air pollution remains quite limited, and further studies need to be conducted.

3.4. $NO_x + SO_2$

The main epidemiological studies that explored the potential link between NO_x and SO_2 exposure and childhood obesity are presented in Table 5 [38,49,53,55,56]. In light of China's national cross-sectional study, each increase of 10 µg/m³ of NO_2 was associated with a heightened prevalence of FBG among the 10–18 age group [38]. Moreover, in another study by Zhang et al., exposure to NO_2 was associated with an increased BMI Z-score, waist circumference, and weight-to-height ratio and a greater share of both general and central obesity; yet, NO_2, being a gaseous pollutant, showed a weaker relationship than that of particulate matter. However, a study by Fioravanti et al. showed no correlation between air pollutant levels and overweight or obesity in children in an Italian birth cohort study with the lowest cohort size among the analyzed articles despite a seemingly high concentration of 69.8 µg/m³ [53]. Similar results were shared in a study examining exposure to traffic-related air pollution during fetal life and child obesity in 4-year-olds in Sweden. There was no correlation between NO_x concentration and overweightness or obesity at the follow-up; moreover, an interesting finding was weak evidence of a link between NO_x levels and being underweight [55]. This might be attributed to the low and medium pollution levels in this country and the study including only one constituent of traffic-related air pollution. A study investigating long-term exposure to NO_2 and SO_2 among children in Hong Kong includes four follow-ups at 9, 11, 13, and 15 years. The trajectory of weight is different, with a higher BMI at 9,13 and 15 years due to heightened exposure to NO_2, whereas lower BMI values at 13 and 15 years were linked to low SO_2 exposure [56].

Table 5. Associations between $NO_x + SO_2$ exposure and childhood obesity.

Author, Year	Location	Age [Years]	Cohort Size	Biomarkers	Main Findings
Fioravanti, 2018 [49]	Italy	0 with a follow-up at 4 and 8	500	waist circumference, waist-to-hip ratio, total and HDL cholesterol	No evidence of an association was found between exposure to air pollutants and overweight/obesity in children.

Table 5. Cont.

Author, Year	Location	Age [Years]	Cohort Size	Biomarkers	Main Findings
Zhang, 2021 [53]	China	7–18	44,718	BMI Z-score, waist circumference, and WHtR	Exposure to NO_2 was associated with an increased BMI Z-score, waist circumference, and WHtR and a higher prevalence of both general and central obesity. Generally, stronger associations were observed for particles than for gaseous pollutants, e.g., NO_2.
Frondelius, 2018 [55]	Sweden	fetal life and 4	5815	body mass index adjusted for Swedish children	No marked associations between traffic-related air pollution (NO_x) exposure during fetal life and overweight and obesity at age four in Malmö, Sweden, an area with low to medium pollution levels, averaging around 20 $\mu g/m^3$ between 1999 and 2005. Weak evidence of an association between NO_x and underweight.
Huang, 2018 [56]	Hong Kong	infants, follow-up at 9, 11, 13, 15	8327	BMI	A higher exposure to NO_2 in childhood was associated with a higher BMI at ~9, ~13, and ~15 years, a lower exposure to SO_2 in utero was associated with a lower BMI at ~13 and ~15 years, and a lower exposure to SO_2 in childhood was associated with a lower BMI at ~15 years. These sex-specific findings concern the relation of air pollution constituents with adiposity.
Zhang, 2021 [38]	China	10–18	9897	glucose oxidase, TG, FBG, HDL-C, abdominal obesity	The odds ratio of Metabolic Syndrome was associated with a 10 $\mu g/m^3$ increase in the two-year average of 1.33; for abdominal obesity, a higher increase in PM_1 and NO_2 was associated with the prevalence of FBG.

3.5. PAHs

The main epidemiological studies exploring the association between childhood obesity and the exposure to PAHs are presented in Table 6 [57–65]. A study investigating the consequences of the exposure of 186 participants aged 6–18 to polycyclic aromatic hydrocarbons in Iran has reached a conclusion that most of the evaluated PAHs enhanced the risk of cardiometabolic risk factors and excess weight. Specifically, exposure to the compounds 2-naphtol, 9-phenanthrol, and $\sum$ OH-PAH was associated with an increased risk of obesity for participants without cardiometabolic risk factors [57,58].

The urinary PAHs concentration and a higher WHtR, an indicator of central obesity even at 3–5 years, were linked in a Canadian study with a sample size of 3667. Surprisingly, in the same age group, the BMI and the matrix were not associated. Overall, among the total study population between 3 and 18 years of age, the participants placed in the highest quadrille for total PAH metabolites or naphthalene only had a three-times-higher risk of developing central obesity than those in the lowest quartile [60,61]. An American study from 2019 supports the previous findings and suggests a positive association of air PAH contamination with childhood BMI and BMI Z-scores at the ages of 5 to 10. Moreover, the growth trajectory of study participants was observed to increase across follow-up visits until age 11 [59].

Higher ambient PAH contamination influenced the levels of HbA1c, systolic blood pressure, and oxidative stress in the US, with a cohort size of 299, who were aged 6–8 years.

It was found that both short- and long-term outdoor residential exposures to traffic-related air pollution including PAHs are associated with biomarkers indicative of a risk for metabolic syndrome [63].

Another study investigated the relationship between indoor air pollution exposures and obese anthropometric indices among Chinese schoolchildren. The study suggests that exposure to more than or equal to three types of indoor air pollution including PAHs increases z-BMI and the overall risk of overweight or obesity. Moreover, the authors discovered a dose–response relationship between the exposure and the aforementioned indices [63].

The only study that has not found an association between PAHs and higher childhood adiposity had the smallest sample size of 198 and monitored relatively low levels of elemental carbon attributable to traffic only during the prenatal period. The follow-up was performed after 7–8 years [61]. Notwithstanding the foregoing, its differing results may have been largely dictated by severe limitations.

Table 6. Associations between PAHs exposure and childhood obesity.

Author, Year	Location	Age [Years]	Cohort Size	Biomarker	Main Findings
Poursafa, 2018 [57]	Iran	6–18	186		An increased risk of cardiometabolic risk factors and excess weight was associated with exposure to most of the evaluated PAHs. Exposure to 1-hydroxypyrene was associated with a higher risk of cardiometabolic risk factors in participants with excess weight. Exposure to 2-Naphtol was also associated with a higher risk of cardiometabolic risk factors in both groups, but the associations were not significant ($p < 0.1$). For participants without cardiometabolic risk factors, exposure to 2-naphtol, 9-phenanthrol, and $\sum$ OH-PAH was associated with an increased risk of obesity.
Bushnik, 2020 [58]	Canada	3–18	3667	Urinary PAHs and Waist-to-Height Ratio	Overall, those in the highest quartile for naphthalene or total PAH metabolites had three times greater odds of having central obesity compared with those in the lowest quartile. Urinary PAH metabolites are associated with WHtR, an indicator of central obesity and a predictor of health risks associated with obesity in children as young as 3–5. Urinary PAH metabolites were associated with measures of obesity in children as young as 3–5 years. While there is considerable interest in evaluating the potential role of early-life exposures in disease, PAHs and air pollution more broadly remain understudied risk factors for later-life obesity and its associated comorbidities.
Sears, 2019 [62]	USA	newborns	198 (HOME) and n = 459 (CCAAPS)		Did not find that traffic-related air pollution exposure was associated with a lower birthweight or higher childhood adiposity at an age of 7–8 years in these two cohorts or the pooled sampled. The results should be cautiously interpreted given prior research and the limitations of our study, including the modest sample size, the relatively low ECAT concentrations, and our ability to examine ECAT only during the prenatal period.

Table 6. Cont.

Author, Year	Location	Age [Years]	Cohort Size	Biomarker	Main Findings
Shi, 2022 [59]	USA	5–14	535	BMI, BMI-Z score	Positive association of air PAH contamination with childhood BMI at the age of 5–10. The incidence of obesity was 20.5% at the age of 5 and 33% at age of 11. In addition, the growth trajectory increased across follow-up visits until age 11.
Bushnik, 2023 [63]	Canada	3–18	3667	BMI, WC, and WHtR	BMI, WC, and WHtR were positively associated with total PAH and naphthalene metabolites in the total population aged 3–18 and in the age groups 6–11 and 12–18. In 3–5-year-olds, WHtR, but not BMI, was significantly associated with total PAH, naphthalene, and phenanthrene metabolites. Overall, those in the highest quartile for naphthalene or total PAH metabolites had three-times-greater odds of having central obesity compared with those in the lowest quartile. Urinary PAH metabolites are associated with WHtR, an indicator of central obesity and predictor of health risks associated with obesity, in children as young as 3–5.
Mann, 2021 [60]	USA	6–8	299	HbA1c	Children exposed to higher PAH contamination had an increased level of included HbA1c, systolic blood pressure, and oxidative stress. The results suggested that both short- and longer-term estimated individual-level outdoor residential exposures to several traffic-related air pollutants, including ambient PAHs, are associated with biomarkers of risk for metabolic syndrome and oxidative stress in children.
Li, 2021 [64]	USA	12–19	827	FBG	Among 827 adolescents, 183 (22.13%) had metabolic syndrome. The levels of 2-hydroxynaphthalene (2-NAP), 2-hydroxyphenanthrene (2-PHE), 2-hydroxyfluorene (2-FLU), 1-hydroxynaphthalene (1-NAP), 3-hydroxyfluorene (3-FLU), and 1-hydroxypyrene (1-PYR) were higher in the group of adolescents with metabolic syndrome. There were positive associations between higher concentrations of 2-NAP and 2-FLU and the odds of metabolic syndrome after adjustment. PAHs may be associated with the odds of metabolic syndrome as well as individual metabolic syndrome components among adolescents.
Kim, 2023 [65]	China	6–12	6499	z-BMI	Indoor air pollution exposures were positively associated with higher obese anthropometric indices and increased odds of overweight/obesity in Chinese schoolchildren. Children exposed to ≥three types of indoor air pollutants had a higher z-BMI and a higher risk of overweight/obesity. A dose–response relationship was discovered between the IAP exposure index and z-BMI as well as overweight/obesity.

4. Discussion

Obesity, being a complex and multifactorial illness defined as "abnormal or excessive fat accumulation that presents a risk to health" by WHO, poses a threat to people at different ages. With a dramatic increase in obesity rates among the general population, the problem of the prevalence of childhood obesity is likely to be an underlying cause for a major incoming health downfall including premature death and disability [65]. Current research has shown that obese children experience both short-term and long-term consequences, e.g., cardiovascular diseases, diabetes, and certain types of cancers, with an earlier onset or greater probability than the general population [48,60,66].

Numerous factors are likely to put children at risk for developing obesity; each and every one of them is dangerous on its own, but researchers suggest that they often come together. An unhealthy diet and a habit of fast food nutrition in particular as well as less physical activity are the main causes of an increased prevalence of obesity, particularly among adolescents living in cities [65,67].

There are socioeconomic factors, including a low socioeconomic status, low parental education, non-parental caregivers, a lower fruit-eating frequency, short sleeping hours, and parental obesity. Maternal-Related Factors even before the childbirth especially seem to play an important role in the process: research has shown that a higher pre-pregnancy BMI directly correlates with childhood obesity [68].

Psychological aspects remain particularly significant causes of obesity: adverse childhood experiences are social determinants of health [66]. Comorbidities are reported to accumulate: unhealthy weight was continuously present among children with comorbidities such as autism spectrum disorders and individuals with sleep and affective problems [69].

Moreover, sleep duration and quality are deemed significant risk factors for childhood obesity. A meta-analysis conducted by Han et al. reported that an increased risk of childhood obesity is accompanied by short sleeping durations [70].

4.1. Mechanisms by Which Air Pollution Affects Obesity

The potential mechanisms linking air pollution exposure to childhood obesity involve complex interplays between environmental factors, physiological responses, and behavioral patterns. The 33 reviewed manuscripts in Table 1–5 show several mechanisms by which air pollution has an impact on obesity. First, airborne pollutants such as PM, SO_2, NO_x, and PAH can induce systemic inflammation and oxidative stress upon inhalation. These inflammatory responses can disrupt metabolic homeostasis, leading to insulin resistance, dyslipidemia, and altered adipokine secretion, all of which contribute to adiposity and weight gain in children [38]. Additionally, exposure to air pollution constituents has been associated with alterations in the gut microbiota composition, which can influence energy metabolism and adipose tissue development [70]. Furthermore, air pollution exposure may also impact neuroendocrine pathways regulating appetite and satiety [38]. The inhalation of pollutants can affect central nervous system function, including regions involved in appetite regulation such as the hypothalamus. The disruption of these regulatory pathways may lead to dysregulated eating behaviors, increased food intake, and, ultimately, weight gain. Moreover, chronic exposure to air pollution has been linked to disruptions in sleep patterns, which can further exacerbate metabolic dysfunction and weight gain in children [71,72].

Beyond physiological mechanisms, our review shows that environmental and socio-economic factors play significant roles in the relationship between air pollution and childhood obesity [73]. Children living in areas with high levels of air pollution often experience limited access to outdoor play spaces and opportunities for physical activity, leading to sedentary lifestyles and reduced energy expenditure. Moreover, socio-economic disparities exacerbate these effects, as low-income communities are disproportionately exposed to higher levels of air pollution and face barriers to accessing healthy food options and healthcare resources [13]. Overall, the studies referred to in Tables 1–5, performed on children living in countries with relatively low pollution levels, showed no association or a weak association between the air pollution and the risk of obesity in children, whereas in developing countries with higher pollution levels, this relationship was prominent.

Exposure to fine particulate matter ($PM_{2.5}$) has been implicated in the development of childhood obesity through several mechanisms. $PM_{2.5}$ inhalation was demonstrated to induce systemic inflammation and oxidative stress. These inflammatory responses trigger the release of pro-inflammatory cytokines and adipokines, disrupting metabolic homeostasis. Chronic inflammation is associated with insulin resistance, dyslipidemia, and impaired glucose metabolism, all of which contribute to adiposity and weight gain in children [74]. Moreover, PM$_{2.5}$ exposure has been linked to alterations in adipose tissue biology. The reviewed research in our study has shown that exposure to PM$_{2.5}$ can lead to adipocyte hypertrophy and hyperplasia, promoting the accumulation of fat mass. Additionally, PM$_{2.5}$-induced inflammation can disrupt adipose tissue function, impairing the secretion of adipokines involved in energy metabolism regulation [75]. Obese children with asthma are more vulnerable to air pollution, especially fine particulate matter [49]. Children with an abnormal body weight and asthma breathe at higher tidal volumes that may increase the efficiency of PM$_{2.5}$ deposition in the lung. This finding may partially explain why obese children with asthma exhibit greater sensitivity to air pollution. PM$_{2.5}$ can also affect gene expression in mitochondria in brown adipose tissue, resulting in an increased production of reactive oxygen species in brown fat stores, which lead to metabolic dysfunction and susceptibility to lipid metabolism and glucose metabolism [49]. Second, the inflammatory response that is triggered by air pollutants can lead to vascular damage as well as insulin resistance and can also have an impact on body weight [47]. Studies also found that the occurrence of sleep-disordered breathing (SDB) was related to exposure to air pollutants [34,39]. Those who lived in regions with high NO$_2$ and PM$_{2.5}$ levels were much more likely to suffer from SDB, which in turn caused mental and physical health disparities including increased weight [50].

Frequent contact with coarse particulate matter (PM$_{10}$) has also been implicated in the development of childhood obesity through various mechanisms, although the effects may differ slightly from those of PM$_{2.5}$. In addition to its effects on adipose tissue, PM$_{10}$ inhalation can also impact respiratory function in children. Respiratory distress caused by PM$_{10}$ exposure may lead to decreased physical activity levels and impaired exercise tolerance, contributing to a sedentary lifestyle and weight gain. Additionally, PM$_{10}$ exposure has been associated with respiratory infections and asthma exacerbations in children, which can lead to decreased lung function and physical activity levels, both of which are risk factors for obesity (Tables 1 and 2).

The presence of ultrafine particulate matter (PM$_1$) presents unique challenges and potential mechanisms in relation to childhood obesity. PM$_1$ particles, being smaller in size than PM$_{2.5}$ and PM$_{10}$, have a greater surface area per unit mass, allowing them to penetrate deeper into the respiratory system and potentially enter the bloodstream directly. This characteristic enhances their ability to induce systemic inflammation and oxidative stress, which are key drivers of metabolic dysfunction and adiposity in children [51]. One significant mechanism by which PM$_1$ may influence childhood obesity is through its impact on adipose tissue biology. Ultrafine particles can infiltrate adipose tissue more readily compared to larger particles, leading to localized inflammation and dysfunction within adipocytes. This disruption can impair adipokine secretion and adipose tissue remodeling, contributing to adiposity and weight gain [50]. Moreover, PM$_1$ particles have been shown to cross the blood–brain barrier and affect central nervous system function. Neuroinflammation and oxidative stress induced by PM$_1$ exposure may disrupt hypothalamic pathways involved in appetite regulation, leading to dysregulated eating behaviors and increased food intake, ultimately promoting obesity in children [52]. Furthermore, PM$_1$ inhalation has been associated with cardiovascular effects, including endothelial dysfunction and impaired vascular reactivity. These cardiovascular effects may exacerbate metabolic dysfunction and adiposity, further contributing to the development of obesity in children. Additionally, similar to other particulate matter fractions, PM$_1$ exposure can exacerbate respiratory conditions such as asthma, leading to decreased lung function and physical activity levels, which are risk factors for obesity [37].

Overall, immature metabolic pathways can increase susceptibility to environmental damage. The mechanisms linking various types of particulate matter (PM) exposure to hypertension are not yet fully understood. It is hypothesized that in the short term, PM exposure disrupts the autonomic nervous system and causes direct local oxidative and inflammatory effects on blood vessels. Over the long term, these effects may combine with chronic, secondary systemic inflammation and oxidative stress, potentially leading to elevated blood pressure. The diameter of PM plays a crucial role in its health impacts, as finer particles can enter the bloodstream directly, triggering a secondary proinflammatory response [35,37,47,48,54].

For NO_x, one significant mechanism by which NO_x may influence childhood obesity is through its role in oxidative stress and inflammation. NO_x exposure can induce the production of reactive oxygen species (ROS) and reactive nitrogen species (RNS) in the body, leading to oxidative damage to cells and tissues. This oxidative stress triggers inflammatory responses, characterized by the release of pro-inflammatory cytokines and chemokines, which can disrupt metabolic homeostasis and promote adiposity. NO_x exposure has also been associated with endothelial dysfunction and impaired vascular health, particularly in children with pre-existing cardiovascular risk factors. Endothelial dysfunction can lead to reduced NO_x bioavailability and impaired vasodilation, contributing to hypertension and metabolic disturbances associated with obesity [51]. Additionally, NO_x exposure may influence adipose tissue biology and energy metabolism. Animal studies have suggested that NO_x exposure can alter adipocyte differentiation and function, leading to adipocyte hypertrophy and adipose tissue inflammation. Furthermore, NO_x-induced inflammation may impair insulin signaling pathways in adipose tissue, exacerbating insulin resistance and metabolic dysfunction. NO_x exposure has also been linked to alterations in gut microbiota composition, which can influence energy harvest from the diet and adiposity. Dysbiosis induced by NO_x exposure may promote inflammation and metabolic disturbances, contributing to obesity development in children [54].

One significant mechanism by which SO_2 may influence childhood obesity is through its pro-inflammatory effects. SO_2 exposure can induce oxidative stress and inflammation in the respiratory system and other tissues. This inflammatory response triggers the release of pro-inflammatory cytokines and chemokines, which can disrupt metabolic homeostasis and contribute to adiposity [41]. Moreover, SO_2 exposure has been linked to respiratory conditions such as asthma exacerbations and airway inflammation in children. Respiratory distress caused by SO_2 exposure may lead to decreased physical activity levels and exercise intolerance, which are risk factors for obesity. Similar to NO_x, SO_2 may also alter adipocyte differentiation and function, leading to adipocyte hypertrophy and adipose tissue inflammation [52]. Furthermore, SO_2-induced inflammation may impair insulin signaling pathways in adipose tissue, exacerbating insulin resistance and metabolic dysfunction. Also similar to NO_2, SO_2 exposure has been associated with endothelial dysfunction and impaired vascular health and may influence the gut microbiota composition, which can impact energy metabolism and adiposity [46].

A potential reason behind PAHs' influence on childhood obesity is their ability to disrupt endocrine signaling pathways. PAHs can act as endocrine disruptors, interfering with hormone synthesis, secretion, transport, and receptor binding. These disruptions can lead to the dysregulation of hormones involved in energy balance and metabolism, such as leptin, adiponectin, insulin, and thyroid hormones, which may contribute to adiposity and weight gain in children [59]. Furthermore, PAHs are known carcinogens and can induce oxidative stress and inflammation in various tissues. Oxidative stress and inflammation triggered by PAH exposure can disrupt metabolic homeostasis, leading to insulin resistance, dyslipidemia, and impaired glucose metabolism, all of which contribute to adiposity and weight gain in children [57]. Additionally, PAHs have been associated with alterations in the gut microbiota composition, which can influence the energy harvest from the diet and adiposity. Dysbiosis induced by PAH exposure may promote inflammation and metabolic disturbances, further contributing to obesity development in children [63]. Lastly, PAH exposure has been linked to respiratory conditions such as asthma exacerbations and airway inflammation in children. Respiratory distress caused by PAH exposure may lead to decreased physical activity levels and exercise intolerance, which are risk factors for obesity. PAHs exposure overall leads to altered DNA methylation levels of genes related to inflammation and immune responses, oxidative stress, cell cycle regulation, and signal transduction [62].

4.2. The Link between Neonatal Exposure and Childhood Obesity

Maternal exposure to air pollution during pregnancy is a source of various negative health outcomes after birth. While children have certain barriers protecting the respiratory system from absorbing the particles, the fetus relies solely on placental blood exchange, which leads to a higher concentration and longer exposure. The direct placental translocation of chemical particles might impede brain development, raise the risk of autoimmune diseases and allergies, and initiate oxidative stress pathways, resulting in endocrine abnormalities such as diabetes or obesity in children. Studies have shown that mothers living in polluted environments tend to give birth to offspring of an abnormal body mass (significantly low in the first few weeks and rapidly growing after) and heightened blood pressure. Particles absorbed by the placenta and transported by the umbilical blood initiate the creation of reactive oxygen species, which strongly influence the mitochondria and ionic balance across cytoplasmic membranes. The results are visible as delayed nerve impulses, incorrect detoxification, and cell death. Moreover, disruptions of glucose metabolism, decreased heart functions, and insulin resistance directly lead to overweight and obesity in children. At the same time, our review has shown that longitudinal studies on mother–child pairs in the context of exposure to air pollution are scarce.

5. Conclusions and Future Management Strategies

From systemic inflammation and the disruption of metabolic homeostasis to alterations in adipose tissue biology and neuroendocrine pathways, air pollution exerts a profound impact on childhood obesity through various pathways.

Addressing environmental and socio-economic determinants of childhood obesity is of crucial importance. Children living in areas with high levels of air pollution face unique challenges in maintaining healthy lifestyles, including limited access to outdoor play spaces, healthy food options, and healthcare resources. Efforts aimed at reducing air pollution levels and promoting healthy lifestyle behaviors are crucial for mitigating the impact of air pollution on childhood obesity [13].

Moving forward, longitudinal studies and interdisciplinary approaches, especially in places with higher levels of air pollution, are needed to address the complex interplay between environmental, social, and individual factors influencing childhood obesity. It is therefore crucial to conduct preclinical experimental studies, as understanding the molecular mechanisms underlying the toxic effects of air pollutants is essential for developing effective preventive and therapeutic strategies. Collaborative efforts between researchers, policymakers, healthcare professionals, and community stakeholders are essential for developing effective strategies for combatting childhood obesity in the context of air pollution [7,44].

Overall, the multifaceted nature of the relationship between air pollution and childhood obesity underscores the importance of adopting a holistic approach to addressing both environmental and socio-economic determinants of health. Based on the reviewed manuscripts, efforts to mitigate air pollution levels and promote healthy lifestyle behaviors are crucial for preventing childhood obesity and improving the long-term health outcomes of children worldwide.

Author Contributions: Conceptualization, K.Z.; methodology, M.J. and K.Z.; software, M.J. and K.Z.; validation, K.Z. and M.J.; formal analysis, A.K. and B.S.; investigation, A.K., B.S., K.Z., and M.J.; resources, K.Z. and M.J.; data curation, B.S. and A.K.; writing—original draft preparation, B.S. and A.K.; writing—review and editing, M.J. and K.Z.; visualization, A.K. and B.S.; supervision, K.Z.; project administration, K.Z. and M.J.; funding acquisition, K.Z. and M.J. All authors have read and agreed to the published version of the manuscript.

Funding: The manuscript was co-financed by the state budget under the program of the Polish Minister of Education and Science under the name "Excellent Science" project no. DNK/SP/548321/2022.

Institutional Review Board Statement: Not applicable.

Informed Consent Statement: Not applicable.

Data Availability Statement: Not applicable.

Conflicts of Interest: The authors declare no conflicts of interest.

References

1. Wang, Y.; Lim, H. The Global Childhood Obesity Epidemic and the Association between Socio-Economic Status and Childhood Obesity. *Int. Rev. Psychiatry* **2012**, *24*, 176–188. [CrossRef] [PubMed]
2. Leung, A.K.C.; Wong, A.H.C.; Hon, K.L. Childhood Obesity: An Updated Review. *Curr. Pediatr. Rev.* **2024**, *20*, 2–26. [CrossRef] [PubMed]
3. Chrissini, M.M.; Panagiotakos, D.B. Public Health Interventions Tackling Childhood Obesity at European Level: A Literature Review. *Prev. Med. Rep.* **2022**, *30*, 102068. [CrossRef]
4. Phelps, N.H.; Singleton, R.K.; Zhou, B.; Heap, R.A.; Mishra, A.; Bennett, J.E.; Paciorek, C.J.; Lhoste, V.P.; Carrillo-Larco, R.M.; Stevens, G.A.; et al. Worldwide Trends in Underweight and Obesity from 1990 to 2022: A Pooled Analysis of 3663 Population-Representative Studies with 222 Million Children, Adolescents, and Adults. *Lancet* **2024**, *403*, 1027–1050. [CrossRef]
5. Rank, M.; Siegrist, M.; Wilks, D.C.; Haller, B.; Wolfarth, B.; Langhof, H.; Halle, M. Long-Term Effects of an Inpatient Weight-Loss Program in Obese Children and the Role of Genetic Predisposition-Rationale and Design of the LOGIC-Trial. *BMC Pediatr.* **2012**, *12*, 30. [CrossRef] [PubMed]
6. Rosiek, A.; Maciejewska, N.F.; Leksowski, K.; Rosiek-Kryszewska, A.; Leksowski, Ł. Effect of Television on Obesity and Excess of Weight and Consequences of Health. *Int. J. Environ. Res. Public Health* **2015**, *12*, 9408. [CrossRef]
7. Miguel-Berges, M.L.; Mouratidou, T.; Santaliestra-Pasias, A.; Androutsos, O.; Iotova, V.; Galcheva, S.; De Craemer, M.; Cardon, G.; Koletzko, B.; Kulaga, Z.; et al. Longitudinal Associations between Diet Quality, Sedentary Behaviours and Physical Activity and Risk of Overweight and Obesity in Preschool Children: The ToyBox-Study. *Pediatr. Obes.* **2023**, *18*, e13068. [CrossRef]
8. Jeong, E.-Y.; Kim, K.-N. Influence of Stress on Snack Consumption in Middle School Girls. *Nutr. Res. Pract.* **2007**, *1*, 349. [CrossRef]
9. Jiang, J.; Lau, P.W.C.; Li, Y.; Gao, D.; Chen, L.; Chen, M.; Ma, Y.; Ma, T.; Ma, Q.; Zhang, Y.; et al. Association of Fast-Food Restaurants with Overweight and Obesity in School-Aged Children and Adolescents: A Systematic Review and Meta-Analysis. *Obes. Rev.* **2023**, *24*, e13536. [CrossRef]
10. Bellisle, F. Meals and Snacking, Diet Quality and Energy Balance. *Physiol. Behav.* **2014**, *134*, 38–43. [CrossRef]
11. Adolphus, K.; Lawton, C.L.; Champ, C.L.; Dye, L. The Effects of Breakfast and Breakfast Composition on Cognition in Children and Adolescents: A Systematic Review. *Adv. Nutr.* **2016**, *7*, 590S–612S. [CrossRef] [PubMed]
12. Roberts, M.; Tolar-Peterson, T.; Reynolds, A.; Wall, C.; Reeder, N.; Rico Mendez, G. The Effects of Nutritional Interventions on the Cognitive Development of Preschool-Age Children: A Systematic Review. *Nutrients* **2022**, *14*, 532. [CrossRef] [PubMed]
13. Abarca-Gómez, L.; Abdeen, Z.A.; Hamid, Z.A.; Abu-Rmeileh, N.M.; Acosta-Cazares, B.; Acuin, C.; Adams, R.J.; Aekplakorn, W.; Afsana, K.; Aguilar-Salinas, C.A.; et al. Worldwide Trends in Body-Mass Index, Underweight, Overweight, and Obesity from 1975 to 2016: A Pooled Analysis of 2416 Population-Based Measurement Studies in 1289 Million Children, Adolescents, and Adults. *Lancet* **2017**, *390*, 2627–2642. [CrossRef]
14. Butzlaf, I.; Minos, D. Understanding the Drivers of Overweight and Obesity in Developing Countries: The Case of South Africa. In *GlobalFood Discussion Papers 232025*; Georg-August-Universitaet Goettingen, GlobalFood, Department of Agricultural Economics and Rural Development: Goettingen, Germany, 2016.
15. Yin, P.; Brauer, M.; Cohen, A.J.; Wang, H.; Li, J.; Burnett, R.T.; Stanaway, J.D.; Causey, K.; Larson, S.; Godwin, W.; et al. The Effect of Air Pollution on Deaths, Disease Burden, and Life Expectancy across China and Its Provinces, 1990–2017: An Analysis for the Global Burden of Disease Study 2017. *Lancet Planet Health* **2020**, *4*, e386–e398. [CrossRef]
16. Hwang, S.E.; Kwon, H.; Jeong, S.M.; Kim, H.J.; Park, J.H. Ambient Air Pollution Exposure and Obesity-Related Traits in Korean Adults. *Diabetes Metab. Syndr. Obes.* **2019**, *12*, 1365–1377. [CrossRef] [PubMed]
17. Kim, K.H.; Kabir, E.; Kabir, S. A Review on the Human Health Impact of Airborne Particulate Matter. *Environ. Int.* **2015**, *74*, 136–143. [CrossRef] [PubMed]
18. Janssen, F.; Bardoutsos, A.; Vidra, N. Obesity Prevalence in the Long-Term Future in 18 European Countries and in the USA. *Obes. Facts* **2020**, *13*, 514–527. [CrossRef] [PubMed]
19. Campolim, C.M.; Schimenes, B.C.; Veras, M.M.; Kim, Y.-B.; Prada, P.O. Air Pollution Accelerates the Development of Obesity and Alzheimer's Disease: The Role of Leptin and Inflammation-a Mini-Review. *Front. Immunol.* **2024**, *15*, 1401800. [CrossRef]
20. Vonk, J.M.; Roukema, J. Air Pollution Susceptibility in Children with Asthma and Obesity: Tidal Volume as Key Player? *Eur. Respir. J.* **2022**, *59*, 2102505. [CrossRef]
21. Guo, L.H.; Zeeshan, M.; Huang, G.F.; Chen, D.H.; Xie, M.; Liu, J.; Dong, G.H. Influence of Air Pollution Exposures on Cardiometabolic Risk Factors: A Review. *Curr. Environ. Health Rep.* **2023**, *10*, 501–507. [CrossRef]
22. Pan, W.; Wang, M.; Hu, Y.; Lian, Z.; Cheng, H.; Qin, J.J.; Wan, J. The Association between Outdoor Air Pollution and Body Mass Index, Central Obesity, and Visceral Adiposity Index among Middle-Aged and Elderly Adults: A Nationwide Study in China. *Front. Endocrinol.* **2023**, *14*, 1221325. [CrossRef] [PubMed]
23. Kim, J.S.; Chen, Z.; Alderete, T.L.; Toledo-Corral, C.; Lurmann, F.; Berhane, K.; Gilliland, F.D. Associations of Air Pollution, Obesity and Cardiometabolic Health in Young Adults: The Meta-AIR Study. *Environ. Int.* **2019**, *133*, 105180. [CrossRef] [PubMed]

24. Bateson, T.F.; Schwartz, J. Children's Response to Air Pollutants. *J. Toxicol. Environ. Health A* **2008**, *71*, 238–243. [CrossRef] [PubMed]
25. Salvi, S. Health Effects of Ambient Air Pollution in Children. *Paediatr. Respir. Rev.* **2007**, *8*, 275–280. [CrossRef]
26. Bramble, K.; Blanco, M.N.; Doubleday, A.; Gassett, A.J.; Hajat, A.; Marshall, J.D.; Sheppard, L. Exposure Disparities by Income, Race and Ethnicity, and Historic Redlining Grade in the Greater Seattle Area for Ultrafine Particles and Other Air Pollutants. *Environ. Health Perspect.* **2023**, *131*, 077004. [CrossRef]
27. Gao, M.; Carmichael, G.R.; Wang, Y.; Saide, P.E.; Yu, M.; Xin, J.; Liu, Z.; Wang, Z. Modeling Study of the 2010 Regional Haze Event in the North China Plain. *Atmos. Chem. Phys.* **2016**, *16*, 1673–1691. [CrossRef]
28. Ye, L.; Zhou, J.; Tian, Y.; Cui, J.; Chen, C.; Wang, J.; Wang, Y.; Wei, Y.; Ye, J.; Li, C.; et al. Associations of Residential Greenness and Ambient Air Pollution with Overweight and Obesity in Older Adults. *Obesity* **2023**, *31*, 2627–2637. [CrossRef]
29. Michalska, M.; Zorena, K.; Wąż, P.; Bartoszewicz, M.; Brandt-Varma, A.; Ślęzak, D.; Robakowska, M.; He, F. Gaseous Pollutants and Particulate Matter (PM) in Ambient Air and the Number of New Cases of Type 1 Diabetes in Children and Adolescents in the Pomeranian Voivodeship, Poland. *Biomed Res. Int.* **2020**, *2020*, 1648264. [CrossRef]
30. Michalska, M.; Bartoszewicz, M.; Wąż, P.; Kozaczuk, S.; Beń-Skowronek, I.; Zorena, K. PM10 Concentration and Microbiological Assessment of Air in Relation to the Number of Acute Cases of Type 1 Diabetes Mellitus in the Lubelskie Voivodeship. Preliminary Report. *Pediatr. Endocrinol. Diabetes Metab.* **2017**, *23*, 70–76. [CrossRef]
31. Centers for Disease Control and Prevention. Defining Childhood Obesity. 2022. Available online: https://www.cdc.gov/obesity/childhood/defining.html (accessed on 14 August 2024).
32. World Health Organization. Growth Reference Data for 5–19 Years. 2007. Available online: https://www.who.int/tools/growth-reference-data-for-5to19-years/indicators/bmi-for-age (accessed on 14 August 2024).
33. Wells, G.A.; Shea, B.; O'Connell, D.; Peterson, J.; Welch, V.; Losos, M.; Tugwell, P. The Newcastle-Ottawa Scale (NOS) for Assessing the Quality of Nonrandomised Studies in Meta-Analyses. Ottawa Hospital Research Institute. 2000. Available online: http://www.ohri.ca/programs/clinical_epidemiology/oxford.asp (accessed on 14 August 2024).
34. Page, M.J.; McKenzie, J.E.; Bossuyt, P.M.; Boutron, I.; Hoffmann, T.C.; Mulrow, C.D.; Shamseer, L.; Tetzlaff, J.M.; Akl, E.A.; Brennan, S.E.; et al. The PRISMA 2020 Statement: An Updated Guideline for Reporting Systematic Reviews. *BMJ* **2021**, *372*, n71. [CrossRef]
35. Tamayo-Ortiz, M.; Téllez-Rojo, M.M.; Rothenberg, S.J.; Gutiérrez-Avila, I.; Just, A.C.; Kloog, I.; Texcalac-Sangrador, J.L.; Romero-Martinez, M.; Bautista-Arredondo, L.F.; Schwartz, J.; et al. Exposure to PM2.5 and Obesity Prevalence in the Greater Mexico City Area. *Int. J. Environ. Res. Public Health* **2021**, *18*, 2301. [CrossRef] [PubMed]
36. Lister, N.B.; Baur, L.A.; Felix, J.F.; Hill, A.J.; Marcus, C.; Reinehr, T.; Summerbell, C.; Wabitsch, M. Child and Adolescent Obesity. *Nat. Rev. Dis. Primers* **2023**, *9*, 24. [CrossRef]
37. Paz-Aparicio, V.M.; Tapia, V.; Vasquez-Apestegui, B.V.; Steenland, K.; Gonzales, G.F. Intrauterine and Extrauterine Environmental PM2.5 Exposure Is Associated with Overweight/Obesity (O/O) in Children Aged 6 to 59 Months from Lima, Peru: A Case-Control Study. *Toxics* **2022**, *10*, 487. [CrossRef] [PubMed]
38. Zhang, Z.; Dong, B.; Chen, G.; Song, Y.; Li, S.; Yang, Z.; Dong, Y.; Wang, Z.; Ma, J.; Guo, Y. Ambient Air Pollution and Obesity in School-Aged Children and Adolescents: A Multicenter Study in China. *Sci. Total Environ.* **2021**, *771*, 144583. [CrossRef]
39. Wu, Q.Z.; Xu, S.L.; Tan, Y.W.; Qian, Z.; Vaughn, M.G.; McMillin, S.E.; Dong, P.; Qin, S.J.; Liang, L.X.; Lin, L.Z.; et al. Exposure to Ultrafine Particles and Childhood Obesity: A Cross-Sectional Analysis of the Seven Northeast Cities (SNEC) Study in China. *Sci. Total Environ.* **2022**, *846*, 157524. [CrossRef] [PubMed]
40. Wu, Q.Z.; Li, S.; Yang, B.Y.; Bloom, M.; Shi, K.; Knibbs, L.; Dharmage, S.; Leskinen, A.; Jalaludin, B.; Jalava, P.; et al. Ambient Airborne Particulates of Diameter ≤1 μm, a Leading Contributor to the Association Between Ambient Airborne Particulates of Diameter ≤2.5 μm and Children's Blood Pressure. *Hypertension* **2020**, *75*, 347–355. [CrossRef]
41. de Bont, J.; Casas, M.; Barrera-Gómez, J.; Cirach, M.; Rivas, I.; Valvi, D.; Álvarez, M.; Dadvand, P.; Sunyer, J.; Vrijheid, M. Ambient Air Pollution and Overweight and Obesity in School-Aged Children in Barcelona, Spain. *Environ. Int.* **2019**, *125*, 58–64. [CrossRef]
42. Huang, C.; Li, C.; Zhao, F.; Zhu, J.; Wang, S.; Sun, G. The Association between Childhood Exposure to Ambient Air Pollution and Obesity: A Systematic Review and Meta-Analysis. *Int. J. Environ. Res. Public Health* **2022**, *19*, 4491. [CrossRef] [PubMed]
43. Lin, L.; Li, T.; Sun, M.; Liang, Q.; Ma, Y.; Wang, F.; Duan, J.; Sun, Z. Global Association between Atmospheric Particulate Matter and Obesity: A Systematic Review and Meta-Analysis. *Environ. Res.* **2022**, *209*, 112785. [CrossRef]
44. Zheng, J.; Zhang, H.; Shi, J.; Li, X.; Zhang, J.; Zhang, K.; Gao, Y.; He, J.; Dai, J.; Wang, J. Association of Air Pollution Exposure with Overweight or Obesity in Children and Adolescents: A Systematic Review and Meta-Analysis. *Sci. Total Environ.* **2024**, *910*, 168589. [CrossRef]
45. Parasin, N.; Amnuaylojaroen, T.; Saokaew, S. Effect of Air Pollution on Obesity in Children: A Systematic Review and Meta-Analysis. *Children* **2021**, *8*, 327. [CrossRef] [PubMed]
46. de Bont, J.; Díaz, Y.; de Castro, M.; Cirach, M.; Basagaña, X.; Nieuwenhuijsen, M.; Duarte-Salles, T.; Vrijheid, M. Ambient Air Pollution and the Development of Overweight and Obesity in Children: A Large Longitudinal Study. *Int. J. Obes.* **2021**, *45*, 1124–1132. [CrossRef] [PubMed]
47. Tong, J.; Ren, Y.; Liu, F.; Liang, F.; Tang, X.; Huang, D.; An, X.; Liang, X. The Impact of PM2.5 on the Growth Curves of Children's Obesity Indexes: A Prospective Cohort Study. *Front. Public Health* **2022**, *10*, 843622. [CrossRef] [PubMed]

48. Liang, X.; Liu, F.; Liang, F.; Ren, Y.; Tang, X.; Luo, S.; Huang, D.; Feng, W. Association of Decreases in PM2.5 Levels Due to the Implementation of Environmental Protection Policies with the Incidence of Obesity in Adolescents: A Prospective Cohort Study. *Ecotoxicol. Environ. Saf.* **2022**, *247*, 114211. [CrossRef] [PubMed]
49. Fioravanti, S.; Cesaroni, G.; Badaloni, C.; Michelozzi, P.; Forastiere, F.; Porta, D. Traffic-Related Air Pollution and Childhood Obesity in an Italian Birth Cohort. *Environ. Res.* **2018**, *160*, 479–486. [CrossRef] [PubMed]
50. Vanoli, J.; Coull, B.A.; de Cuba, S.E.; Fabian, P.M.; Carnes, F.; Massaro, M.A.; Poblacion, A.; Bellocco, R.; Kloog, I.; Schwartz, J.; et al. Postnatal Exposure to PM2.5 and Weight Trajectories in Early Childhood. *Environ. Epidemiol.* **2021**, *6*, E181. [CrossRef]
51. Zhou, S.; Lin, L.; Bao, Z.; Meng, T.; Wang, S.; Chen, G.; Li, Q.; Liu, Z.; Bao, H.; Han, N.; et al. The Association of Prenatal Exposure to Particulate Matter with Infant Growth: A Birth Cohort Study in Beijing, China. *Environ. Pollut.* **2021**, *277*, 116792. [CrossRef]
52. Moody, E.C.; Cantoral, A.; Tamayo-Ortiz, M.; Pizano-Zárate, M.L.; Schnaas, L.; Kloog, I.; Oken, E.; Coull, B.; Baccarelli, A.; Téllez-Rojo, M.M.; et al. Association of Prenatal and Perinatal Exposures to Particulate Matter With Changes in Hemoglobin A1c Levels in Children Aged 4 to 6 Years. *JAMA Netw. Open* **2019**, *2*, e1917643. [CrossRef]
53. Zhang, J.S.; Gui, Z.H.; Zou, Z.Y.; Yang, B.Y.; Ma, J.; Jing, J.; Wang, H.J.; Luo, J.Y.; Zhang, X.; Luo, C.Y.; et al. Long-Term Exposure to Ambient Air Pollution and Metabolic Syndrome in Children and Adolescents: A National Cross-Sectional Study in China. *Environ. Int.* **2021**, *148*, 106383. [CrossRef]
54. Zhang, X.; Zhao, H.; Chow, W.H.; Bixby, M.; Durand, C.; Markham, C.; Zhang, K. Population-Based Study of Traffic-Related Air Pollution and Obesity in Mexican Americans. *Obesity* **2020**, *28*, 412–420. [CrossRef]
55. Frondelius, K.; Oudin, A.; Malmqvist, E. Traffic-Related Air Pollution and Child BMI—A Study of Prenatal Exposure to Nitrogen Oxides and Body Mass Index in Children at the Age of Four Years in Malmö, Sweden. *Int. J. Environ. Res. Public Health* **2018**, *15*, 2294. [CrossRef] [PubMed]
56. Huang, J.V.; Leung, G.M.; Schooling, C.M. The Association of Air Pollution with Body Mass Index: Evidence from Hong Kong's "Children of 1997" Birth Cohort. *Int. J. Obes.* **2019**, *43*, 62–72. [CrossRef]
57. Poursafa, P.; Dadvand, P.; Amin, M.M.; Hajizadeh, Y.; Ebrahimpour, K.; Mansourian, M.; Pourzamani, H.; Sunyer, J.; Kelishadi, R. Association of Polycyclic Aromatic Hydrocarbons with Cardiometabolic Risk Factors and Obesity in Children. *Environ. Int.* **2018**, *118*, 203–210. [CrossRef] [PubMed]
58. Bushnik, T.; Wong, S.L.; Holloway, A.C.; Thomson, E.M. Association of Urinary Polycyclic Aromatic Hydrocarbons and Obesity in Children Aged 3–18: Canadian Health Measures Survey 2009–2015. *J. Dev. Orig. Health Dis.* **2020**, *11*, 623–631. [CrossRef]
59. Shi, X.; Zheng, Y.; Cui, H.; Zhang, Y.; Jiang, M. Exposure to Outdoor and Indoor Air Pollution and Risk of Overweight and Obesity across Different Life Periods: A Review. *Ecotoxicol. Environ. Saf.* **2022**, *242*, 113893. [CrossRef] [PubMed]
60. Mann, J.K.; Lutzker, L.; Holm, S.M.; Margolis, H.G.; Neophytou, A.M.; Eisen, E.A.; Costello, S.; Tyner, T.; Holland, N.; Tindula, G.; et al. Traffic-Related Air Pollution Is Associated with Glucose Dysregulation, Blood Pressure, and Oxidative Stress in Children. *Environ. Res.* **2021**, *195*, 110870. [CrossRef] [PubMed]
61. Jiang, N.; Bao, W.W.; Gui, Z.H.; Chen, Y.C.; Zhao, Y.; Huang, S.; Zhang, Y.S.; Liang, J.H.; Pu, X.Y.; Huang, S.Y.; et al. Findings of Indoor Air Pollution and Childhood Obesity in a Cross-Sectional Study of Chinese Schoolchildren. *Environ. Res.* **2023**, *225*, 115611. [CrossRef]
62. Sears, C.G.; Mueller-Leonhard, C.; Wellenius, G.A.; Chen, A.; Ryan, P.; Lanphear, B.P.; Braun, J.M. Early-Life Exposure to Traffic-Related Air Pollution and Child Anthropometry. *Environ. Epidemiol.* **2019**, *3*, e061. [CrossRef]
63. Bushnik, T.; Ferrao, T.; Leung, A.A. The Impact of Updated Clinical Blood Pressure Guidelines on Hypertension Prevalence among Children and Adolescents. *Health Rep.* **2023**, *34*, 3–15. [CrossRef]
64. Li, K.; Yin, R.; Wang, Y.; Zhao, D. Associations between Exposure to Polycyclic Aromatic Hydrocarbons and Metabolic Syndrome in U.S. Adolescents: Cross-Sectional Results from the National Health and Nutrition Examination Survey (2003–2016) Data. *Environ. Res.* **2021**, *202*, 111747. [CrossRef]
65. Kim, S.H.; Park, M.J.; Park, S.K. Urinary Concentrations of Polycyclic Aromatic Hydrocarbon Metabolites and Childhood Obesity. *Heliyon* **2023**, *9*, e19335. [CrossRef] [PubMed]
66. Schneider, D. International Trends in Adolescent Nutrition. *Soc. Sci. Med.* **2000**, *51*, 955–967. [CrossRef]
67. Tong, Z.; Zhang, H.; Yu, J.; Jia, X.; Hou, X.; Kong, Z. Spatial-Temporal Evolution of Overweight and Obesity among Chinese Adolescents from 2016 to 2020. *Iscience* **2024**, *27*, 108742. [CrossRef] [PubMed]
68. Zorena, K.; Michalska, M.; Kurpas, M.; Jaskulak, M.; Murawska, A.; Rostami, S. Environmental Factors and the Risk of Developing Type 1 Diabetes-Old Disease and New Data. *Biology* **2022**, *11*, 608. [CrossRef]
69. Woo Baidal, J.A.; Locks, L.M.; Cheng, E.R.; Blake-Lamb, T.L.; Perkins, M.E.; Taveras, E.M. Risk Factors for Childhood Obesity in the First 1000 Days: A Systematic Review. *Am. J. Prev. Med.* **2016**, *50*, 761–779. [CrossRef] [PubMed]
70. Han, S.H.; Yee, J.Y.; Pyo, J.S. Impact of Short Sleep Duration on the Incidence of Obesity and Overweight among Children and Adolescents. *Medicina* **2022**, *58*, 1037. [CrossRef]
71. Afshar-Mohajer, N.; Wu, T.D.; Shade, R.; Brigham, E.; Woo, H.; Wood, M.; Koehl, R.; Koehler, K.; Kirkness, J.; Hansel, N.N.; et al. Obesity, Tidal Volume, and Pulmonary Deposition of Fine Particulate Matter in Children with Asthma. *Eur. Respir. J.* **2022**, *59*, 2100209. [CrossRef]
72. Johnson, N.M.; Hoffmann, A.R.; Behlen, J.C.; Lau, C.; Pendleton, D.; Harvey, N.; Shore, R.; Li, Y.; Chen, J.; Tian, Y.; et al. Air Pollution and Children's Health—A Review of Adverse Effects Associated with Prenatal Exposure from Fine to Ultrafine Particulate Matter. *Environ. Health Prev. Med.* **2021**, *26*, 72. [CrossRef]

73. Chiu, Y.H.; Hsu, H.H.; Wilson, A.; Coull, B.A.; Pendo, M.P.; Baccarelli, A.; Kloog, I.; Schwartz, J.; Wright, R.O.; Taveras, E.M.; et al. Prenatal Particulate Air Pollution Exposure and Body Composition in Urban Preschool Children: Examining Sensitive Windows and Sex-Specific Associations. *Environ. Res.* **2017**, *158*, 798–805. [CrossRef]
74. Gardner, R.; Feely, A.; Layte, R.; Williams, J.; McGavock, J. Adverse Childhood Experiences Are Associated with an Increased Risk of Obesity in Early Adolescence: A Population-Based Prospective Cohort Study. *Pediatr. Res.* **2019**, *86*, 522–528. [CrossRef]
75. Hill, A.P.; Zuckerman, K.E.; Fombonne, E. Obesity and Autism. *Pediatrics* **2015**, *136*, 1051–1061. [CrossRef] [PubMed]

Disclaimer/Publisher's Note: The statements, opinions and data contained in all publications are solely those of the individual author(s) and contributor(s) and not of MDPI and/or the editor(s). MDPI and/or the editor(s) disclaim responsibility for any injury to people or property resulting from any ideas, methods, instructions or products referred to in the content.

MDPI AG
Grosspeteranlage 5
4052 Basel
Switzerland
Tel.: +41 61 683 77 34

Journal of Clinical Medicine Editorial Office
E-mail: jcm@mdpi.com
www.mdpi.com/journal/jcm

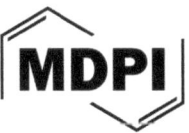

Disclaimer/Publisher's Note: The title and front matter of this reprint are at the discretion of the Guest Editors. The publisher is not responsible for their content or any associated concerns. The statements, opinions and data contained in all individual articles are solely those of the individual Editors and contributors and not of MDPI. MDPI disclaims responsibility for any injury to people or property resulting from any ideas, methods, instructions or products referred to in the content.

www.ingramcontent.com/pod-product-compliance
Lightning Source LLC
LaVergne TN
LVHW072359090526
838202LV00019B/2579